Inclusive and Special Recreation

Inclusive and Special Recreation

Opportunities for Persons with Disabilities

Third Edition

Ralph W. Smith, *The Pennsylvania State University*
David R. Austin, *Indiana University*
Dan W. Kennedy, *The Pennsylvania State University*

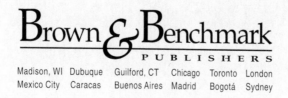

Brown & Benchmark
PUBLISHERS

Madison, WI Dubuque Guilford, CT Chicago Toronto London
Mexico City Caracas Buenos Aires Madrid Bogotá Sydney

Book Team

Publisher *Bevan O'Callaghan*
Project Editor *Scott Spoolman*
Production Editor *Debra DeBord*
Proofreading Coordinator *Carrie Barker*
Art Processor *Renee Grevas*
Production Manager *Beth Kundert*
Production/Costing Manager *Sherry Padden*
Production/Imaging and Development Manager *Linda Meehan Avenarius*
Visuals/Design Freelance Specialist *Mary L. Christianson*
Marketing Manager *Pamela S. Cooper*
Copywriter *M. J. Kelly*

Basal Text *10/12 Times Roman*
Display Type *Helvetica*
Typesetting System *Macintosh*™
QuarkXPress™
Paper Stock *50# Mirror Matte*

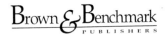

Brown & Benchmark
PUBLISHERS

Vice President of Production and New Media Development *Vickie Putman*
Vice President of Sales and Marketing *Bob McLaughlin*
Vice President of Business Development *Russ Domeyer*
Director of Marketing *John Finn*

A Times Mirror Company

Cover design by Cunningham & Welch Design Group, Inc., Madison, WI.

Cover photograph © B. Busco/The Image Bank

Copyedited by Karen Dorman; proofread by Di Ann Driscoll

Library of Congress Catalog Card Number: 95–76807

ISBN 0–697–15246–4

Printed in the United States of America by Times Mirror Higher Education Group, Inc., 2460 Kerper Boulevard, Dubuque, IA 52001

10 9 8 7 6 5 4 3 2 1

■   ■   ■

*This book is dedicated
to the ones we love.*

CONTENT OVERVIEW

. . .

CONTENTS

■ ■ ■

FOREWORD

■ ■ ■

All experience is an arch, to build upon.

This statement of Henry Brooks Adams in *The Education of Henry Adams* reflects on the foundations of knowledge. In *Inclusive and Special Recreation: Opportunities for Persons with Disabilities,* the authors have carefully provided the groundwork that assists the reader in conceptualizing and developing both the inclusive and special recreation framework and the edifice necessary for sound program development.

The authors, Ralph Smith, David Austin, and Dan Kennedy, have integrated the prevalent thinking of therapeutic recreation, special recreation, leisure education, and related professions into a pragmatic and realistic compendium. They have reflected the evolution and development of recreation services for persons with disabilities over the past 100 years and have provided a rich source for both the student and practitioner in their quest to work hand in hand with individuals with disabilities.

Drs. Smith, Austin, and Kennedy have made numerous individual contributions to inclusive and special recreation in the past three decades. Their work in curriculum development, mainstreaming, attitudinal assessment, playground development, accessible environments, therapeutic recreation education, and sports for persons with disabilities provides the structure necessary for the formulation of this book. The background and experience of the authors have enabled them to incorporate prior and existing recreation practices and provoke thoughts and concerns regarding the future direction of inclusive and special recreation services.

The authors have provided an exciting dimension to the arena of recreation and leisure for individuals with disabling conditions. Their coverage of historical and conceptual approaches, program planning, special program areas, resources, and trends represents the essentials of this thrust. They have built on the cornerstone of inclusive and special recreation a book for all seasons.

Helen Jo Hillman, C.T.R.S.
Former Program Manager
Therapeutic Recreation Services
District of Columbia Department of Recreation

PREFACE

.   .   .

During the past 30 years, there have been many dynamic developments in the field of recreation. Prefaces for the two previous editions of this textbook noted that one of the most exciting of these developments was "the movement of persons with disabilities out of institutions into the mainstream of recreation involvement." Now, with the passage and implementation of the Americans with Disabilities Act in the United States, a new era of recreation involvement is beginning for persons with disabilities. Access to most privately owned businesses, including recreation-related businesses, is now a legal right. Inclusion of persons with disabilities into all aspects of community life is becoming a reality, and recreation providers must offer programs and activities that respond to the needs of *all* consumers.

As society changes, so do textbooks. Thus, we have added the word *inclusive* to our title and revised the textbook to focus on both inclusive and special recreation programming. In Chapter 1, we distinguish between these two concepts, and we have integrated examples of each throughout the remainder of the book. The format and purpose of our textbook remain basically the same as previous editions. We have maintained our programmatic approach, rather than emphasizing disabilities. Moreover, we still believe that a polarity exists between therapeutic recreation and special recreation; we have therefore continued our focus on nonclinical approaches to recreation service delivery that provide opportunities for freely chosen recreation involvement for persons with disabilities.

It is important to note that this textbook was written primarily for undergraduate students, especially those in their first two years of study. As such, it is appropriate for use in community or junior college courses, as well as within four-year baccalaureate programs. Throughout the preparation of this textbook, we tried to keep the needs, interests, and learning styles of undergraduate students foremost in our minds. Whenever possible, we have included examples to illustrate important points, and we have provided useful references and learning activities at the end of each chapter. We have also attempted to write in a style that is appealing to undergraduate students.

This textbook is organized into four distinct parts, and each part is preceded by an introductory statement highlighting its contents. Part I provides an introduction and overview to inclusive and special recreation. The emphasis of this section is on the scope of inclusive and special recreation services, including important concepts and terminology. Part I also includes information on legislation and provides useful facts and techniques related to selected disabling conditions. Part II focuses on actual program planning and implementation and includes detailed descriptions of exemplary inclusive and special recreation programs. Part III offers some examples of program areas (or activities) that have proven effective in meeting the recreational needs of people with disabilities. The final section, Part IV, provides valuable information on community resources that relates to inclusive and special recreation services. This section also outlines current trends in inclusive recreation. At the conclusion of this textbook, we have inserted several appendices containing materials and resources that should prove useful to recreation students and educators as well as to practitioners.

As with previous editions of this textbook, the third edition reflects a combined effort on the part of each author. Dr. Smith had primary responsibility for Chapters 4, 5, 9, 10, and 11; Dr. Austin for Chapters 1, 2, 6, 12, and 13; and Dr. Kennedy for Chapters 3, 7, and 8. Dr. Smith is now listed as the primary author because he has assumed logistical coordination of the project.

We would like to express our sincere gratitude to the many people who have assisted in the preparation of all editions of this textbook. The reactions, insights, suggestions, and efforts of the following people were instrumental in the completion and revision of this book: David Beaver, Challenge Publications; Boni Boswell, East Carolina University; Erin Broadbent, National Park Service; Barbara (Sam) Browne, formerly with the Cincinnati Recreation Commission; Tammy Buckley and Christine Camps, The Pennsylvania State University; Mary Cece and Lois Gill, formerly with the University of Maryland; Peg Connolly, National Council for Therapeutic Recreation Certification; Cliff Crase, Paralyzed Veterans of America; Michael Crawford, University of Missouri; Mary Crooks and Dorothy Lougee, Parks and Recreation Department, Lincoln, Nebraska; Eileen Cuskaden, Edie Ferrante, and Janet Rice, Very Special Arts; Susan Drenkhahn, Carmel Community, Inc., Chandler, Arizona; Jeanne (Hap) Feeley, formerly of the Pennsylvania Easter Seal Society; Julie Forker, Maryland-National Capital Park and Planning Commission; Catherine Fowler, mother of Claudia Fowler; Arnold Grossman, New York University; Gene Hayes, University of Tennessee at Knoxville; Doug Herbert, formerly of Very Special Arts; Helen Jo Hillman, formerly with the District of Columbia Department of Recreation; Jerry D. Kelley, International Alliance on Disability, Washington, D.C.; Terry Kinney, Temple University; C. Wayne Korinek, Parks, Recreation, and Library Department, Phoenix; Robin Kunstler, Lehman College, New York; Stan Labanowich, University of Kentucky; Greg Lais, Wilderness Inquiry; Michal Ann Lord, formerly with the Austin Parks and Recreation Department; David Morgan Lovis, Theatre Unlimited; Steven Mason, formerly with the District of Columbia Special Olympics; John McGovern, formerly with the West Suburban Special Recreation Association, Elmwood Park, Illinois;

Thomas McPike, Chicago Park District; Lee Meyer, University of North Carolina; Brett Millar, Barrie & District Association for People with Special Needs, Ontario; Anna Miller and Glori Steifler, formerly of the League for the Handicapped, Baltimore; Bob Myers, formerly with the Montgomery County Health Department, Silver Spring, Maryland; Jed Nitzberg, The Hospital for Sick Children, Washington, D.C.; Lynn Parfitt, Maine–Niles Association of Special Recreation, Illinois; David Park, National Park Service; Janet Pomeroy, RCH, Inc., San Francisco; Lou Powell, University of New Hampshire; Lawrence Reiner, Northeast DuPage Special Recreation Association, Elmhurst, Illinois; Gary Robb, Ed Hamilton, and Don Rogers, Bradford Woods, Indiana; Lyn Rourke, Courage Center, Golden Valley, Minnesota; Stuart Schleien, Carla Tabourne, Jonathan Balk, Ronald Jenkins, Jennifer Mactavish, and Kathy Strom, University of Minnesota; James Schmutz, District of Columbia Special Olympics; Chris Smith, Pennsylvania Special Olympics; Kevin Smith, Department of Leisure Services, City of Miami; Bob Szyman, St. Louis Wheelchair Athletic Association; Byron Welker, Northern Indiana Children's Hospital, South Bend; Billie Wilson, Montgomery County Department of Recreation; and many students from Indiana University, The Pennsylvania State University, and the University of Maryland.

We would like to give a special thanks to our families for their understanding and support throughout the preparation and revision of this textbook. We sincerely hope that the finished product is worthy of the many sacrifices. We would also like to thank Scott Spoolman, Project Editor at Brown & Benchmark Publishers, and Susie Butler of SJB Consulting for their assistance.

Two people who were instrumental in the first edition of this book, Bobbi Kreisberg (Hospital for Sick Children) and Fred Humphrey (University of Maryland), died prior to publication of the third edition. We miss you, Bobbi and Fred.

Ralph W. Smith
David R. Austin
Dan W. Kennedy

Inclusive and Special Recreation

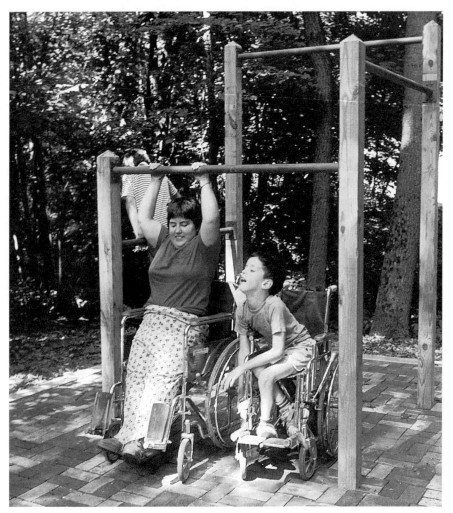

(Photo courtesy of Bradford Woods, Indiana University)

PART ONE

INTRODUCTION AND OVERVIEW

The public recreation and parks profession has long prided itself on its ability to contribute to the well-being and quality of life of the citizenry. Yet, as problems of persons with disabilities have become increasingly more visible in society, it has become apparent that this profession has had only a tenuous grasp on the nature of problems that citizens with disabilities face during their leisure and on the need for the full inclusion of persons with disabilities by leisure service providers. Fortunately, there is a vital movement among leisure service providers to establish services that meet the recreational needs of persons who have disabilities. The Americans with Disabilities Act has provided stimulus for this movement.

Although the provision of recreation services for persons with disabilities is a comparatively new area of interest for public recreation and parks, one can see origins of concern for people with special needs dating back to the beginnings of organized recreation in America. Chapter 1, Introduction, reviews both historical and philosophical bases for the provision of leisure services for individuals with disabilities. Views of authorities such as Carter, Kelley, Meyer, Robb, Pomeroy, and Stein and Sessoms are presented, and conclusions are drawn that suggest that a harmonious arrangement for the cooperation of general leisure service professionals and therapeutic recreation specialists can become a reality.

Chapter 2, Concepts and Attitudes Underlying Inclusive and Special Recreation Services, presents concepts and attitudes basic to understanding the delivery of services for persons with disabilities. Concepts surrounding the terms *disability, handicap, special populations, special recreation, inclusive recreation, mainstreaming,* and *normalization* are discussed. Chapter 2 concludes with an in-depth approach to attitudes as they relate to serving persons with disabilities. A major segment of the section on attitudes is devoted to alternatives proposed by the National Easter Seal Society and Dattilo and Smith to avoid stigmatized language when referring to individuals with disabilities.

Chapter 3, Legislation Affecting Inclusive and Special Recreation Services, reviews legislation pertaining to equal access to educational and recreation services for those with disabilities. Particular attention is given to the Americans with Disabilities Act.

Although it is critical that we avoid the trap of labeling those with disabilities, we may find information concerning various disabling conditions to be useful. Chapter 4, Disabling Conditions, begins with a discussion of the potential pitfalls and hazards involved in labeling people who have disabilities. This is followed by helpful facts, tips, and techniques associated with specific types of disabilities.

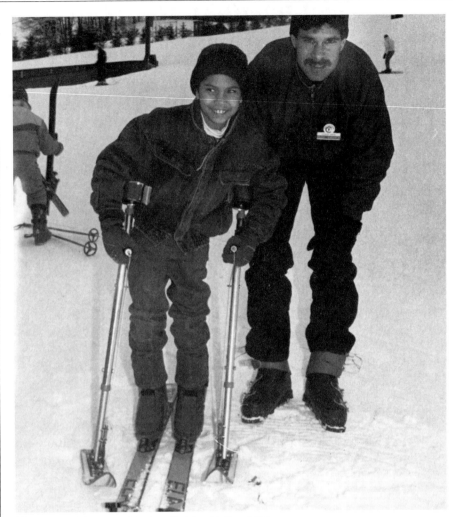

(Courtesy of Courage Center, Golden Valley, MN)

1

Introduction

■ ■ ■

Organized recreation in the United States grew out of social concern for persons attempting to cope with a rapidly changing world created by the Industrial Revolution. Most authorities cite the establishment of a sand play area for disadvantaged children in Boston in 1885 as the beginning of the recreation movement in America. This play area became known as the Boston Sand Gardens. The provision of wholesome recreation was also a central part of the settlement-house movement established to ease the transition to urban living for thousands of persons immigrating to the cities of America during the Industrial Revolution. Settlement houses, such as Jane Addams's Hull House in Chicago, provided playgrounds for children and recreational opportunities for adults to help them adapt to an urban life characterized by overcrowding and poor living conditions.

The beginnings of organized recreation in our nation thus evolved from a humanistic concern for the welfare of those who found themselves with few resources in inhospitable circumstances. Wholesome recreation was viewed as necessary for those disadvantaged individuals who had special needs.

As community recreation grew, it began to lose its focus on meeting the needs of those who were disadvantaged. More affluent sections of cities began to demand and receive community recreation services. Community recreation steadily moved away from its historical roots of serving the disadvantaged to the cause of "recreation for all." Recreation began to be perceived not as a social instrument but as an end in itself, an experience all should enjoy.

Gray (1969), in a now classic article titled "The Case for Compensatory Recreation," has written: "Gradually the social welfare mission weakened and a philosophy which sees recreation as an end in itself was adopted; this is the common view in public recreation agencies throughout the country" (p. 23).

In a similar vein, Sessoms and Stevenson (1981) have written that

> Adult education, recreation, and social group work all have a common heritage. Each is a product of the social welfare reforms that occurred in our cities and industries at the turn of the nineteenth century. Their founders shared a similar belief—they were concerned with the quality of life and believed that through the "proper" use of leisure, it could be achieved. (p. 2)

Like Gray, Sessoms and Stevenson observed that the organized parks and recreation movement has deviated from its original mission. They added,

> With both adult education and social work establishing their turf, recreation services did the same. Although some recreation specialists were concerned with the therapeutic or socially rehabilitative activities or with teaching and developing leisure skills and attitudes, the recreation profession set as its primary concerns the management of recreational environments and the offering of free-time activities. Outdoor recreation and sports programs became its program focus. (pp. 2, 3)

Although having its roots in socially purposeful programs for disadvantaged individuals, the recreation profession appears to have moved away from its initial focus. As community recreation has grown, it has broadened its scope to "recreation for all." However, as Carter and Kelley (1981) have suggested, the idea of recreation for all may have in reality become "recreation for the norm." As community recreation and parks departments have attempted to spread their resources to meet everyone's recreational needs, concern for people with special needs has been lost as a central feature of public recreation and parks.

WHY THE PAST LACK OF LEISURE SERVICES FOR PEOPLE WITH SPECIAL NEEDS?

As might be anticipated, there have been pleas for a return to an extensive concern for leisure services to people with special needs. For example, early in the 1970s, Kraus (1971) wrote of the need for recreation and parks administrators to take leadership for socially purposeful programs, including those to serve elderly individuals and persons with physical and mental disabilities. From another perspective, in 1980 the International City Management Association in its publication, *Managing Municipal Leisure Services* (Lutzin, 1980) called for the development of leisure services for people with special needs. More recently, concerned leaders like Bridge and Hutchison (1988), Dattilo (1991), Howe-Murphy and Charboneau (1987), Schleien and Ray (1988), and others have emphasized the need for providing services that offer the greatest possible amount of physical and social integration.

Yet today we find that persons with physical or mental disabilities, individuals who are old, and others with special needs have been largely underserved by community public recreation and parks departments. Why is this so? Why have so many departments that owe their very existence to the social welfare motive failed to respond to the needs of people with special needs?

Perhaps the lack of services for people with special needs has simply reflected the history of neglect of society in general for those who have not fit society's norms. During the first half of the 20th century, we systematically excluded indigent people and persons with physical or mental disabilities from community participation. Indigent old people were sent to "old folks homes" or "county poor farms." Individuals with mental retardation were placed in large institutions located in rural areas. Likewise, individuals with serious problems in mental health were taken away to "insane asylums." In short, those who deviated from society's norms were effectively removed from the mainstream of society. In light of this, it is not surprising that, as the recreation movement expanded across the United States and Canada, it lost its dedication to individuals from underserved groups.

Pragmatic Reasons for Lack of Service

Surveys of public recreation and parks departments have revealed several reasons for the past absence of services for people with disabilities. These reasons included insufficient budgets, inadequate facilities, lack of skills and knowledge necessary to establish a program, the feeling that other community agencies already provided programs, and a lack of awareness of the need for programs for people with disabilities. Assistance, these agencies felt, would be helpful to them in establishing programs by providing financial aid, additional staff, specially trained staff, additional accessible facilities, inservice training, consultation, and transportation (Austin, Peterson, & Peccarelli, 1978; Edginton, Compton, Ritchie, & Vederman, 1975).

Probably the greatest block to services historically was the reported lack of awareness of the need for these programs, plus the perception that other agencies already provided such programs. These rationalizations allowed administrators of recreation and parks systems to remove themselves entirely from the responsibility of providing recreation for persons with disabilities. Perhaps the broadening of the concept of *therapeutic recreation,* discussed in the next section, prompted administrators to feel less responsible for the provision of recreation for people with disabilities.

A Broadening Concept of Therapeutic Recreation

In the United States during the 1940s and 1950s, there developed recreation services within hospitals and institutions serving persons with various physical and mental disabilities. In some instances, those who provided these services were known as "hospital recreation workers." They identified themselves primarily with the Hospital Recreation Section of the American Recreation Society. Their approach was that of "recreation for the sake of recreation." They believed that recreation existed within their hospitals to promote the general well-being of the patients. Another segment employed in hospitals and institutions identified themselves as "recreation therapists." They formed the National Association of Recreational Therapists. To them, recreation was more than a wholesome activity; it was a tool to treatment and rehabilitation.

These two contrasting groups joined together in the 1960s under the banner of a then relatively new term, *therapeutic recreation.* Therapeutic recreation was used as an umbrella term to generally encompass the perspectives of both the American Recreation Society and the National Association of Recreational Therapists. Ultimately, therapeutic recreation came to be broadly interpreted as including any recreational service to individuals with mental or physical disabilities, in either the hospital or the community, whether for the purpose of providing treatment or for a recreative experience.

Carter and Kelley (1981) have made a persuasive case that the broadening of the concept of therapeutic recreation led to difficulty in establishing community-based recreation services for persons with disabilities. They have written,

> This expanded concept of therapeutic recreation that included community services has had two major consequences for disabled adults and children, consequences that are not necessarily regarded as positive. First, because most disabled and impaired individuals are now living in a noninstitutional setting or are in the process of being mainstreamed back into community life, they do not need, nor do they have any desire to have, "therapy." Furthermore, they have no wish to carry the stigma of being recipients of "therapeutic" recreation services. Therefore, the broadened service delivery perspective that has maintained a "treatment" image runs counter to the desires of many disabled adults and young people to seek a "normal" range of experiences like their nondisabled peers.
>
> Secondly, the therapeutic recreation field claims to be the primary professional group delegated the exclusive responsibility to serve disabled populations. The longer this image is promoted, the more difficult it becomes to convince the community recreation specialist that he must assume responsibility to provide recreation to *all* persons in his community regardless of the extent of their disabilities. (pp. 64, 65)

Carter and Kelley's points seem to be well founded. Most persons with disabilities who live in the community do not require the therapy normally associated with therapeutic recreation, nor do they wish to be stigmatized as being recipients of therapeutic recreation services. Like other citizens, the vast majority of people with disabilities and their families simply want the opportunity to take part in recreation experiences.

The twin concepts of mainstreaming and normalization call for helping people who have disabilities to take part in the mainstream of society within the most normative and least restrictive environment possible. Most persons in our society are not served by therapeutic recreation specialists but by community recreation personnel. It is, then, the responsibility of community recreation professionals to provide recreation services for those who have disabilities. Carter and Kelley feel that only when the therapeutic recreation profession steps aside and acknowledges that community recreation for persons with disabilities is the domain of public recreation and parks departments will the full responsibility be borne by those who have the obligation to meet the recreational needs of our citizens. It seems quite possible that by claiming to be primarily responsible for the entire spectrum of recreation for people with disabilities, therapeutic recreation specialists may in the past have allowed community recreation systems to relinquish their rightful duty to serve these individuals. Times, however, are changing. Federal legislation mandates that access to community recreation services must be offered to people who have disabilities.

People with disabilities enjoy the same recreation activities as most other people in their communities. (Courtesy of Courage Center, Golden Valley, MN)

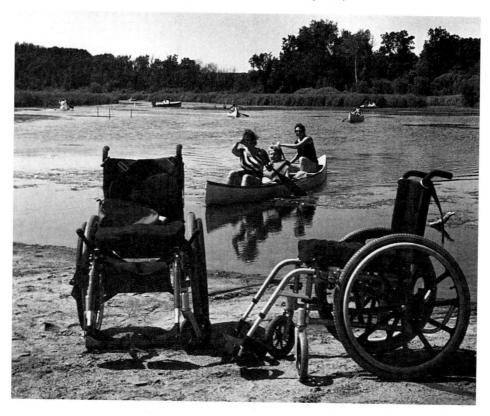

A NEW BEGINNING: THE ADA

With the passage of Public Law 101-336, the Americans with Disabilities Act (ADA), on July 26, 1990, the United States officially recognized the rights of people with disabilities to equal access to all services provided by local, state, and federal government, including recreational services. In fact, the ADA allows full and equal access by persons with disabilities to any place of public accommodation, governmental or private. Private recreation entities include restaurants, bars, theaters, stadiums, auditoriums, convention centers, museums, libraries, parks, amusement parks, zoos, golf courses, gymnasiums, or other places of recreation (*Federal Register*, 1991; Wehman, 1993). Thus, with the advent of the ADA, full accommodation for persons with disabilities is mandated by law. The ADA provides broad civil rights protections and equality of opportunity for Americans with disabilities in all aspects of their lives, including recreation.

While a number of recreation and leisure service providers in the United States recognized their moral obligation to serve persons with disabilities prior to PL 101-336, many more did not. In this regard, it would probably be conceded that Canadians have been ahead of their American counterparts. The ADA marks a beginning for America— a beginning that includes opportunity for full recreation participation for Americans with disabilities.

The ADA defines persons with disabilities as anyone with a physical or mental impairment that substantially limits one or more major life activities or who has a record of such an impairment or is regarded as having such an impairment. Major life activities include: (a) walking, breathing, seeing, hearing, speaking, learning, and working; (b) activities of daily living (e.g., bathing, dressing, getting around the home); and (c) community and home management (e.g., household chores, shopping, getting around the community) (Disabilities Statistics Program, 1992).

It is estimated that of the more than 43 million Americans with disabilities, 36.1 million are limited in major activity. This is more than 14% of the U.S. population. Only 2.3 million of these individuals live in institutions, while the vast majority (33.8 million) live in the community (LaPlante, 1992).

Of all people with disabilities, older individuals are most likely to have impairments that limit the amount or kind of major activities they can perform (LaPlante, 1992). The United States entered the 1990s with more than 30 million people who were 65 years of age or older (Godbey, 1989). There is every indication that the number of older people and those with disabilities will continue to grow as we move into the 21st century (Pegels, 1988). In sum, it is clear that, in the United States, there are significant and growing numbers of persons with disabilities who need to be provided equal access to recreation by public park and recreation agencies, as well as by private recreation providers.

WHAT IS THE RELATIONSHIP OF THERAPEUTIC RECREATION TO SPECIAL RECREATION?

The Purpose

The purpose of therapeutic recreation has long been debated. To clarify the situation, early in the 1980s the National Therapeutic Recreation Society (NTRS), a branch of the National Recreation and Park Association (NRPA), developed the philosophical position that "the purpose of therapeutic recreation is to facilitate the development, maintenance, and expression of an appropriate leisure lifestyle for individuals with physical, mental, emotional, and social limitations" (National Therapeutic Recreation Society, 1982).

The purpose is based on the assumption that

> Leisure, including recreation and play, are [sic] inherent aspects of the human experience. The importance of appropriate leisure involvement has been documented throughout history. More recently, research has addressed the value of leisure involvement in human development, in social and family relationships, and, in general, as an important aspect of the quality of life. Some human beings have disabilities, illnesses, or social conditions which limit their full participation in the normative social structure of society. These individuals with limitations have the same human rights to, and needs for, leisure involvement. (National Therapeutic Recreation Society, 1982)

The NTRS position is strikingly similar to that taken originally by the Hospital Recreation Section of the American Recreation Society (ARS). In the 1950s, ARS had championed the cause of recreation as a need and right of all individuals, including persons with illnesses and disabilities. You may recall that those affiliated with ARS viewed therapeutic recreation as the provision of wholesome recreation experiences for ill and disabled persons. In contrast, the National Association of Recreational Therapists (NART) viewed therapeutic recreation as the provision of recreation as a means to treatment. Those taking the ARS position were very much tied to the recreation movement that stood for "recreation for all." Those affiliating with NART had little association with organized recreation but were more closely aligned with the health and rehabilitation community. Their cause was not recreation; it was health restoration and promotion.

Although the National Recreation and Park Association has since replaced the American Recreation Society, similar arguments can be heard. Those supporting the NTRS/NRPA position still champion the "recreation for all" philosophy of the ARS. Other therapeutic recreation specialists argue just as strongly that the purpose of therapeutic recreation is to use recreation as a purposeful intervention to help clients relieve or prevent problems and to assist them in personal growth in an effort to allow achievement of as high a level of health as possible. Although they realize the tremendous benefits to be achieved in recreation, the therapeutic recreation specialists see recreation as a means to an end, not an end in itself.

The forming of the American Therapeutic Recreation Association (ATRA) in 1984 may be perceived as an attempt by clinically oriented therapeutic recreation specialists to break away from NTRS/NRPA to form a professional association that would foster the delivery of treatment services. In many respects, ATRA seems to have picked up where the National Association of Recreational Therapists left off. The express concern of ATRA is with the application of intervention strategies using recreation to promote independent functioning and to enhance the optimal health and well-being of clients (American Therapeutic Recreation Association, 1993).

A Model for Therapeutic Recreation

The NTRS philosophical statement is fashioned after a model originally proposed by Gunn and Peterson (1977, 1978) and that later appeared in Peterson and Gunn (1984). These authors believe that the purpose of facilitating leisure experiences for persons with disabilities should be carried out through a continuum of services. They divide the continuum into three components: therapy, leisure education, and recreation participation. Therapy is directed toward improvement of functional behavior that may impede leisure involvement. Leisure education teaches new recreational and social skills and allows for the pursuit of various issues in leisure counseling. The last component—recreation participation—concerns the provision of self-directed leisure participation for individuals with disabilities. Thus, the continuum ranges from client dependence during therapy that will remove barriers to leisure behavior, at one end, to independent leisure functioning at the other.

When closely examined, it becomes apparent that the therapy and leisure education components merge. Both deal with facilitating change. Thus, as Meyer (1981) has proposed, the model is made up of two components—treatment and recreation. Meyer has identified five implications of the model: (1) Two different types of practitioners (therapists and adaptive or special recreators) are represented; (2) the adaptive recreators operate within the jurisdiction of community recreation; (3) *therapeutic recreation* is a title that describes a service continuum; (4) therapeutic recreation is not an occupation in itself but a field that represents at least two occupational specialties; and (5) the uniqueness of therapeutic recreation is related primarily to whom it serves (i.e., people with disabilities), rather than what is provided or how it is provided.

Meyer elaborates on these points. He has written,

> The dual representation of therapists and special recreators by NTRS seems to present some ideological as well as practical difficulties. Ideologically, this position suggests that therapeutic recreation is not an occupation per se, which seems to imply that therapeutic recreation is a "field." This same position also seems to suggest that the uniqueness of therapeutic recreation is not so much in what it provides or how it is provided, but rather to whom it is provided. This is less an issue in the treatment component of therapeutic recreation. But, in the special recreation component it approaches a categorical orientation: adapted recreational opportunities for a mentally retarded child, eight years old, is therapeutic recreation . . . while recreation opportunities for a preschool child, four years old, is considered to be "community or general" recreation. . . . Both children require some type of adaptations to facilitate recreation participation. What makes one set of adaptations TR (special recreation) and another set of adaptations general recreation? The purpose of service is the same in both cases. (pp. 13, 14)

Elsewhere, Meyer (1980) has concluded that

> Some might argue that there are not two cadres of practitioners, only one—therapeutic recreators. To reason in this fashion is to ignore the obvious differences between these two subspecializations in regard to purpose, work setting, accountability structure, etc. Therapists

and special recreators function in different worlds. Given such significant differences it is only a matter of time (if it is not already here) when one or the other of these specializations seeks independence from the other. (p. 37)

Others have also taken issue with the concept that therapeutic recreation should be all-encompassing, including both the use of recreation as a purposeful intervention and the provision of opportunities for recreation participation. It is their position that any philosophical approach must establish clear boundaries for the field. Carter and Kelley (1981), for example, draw a distinction between recreation and therapeutic recreation. They have written,

> The primary purpose of recreation is to provide programs and services to make possible individualized recreation experiences. . . . The primary purpose of therapeutic recreation is to assist the individual in achieving optimal healthy functioning and independence through interventions designed to bring about a desired change in behavior. To the community recreation specialist, the recreation experience can be viewed as an "end unto itself," requiring no other justification. To the recreation therapist the recreation activity is a means by which remediation, restoration, or rehabilitation objectives can be achieved. (p. 65)

Austin (1991), like Meyer (1980) and Carter and Kelley (1981), has also questioned the inclusion of the special recreation component under the domain of therapeutic recreation. He has written,

> I object to the suggestion that a *primary* role of the therapeutic recreation specialist is that of a recreation leader or supervisor for the provision of recreation opportunities for members of special population groups. If the major function of special recreation is the provision of opportunities for self-directed leisure, then those charged with the responsibility for the delivery of leisure services—community recreation personnel—should operate special recreation programs. (p. 131)

Austin concludes by stating that therapeutic recreation specialists are not "recreators for special populations," but are rather helping professionals who intervene in their clients' lives through purposeful intervention directed through the application of the *therapeutic recreation process,* involving (1) individual client assessment, (2) individual program planning, (3) implementation of the program, and (4) evaluation of the effect of the program.

A parallel point of view has been taken by Carter, Van Andel, and Robb (1985). In their introductory textbook, they have written that therapeutic recreation

> refers to the specialized application of recreation for the specific purpose of intervening in and changing some physical, emotional, or social behavior to promote the growth and development of the individual. Therapeutic recreation may be viewed as a process or systematic use of recreation activities and experiences to achieve specific objectives. This process is not limited to certain categories (of individuals) or a particular setting. (pp. 15, 16)

Robb (1980) has expressed a similar view. He has stated,

> The position (defining therapeutic recreation as the application of the therapeutic recreation process) seems to be the best approach . . . to enhance organizational understanding,

eliminate encroachment, and spell out jurisdictional boundaries. In my discussion with leaders of the park and recreation field, I believe many would welcome this delimitation. Acceptance of this position would eliminate conflicts within the TR field. Persons currently working with special populations in a service capacity through recreation experiences . . . could identify with the general recreation field. Perhaps this identification would provide the impetus and leadership needed for the broader field to accept the responsibility of serving all people. (p. 46)

Thus, Robb believes therapeutic recreation should maintain a singularity of purpose by employing the therapeutic recreation process as a means to helping clients. By so restricting therapeutic recreation, he expects the general field of parks and recreation would react by assuming its rightful responsibility for the provision of recreation for people who have disabilities.

Therapeutic Recreation and Inclusive Recreation: A Polarity

In the field of therapeutic recreation, two philosophical points of view have emerged. One defines therapeutic recreation primarily as the provision of leisure services for those people who have some type of limitation. This position has been adopted by the National Therapeutic Recreation Society, a branch of the National Recreation and Park Association. The other view holds that therapeutic recreation should restrict itself to the application of purposeful interventions employing the therapeutic recreation process, and should, therefore, relinquish the provision of community recreation for people with disabilities to community recreation and parks personnel.

At this point, we take the position that a polarity does exist. We believe that inclusive recreation (i.e., recreation including persons with disabilities) and therapeutic recreation (i.e., recreation as a clinical intervention directed toward treatment or rehabilitation aims) stand as two separate entities. This book examines inclusive recreation services, *not* therapeutic recreation. Further, we believe the time has come to embrace new wording to describe the full inclusion of persons with disabilities into the recreation mainstream. We propose *inclusive recreation* be used because it is a broader term than special recreation and it better reflects equal and joint participation of persons with and without disabilities. The term *special recreation* can continue to be employed to describe special or adapted activities, such as the Special Olympics and wheelchair sports, through which specific needs are met.

It is our intent to bring about an appreciation of the importance of inclusive recreation services for persons with disabilities, as well as a knowledge of how to develop and deliver special recreation services. We have made a concerted effort to provide a nonclinical textbook that deals with the provision of inclusive recreation and special recreation services to persons with disabilities.

LEADERSHIP WITH PERSONS WHO HAVE DISABILITIES

Stein and Sessoms's (1977) *Recreation and Special Populations* has been an important book in the movement to bring recreation services to "special populations,"[1] including persons with disabilities. In the view of Stein and Sessoms, professionals from the general recreation and parks field should provide community-based recreation services for people with special needs. They have written,

> If such concern (for special populations) is to be converted into new and expanded community service, it must be accompanied by a growing cadre of professional recreation leaders and volunteers who have gained some awareness and understanding of the leisure problems of these disadvantaged people and who are oriented to the possibilities of providing leisure opportunities aimed at resolving their needs. Here, it is important to understand, our focus is on present and future recreators who are trained for general community service rather than on those leaders who might be considered specialists in working with a specific population. (pp. 15, 16)

Stein and Sessoms go on to state:

> Experience has demonstrated that a professional recreator who is effective in working with people in general can be equally effective in working with people from a special population. The only provisions beyond his professional skills and understanding are 1) that he be properly oriented to any unique psychological, social, or physical difficulties and possible limitations that may sometimes be faced by persons within a given population; and 2) that he be endowed with the attitudinal capacity to work with such people. Remember, we are discussing the ability to work with *people*—nothing more! Therefore, we should recognize that such orientation and attitudinal capacity are essential in working with *any* segment of a general population, whether considered special or not. (p. 16)

Bullock, Wohl, Webreck, and Crawford (1982) have suggested that existing general recreation staff can be given training to enable them to work with participants who have disabilities. Specific areas of training prescribed by Bullock and his colleagues include

1. Characteristics of various disabilities, noting possible limitations and special considerations (emergency and health care procedures should also be outlined here).
2. General activity and equipment modification techniques.
3. Overview of the least-restrictive-environment concept and how it is being implemented in the department.
4. Assessment of existing attitudes of recreation professionals toward individuals with handicapping conditions.
5. Creation of peer acceptance.
6. Use of instructional aides and volunteers.
7. Location of additional resource information for a specific disability. (pp. 106, 107)

---

1. Historically, the term *special populations* has been used to describe people who have special needs because of some physical, mental, or psychological difficulty. Except when citing others, the authors of this text have avoided using this term for reasons outlined in Chapters 2 and 4.

The *LIFE Resource Manual* (1993), developed by the Center for Recreation and Disability Studies at the University of North Carolina at Chapel Hill, offers an excellent resource for staff training.

Thus, authorities have proposed that general community recreation professionals can and should assume responsibility for inclusive recreation opportunities. But what specific skills and knowledge are needed to work in community recreation with people who have special needs? Perhaps a study covered in the next section will help to answer this question.

COMPETENCIES NEEDED TO WORK WITH PERSONS WHO HAVE DISABILITIES

Austin and Powell (1980) conducted an investigation to determine what competencies entry-level general community recreation professionals should possess to enable them to serve participants with disabilities. They first found 142 colleges and universities in the United States and Canada that offered a course in recreation for special populations for general recreation and parks students. Instructors of the relevant course at 62 of the institutions of higher education, along with 27 administrators of community-based recreation programs for persons with special needs, participated in a competency identification study. These instructors and administrators identified 86 competencies they felt were necessary for entry-level recreation personnel to work with people who have disabilities.

The 86 competencies identified by Austin and Powell were organized according to clusters of similar competencies. The highest-ranked cluster dealt with competencies related to attitudes (rated 4.26 on a 5-point scale). Other high-ranking areas of competence were facility design and accessibility (4.17), orientation to recreation for persons with disabilities (4.15), leadership and supervision (4.09), and mainstreaming (3.94). The rankings for all 16 clusters of competencies are shown in Table 1.1.

To present the nature of specific competencies, a representative sample was listed under each of the highest ranked clusters. First, under the *attitudes* cluster are competencies such as the following:

- Understands how positive attitudes toward persons with disabilities may be developed within recreational programs
- Demonstrates awareness of personal attitudes toward persons with disabilities
- Understands various societal attitudes toward persons with disabilities

Under the cluster on *facility design and accessibility* are competencies such as the following:

- Understands the frustrations experienced in an inaccessible environment
- Describes physical barriers to accessibility and how they can be eliminated
- Identifies resources available on the design of barrier-free recreational environments

Table 1.1 Areas of Competency

Cluster	Mean Score
Attitudes	4.26
Facility design and accessibility	4.17
Orientation to recreation for persons with disabilities	4.15
Leadership and supervision	4.09
Mainstreaming	3.94
Program design	3.92
Aids, appliances, safety procedures	3.89
Trends and issues	3.84
Leisure education	3.80
Professionalism	3.79
Resources and services	3.75
Advocacy and legislation	3.75
Training	3.73
Equipment and supplies	3.69
Characteristics of persons with disabilities	3.50
Funding sources	3.26

Source: D. R. Austin and L. G. Powell. Competencies needed by community recreators to serve special populations. In D. R. Austin, Ed., *Directions in Health, Physical Education, and Recreation; Therapeutic Recreation Curriculum: Philosophy, Strategy, and Concerns* (Bloomington: Indiana University School of Health, Physical Education and Recreation, 1980), p. 34.

Representative of the cluster on *orientation to recreation for persons with disabilities* are competencies dealing with philosophical understandings, including the following:

■ Develops a personal/professional philosophy of recreation for persons with disabilities in community settings

■ States a rationale for the provision of community recreation for persons with disabilities

■ Knows role of recreation services for persons with disabilities in the community recreation department

The *leadership and supervision* cluster contains competencies such as the following:

■ Recognizes the importance of considering individual needs and interests during program leadership

■ Knows principles of instruction useful for executing recreation activities for special populations

■ Knows how to facilitate integrated recreational groups (create an atmosphere conducive to mainstreaming)

The *mainstreaming* cluster contains the following competencies, among others:

- Understands concepts of mainstreaming
- Understands concepts of normalization
- Describes approaches to mainstreaming in community recreation

The competencies identified by Austin and Powell's (1980) experts constitute a listing of basic skills and knowledge necessary for entry-level professionals assuming positions in recreation and parks departments. This information, coupled with that provided by others such as Pomeroy (1974), Bullock et al. (1982), and Schleien and Ray (1988) could serve as a basic foundation for preservice and in-service training of community recreation professionals.

COMMENT ON LEADERSHIP RESPONSIBILITY IN COMMUNITY RECREATION

Public recreation and parks agencies must return to their professional heritage of concern with recreation for persons with special needs. As the suppliers of public recreation and parks services, it seems clear that they have the responsibility to offer recreation services for persons with disabilities, since it is their duty to serve the recreational needs of their jurisdictions at large. But it is particularly important that public recreation and parks agencies reach out to underserved segments of the population, including persons with physical or mental disabilities and older persons.

Further, we believe that inclusive and special recreation programs should be largely organized and led by general recreation professionals. If such programs are to be an integral part of the organization's offerings, they should be provided by the regular professional staff. The exception to this would be in programs with therapeutic intent. These are programs directed toward facilitating change through meeting specific objectives. Use of the therapeutic recreation process to effect specific outcomes calls for the knowledge and skills possessed by a professional prepared as a therapeutic recreation specialist. Therefore, we envision therapeutic recreation specialists working in recreation and parks agencies in programs that are aimed at therapeutic objectives, with general recreation professionals delivering opportunities for leisure experiences. There appears to be no reason why general recreation professionals and therapeutic recreation specialists should not function together in the cause of providing necessary services for persons with disabilities.

With the passage of the Americans with Disabilities Act (ADA), it is also the law of the land in the United States that recreation providers allow access to their services by persons with disabilities. The ADA, however, goes beyond governmental recreation agencies to also cover all public recreation accommodations including sport, resort, and commercial recreation enterprises. Therefore, we urge students preparing for careers in any aspect of public or private recreation to ready themselves for the important task of serving persons with disabilities.

Finally, we believe that both public and private recreation providers should offer inclusive services so that persons with disabilities have access to enjoy recreation experiences as others do. Physical and social barriers must be removed and accommodations made to permit free and equal access to recreation by persons with disabilities. Means must be provided for persons who are disabled and nondisabled to recreate together harmoniously.

SUMMARY

The organized recreation movement grew out of a social welfare concern reflected by the establishment of the Boston Sand Gardens and recreation programs in settlement houses. Eventually, however, public recreation lost its focus on individuals with special needs as a new philosophy developed that viewed recreation as an end in itself, rather than as a means to reach social ends.

It has been suggested that a broadened concept of therapeutic recreation (TR), which viewed TR as encompassing all recreation for persons with disabilities, further contributed to a perception that public recreation and parks did not have a responsibility for providing services for persons with disabilities, because these services were being provided by those identified as therapeutic recreation specialists. This broad view of therapeutic recreation has been challenged by several authors who have taken the position that inclusive and special recreation services rightfully fall within the domain of public recreation and parks. The Americans with Disabilities Act now makes it mandatory that all recreation providers (both public and private) make their facilities and programs accessible to persons with disabilities. The final segment of the chapter discussed in-service training needs and necessary competencies for recreation professionals to offer leisure opportunities for those persons who have disabilities.

SUGGESTED LEARNING ACTIVITIES

1. Prepare a two- to four-page paper in which you provide support for the idea that organized recreation evolved out of humanistic concerns.
2. In a discussion group, list reasons why communities fail to offer leisure services to people with special needs. Which reason or reasons do most of the group members consider most prominent?
3. Interview a parks and recreation administrator in your home town on the subject of community recreation for people with disabilities. Ask why the community offers (or fails to offer) leisure services for people with special needs. Prepare a two- to three-page report on your interview.
4. Prepare a two- to three-page paper on the relationship between therapeutic recreation and special recreation services. Arrive at your own personal position regarding the relationship.

5. Prepare a two-page paper in which you agree or disagree with this statement: "Existing general recreation staff can be given training to enable them to work with participants with disabilities."

6. Examine the 16 critical competencies listed in the chapter. Then do a three- to five-page self-assessment paper based on the critical competencies.

7. In class, discuss how you believe general recreation professionals and therapeutic recreation specialists can function together in the provision of community recreation for persons with disabilities.

REFERENCES

American Therapeutic Recreation Association. *Recreational Therapy: An Integral Aspect of Comprehensive Healthcare.* Hattisburg, MS: American Therapeutic Recreation Association, 1993.

Austin, D. R. *Therapeutic Recreation Processes and Techniques* (2nd ed.). Champaign, IL: Sagamore Publishing, 1991.

Austin, D. R., J. A. Peterson, & L. M. Peccarelli. The status of services for special populations in park and recreation departments in the state of Indiana. *Therapeutic Recreation Journal, 12*(1), 50–56, 1978.

Austin, D. R., & L. G. Powell. Competencies needed by community recreators to serve special populations. In D. R. Austin, Ed. *Directions in Health, Physical Education, and Recreation, Therapeutic-Recreation Curriculum: Philosophy, Strategy, and Concepts.* Bloomington, IN: Indiana University School of Health, Physical Education, and Recreation, 1980, pp. 33, 34.

Bridge, N. J., & P. Hutchison. Leisure, integration, and community. *Journal of Leisurability, 15*(1), 3–15, 1988.

Bullock, C. C., R. E. Wohl, T. E. Webreck, & A. M. Crawford, Eds. *Leisure Is for Everyone Resource and Training Manual.* Chapel Hill: University of North Carolina Curriculum on Recreation Administration, 1982.

Carter, M. J., & J. D. Kelley. Recreation programming for visually impaired children. In J. D. Kelley, Ed. *Recreation Programming for Visually Impaired Children and Youth.* New York: American Foundation for the Blind, 1981, pp. 63–79.

Carter, M. J., G. E. Van Andel, & G. M. Robb. *Therapeutic Recreation: A Practical Approach.* St. Louis: Times Mirror/Mosby College Publishing, 1985.

Dattilo, J. Leisure and TASH resolutions: A review of the literature and recommendations for future directions. In L. Meyer, C. Peck, & L. Brown, Eds. *Critical Issues in the Lives of People with Severe Disabilities.* Seattle: The Association for Persons with Severe Handicaps, 1991.

Disability Statistics Program. *Disability Statistics Abstract: People with Functional Limitations in the U.S.* San Francisco: Disability Statistics Program, University of California, 1992.

Edginton, C. R., D. M. Compton, A. J. Ritchie, & R. K. Vederman. The status of services for special populations in park and recreation departments in the state of Iowa. *Therapeutic Recreation Journal 9*(3), 109–116, 1975.

Federal Register, 54(144), July 26, 1991.

Godbey, G. C. *The Future of Leisure Services: Thriving on Change.* State College, PA: Venture, 1989.

Gray, D. E. The case of compensatory recreation. *Parks and Recreation, 4*(4), 23, 24ff, 1969.

Gunn, S. L., & C. A. Peterson. Therapy and leisure education. *Parks and Recreation, 12*(11), 22ff, 1977.

Gunn, S. L., & C. A. Peterson. *Therapeutic Recreation Program Design: Principles and Procedures.* Englewood Cliffs, NJ: Prentice-Hall, 1978.

Howe-Murphy, R., & B. G. Charboneau. *Therapeutic Recreation Intervention: An Ecological Perspective.* Englewood Cliffs, NJ: Prentice-Hall, 1987.

Kraus, R. *Recreation and Leisure in Modern Society.* New York: Appleton-Century-Croft, 1971.

LaPlante, M. P. *Disability Statistics Abstract: How Many Americans Have a Disability?* San Francisco: Disability Statistics Programs, University of California, 1992.

LIFE Resource Manual. Chapel Hill, NC: Center for Recreation and Disability Studies, University of North Carolina at Chapel Hill, 1993.

Lutzin, P. B. Serving the handicapped and elderly. In S. G. Lutzin, Ed. *Managing Municipal Leisure Services.* Washington, DC: International City Management Association, 1980, p. 152.

Meyer, L. E. Three philosophical positions of therapeutic recreation and their implications for professionalization and NTRS. In *Proceedings of the First Annual Post-Doctorate Institute.* Bloomington: Indiana University Department of Recreation and Park Administration, 1980, pp. 28–42.

Meyer, L. E. Three philosophical positions of therapeutic recreation and their implication for professionalism and NTRS/NRPA. *Therapeutic Recreation Journal, 15*(2), 7–16, 1981.

National Therapeutic Recreation Society. Philosophical position statement of the National Therapeutic Recreation Society, 1982.

Pegels, C. C. *Health Care and the Older Citizen.* Rockville, MD: Aspen, 1988.

Peterson, C. A., & S. L. Gunn. *Therapeutic Recreation Program Design: Principles and Procedures* (2nd ed.). Englewood Cliffs, NJ: Prentice-Hall, 1984.

Pomeroy, J. One community's effort. Paper presented at the Institute on Community Recreation for Special Populations sponsored by North Texas State University and the Texas Recreation and Park Society, Arlington, TX, July 19, 1974.

Robb, G. M. A practitioner's reaction to three philosophical positions of therapeutic recreation and their implications for professionalization and NTRS. In *Proceedings of the First Annual Post-Doctorate Institute.* Bloomington: Indiana University Department of Recreation and Park Administration, 1980, pp. 43–52.

Schleien, S. J., & M. T. Ray. *Community Recreation and Persons with Disabilities: Strategies for Integration.* Baltimore: Paul H. Brookes, 1988.

Sessoms, H. G., & J. L. Stevenson. *Leadership & Group Dynamics in Recreation Services.* Boston: Allyn and Bacon, 1981.

Stein, T. A., & H. D. Sessoms. *Recreation and Special Populations* (2nd ed.). Boston: Holbrook Press, 1977.

Wehman, P. *The ADA Mandate for Social Change.* Baltimore: Paul H. Brookes, 1993.

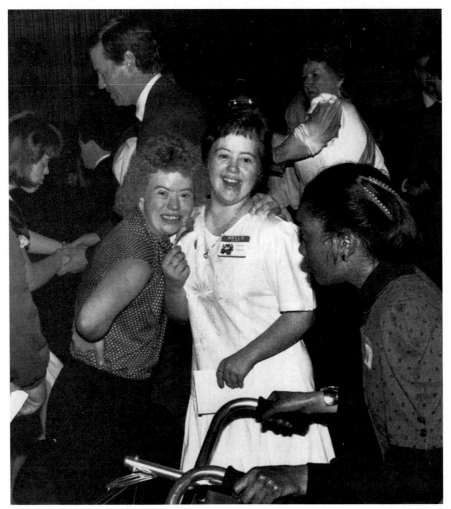

(Courtesy of Maryland-National Capital Park and Planning Commission, Special Populations Division; Photo by Steve Abramowitz)

2

Normalization

Another important term is *normalization*. This term refers to the provision of relatively normal experiences so that individuals with disabilities can maintain or develop traits and behaviors that are as culturally normative as possible (Wolfensberger, 1972). In Wolfensberger's words, normalization is

> the utilization of means which are as culturally normative as possible, in order to establish and/or maintain personal behaviours and characteristics which are as culturally normative as possible. (p. 28)

The term *normalization* does not imply that *all* people with disabilities should be participating in regular community recreation programs. Following the concept of normalization does not preclude the provision of special, segregated programs. Normalization does, however, imply that special recreation programs be as normal as possible and that relatively normal behaviors be expected from participants, to the greatest possible degree.

For example, segregated athletic participation should be as close as possible to the way the sport is normally played. Modifications need to be minimal so that as normal an athletic experience as possible can be gained by the participants. Another example involves planning activities to fit the range of participants. Activities should be age appropriate. Adults who have mental retardation should not be expected to take part in childish games. They should be able to enjoy normal adult activities that are suited to their skills rather than forced into activities designed for children.

As a general rule, the least possible modification of activities is best. Ideally, activities should not be modified at all, or should be changed as little as possible. At the same time, appropriate behavior should be expected from participants, to the greatest extent possible. In so doing, they will be able to develop skills that allow them to fit into regular recreation activities in the community. The expectation of socially normative behavior allows participants to adjust to normal community programs.

We hope that ultimately there will be a diminished need for special recreation programs as persons with special needs are able to take part in regular community programs. In regard to this point, Spinak (1975) has written,

> The long term objective for recreation programming for [people with disabilities] would hopefully be a gradual phasing-out process of "special" programs—but not to the point of termination. As [citizens with disabilities] begin to get a better grip on independence and integration, their need for special group programs should diminish. This idea is based on the belief that many [individuals with disabilities] will be able to accept the normalizing process. Undoubtedly, there will be those who are incapable of taking on full or even semi-independence for any one of many reasons. For these individuals, special recreation programs will have to be retained. Many of those who become self-sufficient will still maintain a need for generically-focused social and recreation activities. For them as well, special recreation programs should be kept available. (p. 34)

ATTITUDES

What Are Attitudes?

Attitude theorists almost inevitably include an affective component in defining the term *attitude*. That is, they see attitudes as reflecting the degree of favorableness, or unfavorableness, an individual feels toward an attitude object. Said another way, our attitudes are a gauge of our liking for someone or something (Sabini, 1992; Weber, 1992; Worchel, Cooper, & Goethals, 1991).

Attitudes are generally thought to be based on beliefs, thoughts, or ideas held toward attitude objects, whether the objects are persons, groups, places, or things. While attitudes may certainly influence behavior, they deal exclusively with how individuals *feel* toward an object, not with how they act.

Thus, in summary, we may say that attitudes rest on learned beliefs and reflect an individual's degree of liking for the attitude object. While attitudes may have a strong effect on behavior, there does not appear to be a one-to-one correspondence between attitudes and behaviors. Attitudes deal with the degree of liking for an object. Behaviors deal with our actions.

Language and Attitudes Toward Persons with Disabilities

The words we use in our everyday language tend to reflect our attitudes. Use of the terms *the disabled* or *the handicapped* are offensive to many persons because their use implies that the individuals placed in these categories are not unique human beings but are the same as all others so categorized. It is just as misleading to categorize people with disabilities as "the disabled" as it would be to categorize those enrolled in elementary schools, high schools, vocational schools, and colleges as "the students." Of course they are all students, but there the similarity ends. Their only similarity is that they are studying in educational institutions. Yet once labeled one of "the students," a young adult may be perceived differently when encountered by university personnel or the local police, or when attempting to cash a check at a place of business or obtaining housing in the community.

Likewise, the only similarity among those with disabilities is that they differ from most others in having a disability. Even in regard to their disabilities, there is a tremendous degree of variability among those who have disabilities. Certainly orthopedic disabilities are very different from learning disabilities or mental impairments. Hearing impairments differ greatly from emotional disturbances, and so on. However, once we label a person as handicapped, there is a tendency not to think of him or her as an individual with unique potentials. Instead we restrict our thinking about the individual to the labeled condition. Our stereotyped thinking minimizes our perceptions of the person's uniqueness as a human being. We focus our perceptions on categorical differences, rather than on the individual. It was in recognition of this problem that former President Reagan's

May 10, 1988, Executive Order 12640 changed the name of the 41-year-old President's Committee on Employment of the Handicapped to the President's Committee on Employment of People with Disabilities.

Because labeling a person does tend to restrict everyone's thinking, in this book we have attempted to avoid using the terms *the handicapped* or *the disabled*. Instead, we have used phrases such as "persons with disabilities" and "persons with special needs." In so doing we hope to remind ourselves and the reader of the fact that those who have a disability are, first and foremost, individual human beings much more similar to us than different. Appropriate use of terminology regarding persons who have disabilities should not be minimized. It is of fundamental importance in establishing the inherent worth and dignity of *all* human beings. Emphasizing this point, Mary Johnson, editor of the often-controversial publication *The Disability Rag* has identified language and words as probably the biggest limitation facing persons with disabilities (Rag Time, 1989).

Guidelines concerning appropriate terminology in portraying persons with disabilities have been provided by the National Easter Seal Society (NESS) (1981), Dattilo and Smith (1990), and Dattilo (1994). Based on these works, the following principles are offered:

1. Emphasize the uniqueness and worth of each individual by considering the person first. When generic references to a disabling condition are necessary, the word *disability* is more appropriate than the word *handicapped*.

Following this guideline, phrases such as *person with a disability* or *individual who has a disability* are appropriate, since these place the person or individual first. It would be inappropriate to refer to persons with disabilities as *the disabled*, since this places the emphasis on the noun *disabled* and implies that the person's total identity is tied to his or her disability. Also, this guideline suggests avoiding the use of the term *disabled* as an adjective, such as in *disabled persons*.

2. Because the person is not the condition, reference to the person in terms of the condition he or she has is inaccurate as well as demeaning. (NESS, p. 284)

We should never refer to someone as an *epileptic* or a *CP*. Instead, we should refer to him or her as "a person who has epilepsy" or "a person who has cerebral palsy." The individual is, of course, much more than a person who happens to have epilepsy or cerebral palsy or any other disorder. Moreover, the use of acronyms (e.g., CP, MR) should be avoided whenever possible because they emphasize the condition rather than the person. Also, for some who are unaware of their meaning, acronyms may add negative connotations to a disabling condition.

3. Some categorical terms are used correctly only when communicating technical information—for example, hard of hearing, deaf, partially sighted, and blind. (NESS, p. 284)

Rather than using expressions such as *partially sighted* or *deaf*, it is more appropriate to use the expressions *persons who have partial vision* or *individuals who have a partial hearing loss*. Such expressions not only place the emphasis on the person but more accurately reflect the disabilities.

It is sometimes necessary to use the person's disability as an adjective; however, such terminology should be avoided, if possible. (Photo by Lawrence M. Levy)

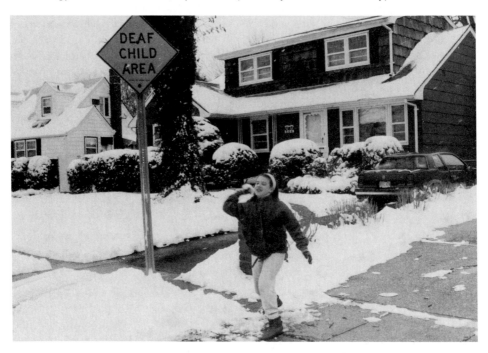

Avoid using words or terms that are negative, judgmental, or paternalistic (including use of otherwise acceptable terms in an appropriate context). Instead, use objective descriptions to emphasize each individual's abilities. Terms such as *afflicted with, crippled, invalid,* and *victim* should be avoided. Instead of saying *afflicted with,* say "the individual has an affliction." Rather than using the negative term *crippled,* use an expression such as *the person with a physical disability,* and so on. Also, it is more empathetic and accurate to use the phrase *a woman who uses a wheelchair* instead of such terms as *confined to* or *wheelchair-bound.* Words such as *defect* or *defective* reinforce negative ideas about persons with disabilities. As the Easter Seal Society guidelines stipulate, it is permissible for us to use the terms *defect* or *defective* in describing an object—but not in describing human beings. Instead of *birth defect,* we can say *disability present at birth* or *born with.* Other terms that cause difficulty if used incorrectly are *diagnose, disease,* and *patient.*

Paternalistic terms may belittle individuals, such as referring to adults as *kids,* or they may overemphasize routine achievements by using terms like *brave* or *courageous.*

4. When it is necessary to make a distinction, use the phrase *people without disabilities.*

Particularly offensive to many people with disabilities is the use of the term *normal* to apply to individuals without apparent disabilities. As Dattilo and Smith stated, such usage implies that a disability is the single distinguishing factor that divides people into two primary categories: "normal" and "disabled." The preferred phrase is *people without disabilities;* however, the term *nondisabled* may also be acceptable and is used periodically within this book. Another term for a person without a disability is *TAB*. This term is an acronym for "temporarily able-bodied" and is intended to make persons without disabilities aware they may experience a disabling condition at some point in their lives. TAB, however, is not a widely known expression and should be avoided unless it is specifically used to illustrate the point that anyone may experience a disability.

It is important to note that appropriate terminology related to disability is constantly changing. A term that is considered appropriate at one point in time may later be considered inappropriate or even offensive. Conversely, as Dattilo (1994) has written:

> Words that are currently creating controversy, and have yet to receive a general consensus, may be the words of choice in the future. In all situations, listen to your constituents to determine the terms and phrases they most prefer and attempt to understand their reasons for these choices. (p. 73)

Means to Attitude Change

Attitude change is generally perceived to be brought about through two means. One is through the use of *persuasive communication.* The second is through *exposure.*

Persuasive Communication. Authorities generally agree that attitudes are changed by means of one of two routes to persuasion. These are the *central route* and the *peripheral route.* When people carefully scrutinize presentations, they are using the central route. People concern themselves with carefully considering the arguments contained in the message and how strong they are. Attitudes generally change to the extent that arguments are strong. People tend to follow the central route in instances when they care about a particular issue. When the topic is less important, people are more likely to follow the peripheral route. Using the peripheral route, individuals are more affected by the mood they are in and tend to pay more attention to factors such as the communicator's attractiveness and likability. Celebrities are often used to persuade via the peripheral route (Cooper & Aronson, 1992; Sabini, 1992; Worchel, Cooper, & Goethals, 1991).

Therefore, to alter attitudes toward serving persons with disabilities, certain principles should be followed. If the audience sees the issue as important, strong arguments need to be put forth to ensure a persuasive communication. On the other hand, if the audience does not perceive the topic as being important, the presenter should be chosen carefully, because the attributes of the communicator (e.g., attractiveness) may have a significant effect, and care should be taken to put audience members in a good mood.

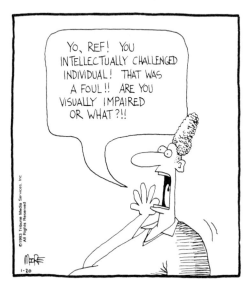

Politically correct heckling

A related strategy is to ask audience members to *role-play*. If persons are asked to play the role of someone who holds a position differing from theirs, they often will alter their beliefs to correspond with the role assumed. Some research has found that role playing produces greater attitude changes than receiving a presentation (Worchel, Cooper, & Goethals, 1991). Although there is a lack of empirical evidence in the literature indicating the use of role playing in changing attitudes toward serving individuals with disabilities, it would appear to be an effective method.

Altering Attitudes Toward Persons with Disabilities. Both role playing and presentations have been successfully employed to alter general attitudes toward individuals with disabilities. Researchers at the University of Illinois (Clore & Jeffery, 1972) found that role-playing a wheelchair user by traveling on campus for an hour brought about more positive attitudes toward persons with disabilities. Such realistic experiences should not be confused, however, with simulations in which individuals without disabilities take part in recreational activities while simulating disabilities. Donaldson (1980), after reviewing the research, has stated, "the present fad of game-type disability simulations may have little effect in helping participants see [persons with disabilities] in less stereotypic ways" (p. 511).

Presentations have sometimes been effective in changing global attitudes toward persons with disabilities. One study (Austin, Powell, & Martin, 1981) involved the use of a class presentation that positively influenced the attitudes recreation and leisure studies students held toward individuals with disabilities. Results of studies involving such presentations, however, have been equivocal. To date, the exact factors that contribute to positive changes have not been identified. Further research is needed to determine more precisely the factors that facilitate positive changes resulting from presentations directed toward altering attitudes about persons with disabilities.

Exposure. Zajonc (1968) conducted the now-classic "black bag" social psychology study. Zajonc exposed university students in a speech class to an unknown person hidden inside a large black bag. The person in the black bag sat quietly on a table in the rear of the classroom during the entire semester. At the beginning, students were hostile toward the black bag but grew to like it by the end of the term. It was reasoned that mere exposure to an object (in this case, the black bag) was sufficient to bring about attitude enhancement. In other words, attitudes are enhanced by mere exposure to, or contact with, an attitude object.

Exposure as a Means to Alter Attitudes Toward Persons with Disabilities. Research has revealed that mere contact with individuals who have disabilities, unlike contact with black bags, does not necessarily produce more positive attitudes toward these individuals. In fact, negative attitudes may result if nondisabled persons experience tension or anxiety, or perceive information that reinforces existing stereotypes (Donaldson, 1980). Since uninitiated people may feel uncomfortable with persons who have disabilities, it is of utmost importance to structure the situation so that nondisabled persons experience pleasant feelings during their exposure to persons with disabilities. It is likewise important that old stereotypes are not reinforced but instead are changed as a result of the contact. Recreational situations should provide an ideal setting for altering attitudes through exposure to persons with disabilities. A pleasant recreation environment offers an ideal situation in which persons without disabilities can interact with individuals who provide healthy, positive images of persons with disabilities. An example of this is college students working in recreational sports programs with skilled athletes who are disabled.

Austin and Lewko (1979) reported that camp staff working with campers who had disabilities became markedly more positive in their attitudes from the beginning to the end of a six-week summer camp. They attributed their results, in part, to the positive environment. They wrote,

> The positive social-recreational climate normally found in the informal camp setting would seem to facilitate the development of positive attitudes toward [people with disabilities]. (p. 5)

In retrospect, while the mere contact hypothesis was perhaps naive, it has led us to more research that has revealed that, under certain conditions, contact with persons who have disabilities can lead to more positive attitudes. Nevertheless, even though exposure may produce a positive effect on general attitudes toward people with disabilities, global attitudes have not been found to correlate with specific behaviors, such as providing recreation services for people with special needs. The following section covers work that questions our traditional thinking regarding attitudes and behavior.

A Myth?

Several authors in the field of leisure and recreation (e.g., Howe-Murphy & Charboneau, 1987; Schleien & Ray, 1988) have proclaimed that negative attitudes toward persons with disabilities cause barriers to the provision of recreation services for these persons. However, Ajzen (1988) has argued convincingly that attitudes toward any given object (e.g., persons with disabilities) can predict only a *general pattern* of behavior, and not a *specific* behavior. Thus a general measure of attitude (i.e., a score on a scale measuring attitudes toward persons with disabilities) would not be useful in predicting a specific behavior, such as providing recreation services for persons with disabilities.

Following the conceptual framework provided by Ajzen (1988), we would be unwise to believe that if we alter attitudes toward persons with disabilities in a positive way, we can expect those holding more favorable attitudes to be more likely to provide special recreation services. Ajzen stipulates that, to predict a *specific behavior,* one needs to know the *specific attitude* related to that behavior. To predict whether a community parks and recreation professional would provide services designed for persons with disabilities, we would need to know his or her specific attitude toward serving them, not what general attitude he or she holds toward individuals who have disabilities.

There are, of course, factors other than attitudes that could influence whether persons with disabilities would be served by community parks and recreation specialists. Factors such as social norms, influences from other people, consequences of the behaviors, and personality traits have been used in predicting behavior (Ajzen, 1988; Ajzen & Fishbein, 1980). Another factor influencing behavior is the amount of experience a person has had with the attitude object (Fazio & Zanna, 1978; Regan & Fazio, 1977). Findings suggest that behaviors can be predicted from attitudes when the person has had previous experience with the attitude object. For example, an individual who has had experience in the provision of recreation for persons with special needs would be more apt to act in accord with his or her attitudes toward serving persons with disabilities than would a person without previous experience.

Thus, the traditional model in which it was supposed that improvement in general attitudes toward persons with disabilities would result in increased provision of recreation services to persons who have disabilities has not found support in modern attitude literature. The level of specificity of the attitude and other factors (e.g., social norms, previous experiences) need to be taken into consideration when attempting to predict any behavior, including the provision of recreation services to persons who have disabilities.

Rynders, J. E., & S. J. Schleien. *Together Successfully.* Arlington, TX: Association for Retarded Citizens of the United States, 1991.

Sabini, J. *Social Psychology.* New York: W.W. Norton & Company, 1992.

Schleien, S., & M. T. Ray. *Community Recreation and Persons with Disabilities: Strategies for Integration.* Baltimore, MD: Paul H. Brooks, 1988.

Smith, R. *Programming for Handicapped Individuals in Public Park and Recreation Settings.* Washington, DC: Hawkins and Associates, 1980.

Spinak, J. Normalization and recreation for the disabled. *Leisurability, 2*(2), 31–35, 1975.

Stein, J. U. Mainstreaming in recreational settings: It can be done. *Leisure Today.* In *Journal of Physical Education, Recreation and Dance, 56*(5), 3, 52, 1985.

Weber, A. L. *Social Psychology.* New York: HarperCollins Publishers, 1992.

Wehman, P. *The ADA Mandate for Social Change.* Baltimore: Paul H. Brookes, 1993.

Wolfensberger, W. *Normalization.* Toronto: National Institute on Mental Retardation, 1972.

Worchel, S., J. Cooper, & G. R. Goethals. *Understanding Social Psychology* (5th ed.). New York: Brooks/Cole, 1991.

Zajonc, R. B. Attitudinal effects of mere exposure. *Journal of Personality and Social Psychology, 9*(2), 1–27, 1968.

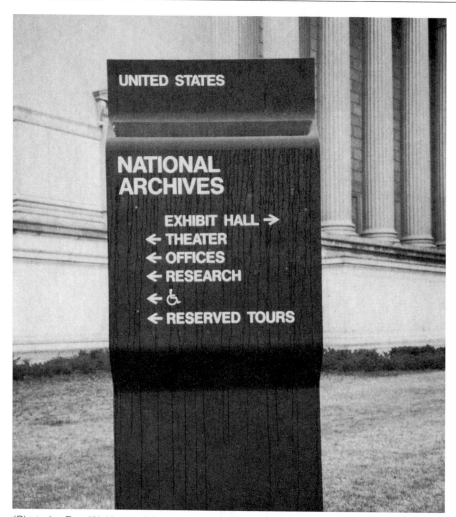

(Photo by Dan W. Kennedy)

3

Legislation Affecting Inclusive and Special Recreation Services

■ ■ ■

Over the past three decades, concern for equal rights for individuals who have disabilities has been developing and changing. Legislation pertaining to equal access, as well as rights to educational and recreational services, has evolved. This chapter presents a selection of legislative acts that, to varying degrees, have affected the delivery of recreation services to persons with disabilities who reside in the United States. The Americans with Disabilities Act of 1990 is showcased in the first section, followed by accessibility legislation, rehabilitation acts, education legislation, and other legislative efforts that have set the tone for many of the recent developments in the delivery of recreation and park programs and services to individuals with disabilities.

THE AMERICANS WITH DISABILITIES ACT OF 1990, PL 101-336

Attention to persons with disabilities has since World War II led to better health care, the right to vote, and the right to a free, appropriate, public education. Although legislation in the 1970s in America was passed to prohibit discrimination on the basis of disability, discrimination continued in an array of areas, including employment, transportation, and *recreation.*

How Does Discrimination Manifest Itself in Recreation Programs and Services?

- It may occur when a person with a disability or family member of the person inquires about enrolling in a particular program and is referred inappropriately elsewhere.
- It occurs when parks, playgrounds, and other recreation facilities and equipment are not designed for accessibility and usability.
- It occurs when camp personnel refuse to accommodate a child with a mild impairment.
- It occurs when individuals with disabilities are not granted a job interview because they possess an impairment.

What Is the Purpose of the Americans with Disabilities Act?

Legislation providing a clear goal of eliminating discrimination against persons with disabilities was first introduced to the 100th Congress in 1988, and was known as the Americans with Disabilities Act (ADA). It was signed into law in July, 1990. ADA is designed to increase significantly the opportunity for millions of Americans with disabilities to participate more fully in the activities and to benefit from the services generally available to all other Americans.

The bill represents a major expansion of the rights of individuals with disabilities. As have other civil rights measures, the requirements of the ADA apply to both public and private employers and to providers of public services. This encompasses a multitude of services including shopping, going to the movies, and participating in *recreation and park services*. As McGovern (1992) states:

> Make no mistake about it, the ADA IS a civil rights law. Congress intended that the ADA will extend the protections of the 1973 Rehabilitation Act to all 33,000 units of government, and all organizations and businesses in this country that affect the availability of goods, services, and facilities for the general public. (p. 7)

Recreation specialists need to be advocates for the civil rights of persons with disabilities and determine how the various aspects of the legislation affect programs and services. Nondiscriminatory practices are vital to the integration of persons with disabilities within the mainstream of American life. As noted by Schleien and Ray (1988), the community recreation professional must ensure that the philosophical position of the agency is nondiscriminatory in practice, policy, and attitudes.

Who Is Protected by the ADA?

All individuals with disabilities are protected. The ADA definition of *individual with a disability* is very specific. A person with a disability is an individual who:

- has a physical or mental impairment that substantially limits one or more major life activities;
- has a record of such an impairment; or
- is regarded as having such an impairment.

In order for the requirements under the ADA to be applied, the disability has to result in a substantial limitation of one or more major life activities, such as caring for one's self, performing manual tasks, walking, seeing, hearing, speaking, breathing, learning, working, and *participating in community activities*.

Table 3.1 Americans with Disabilities Act Overview

Title	Category	Effective Date	Enforcement
I	Employment	1/26/92	Equal Employment Opportunity Commission
IIA	Government services	1/26/92	U.S. Department of Justice*
IIB	Public transit	8/26/92	U.S. Department of Transportation
III	Public accommodations	1/26/92	U.S. Department of Transportation
IV	Telecommunications	7/26/93	Federal Communications Commission

*Complaints may be filed with the state, with the U.S. Department of Justice or a designated federal agency (e.g., for parks and recreation, the Department of Interior), or in federal court.

Who Must Comply with the ADA?

There are five titles within the ADA (see Table 3.1). Title V includes miscellaneous provisions and is not referenced in Table 3.1. Title I covers nondiscrimination in employment activities; Title II requires states and local government entities, programs, and transportation to be made accessible to and usable by persons with disabilities; Title III covers the accessibility and availability of programs, goods, and services provided to the public by private entities; and Title IV requires that telecommunications services be made accessible to persons with hearing and speech impairments.

For example, private employers, state and local governments, employment agencies, labor unions, and joint labor-management committees must comply with Title I of the ADA. An employer cannot discriminate against *qualified* applicants and employees on the basis of disability. Title III of the Act applies to privately operated entities including restaurants, public buildings, *parks,* and *other places of recreation.*

What Does the ADA Require of Businesses and Organizations?

The ADA requires businesses and organizations to afford individuals with disabilities a full and equal opportunity to enjoy the goods, services, facilities, privileges, and advantages of accommodations generally provided to their clientele. Businesses and organizations must provide these services to individuals with disabilities *in the most integrated*

FOUR RULES FOR COMPLIANCE
WITH THE ADA

1. No medical questions on application forms

2. Focus on individual ability, not disability.

3. Don't treat persons with disabilities differently from other people.

4. Provide reasonable accommodation where it is necessary so long as it doesn't pose an undue hardship.

---

setting appropriate to the needs of those individuals. Therefore, all recreation programs, services, and activities must be available in the most integrated setting possible. To ensure the provision of services in the most integrated setting, the ADA requires the following of covered businesses:

- that they make reasonable modifications in policies, practices, and procedures when necessary to afford services to individuals with disabilities, unless these modifications would fundamentally alter the nature of the services;

- that they provide auxiliary aids and services to ensure that individuals with disabilities are not excluded, denied services, segregated, or otherwise treated differently from other individuals, unless the auxiliary aid or service would fundamentally alter the nature of the service or would result in an undue burden;

- that they remove architectural and communication barriers that are structural, if the removal of these barriers is readily achievable;

- that they design new facilities so that they are readily accessible to individuals with disabilities unless accessibility is structurally impractical; and

- that, when undertaking an alteration of an existing structure, they design alterations in a manner that, to the maximum extent feasible, provides accessibility. The regulations specifically focus on accessibility in entrances, hallways, bathrooms, telephones, and drinking fountains.

What Does the ADA Mean to Providers of Recreation and Parks Services?

As indicated earlier, community-based recreation agencies must ensure that the philosophical position of their organization is nondiscriminatory in practice, policy, and attitudes. If this occurs in both hiring practices and in the delivery of recreation and leisure services to persons with disabilities, then the intent of the law is met.

More specifically, when hiring individuals with disabilities, recreation and parks agencies must treat such persons the same as persons without disabilities and provide reasonable accommodation where it is necessary so long as it doesn't pose an undue hardship. For instance, the chairs in a recreation room may need to be reorganized to accommodate individuals in wheelchairs.

With regard to offering recreation and parks programs and services to persons with disabilities, these individuals cannot be excluded, denied, or otherwise treated differently from other individuals, unless the service or program would fundamentally alter the nature of the service or would result in an undue burden. For example, the recreation agency may have to provide or help provide transportation to and from a program site, or the parks and recreation agency may need to create a path in a park between playground apparatus to make the areas accessible and usable by children with disabilities.

The Title II requirements are of primary interest to recreation and leisure agencies. According to McGovern (1992), the key to the Title II requirements is the determination of whether an individual with a disability could meet *essential eligibility* requirements for the use or enjoyment of parks and recreation agency programs and services. For example, if an individual with a disability meets the essential eligibility requirements under the ADA, a parks and recreation department must consider revising requirements for registration and eligibility for participation in programs, removing architectural barriers, providing additional communications media to reach visual and hearing impaired individuals, and providing additional services to accommodate special needs.

McGovern (1992) suggests that *essential eligibility* is likely to include capacity, charges, and conduct.

> Has this individual registered for the service, program, or activity before it was closed because it was at capacity?
>
> Will the individual pay the usual fees for the program?
>
> Will the individual follow reasonable rules of conduct? (p. 10)

Four additional factors that may modify eligibility are *residency, relative skill, safety,* and *age*. As McGovern points out, it is important that modifications apply to all registrants.

Finally, architectural and communication barriers must be removed so that persons with disabilities have access to programs and services. This can include providing access to buildings, restrooms, telephones, and drinking fountains. Recreation and parks agencies also need to make their programs accessible. This may involve modifying program materials. For example, an individual with a visual impairment may want to play bridge. In this instance a special deck of cards with raised numbers may be necessary. If a person with a hearing impairment wants to view a movie, effort must be made to accommodate the person by doing such things as raising the volume, providing an amplifier, having an interpreter, or using closed captions. However, if one or more of these options puts an undue burden on the agency, then they do not have to comply. The ADA defines *undue hardship* as an accommodation that is unduly costly, extensive, substantial, or disruptive, or would fundamentally alter the nature or operation of the business or activity.

ACCESSIBILITY

The Architectural Barriers Act of 1968, PL 90-480

Public Law 90-480 is commonly known as the Architectural Barriers Act. It has been amended twice since its initial enactment in 1968: once to cover construction of transportation facilities in the Washington metropolitan area in 1970; and in 1976, to strengthen the language of the original bill and to include buildings of the United States Postal Service under PL 90-480 coverage.

While PL 90-480 does not reference recreation, it has had a significant impact on the provision of recreational opportunities for persons who are disabled. In essence, the act ensures that certain buildings financed with federal funds are so designed and constructed as to be accessible to and usable by those with disabilities. By 1973, all 50 states had passed similar legislation, and many local governments had passed local ordinances relating to accessibility.

The standards used in PL 90-480 are those developed in 1961 by both the President's Committee on Employment of the Handicapped and the National Easter Seal Society. These guidelines were published in a document entitled *American National Standard Specifications for Making Buildings and Facilities Accessible to and Usable by Physically Disabled People* and were adopted by the American National Standards Institute (ANSI). The specifications, of course, focus on access to buildings and facilities. Definitions are presented, along with wheelchair specifications, and site development (grading, walks, parking lots). Specifications for items such as ramps, entrances, toilet rooms, and public telephones are highlighted. (See Chapter 6 for detailed information on accessibility standards.)

There are several guidelines and legislative acts prepared by governmental bodies that relate to PL 90-480. For example, The Rehabilitation Act of 1973 (PL 93-112) established the Architectural and Transportation Barriers Compliance Board to ensure adherence to PL 90-480. The Veterans Administration (VA) in its VA Construction Standard CD-28 (1973), entitled "Accommodations for the Physically Handicapped," designates some of the ways that VA facilities need to be altered or designed to accommodate disabled persons. The Building Officials and Code Administrators Building Code was modified in June, 1974, to add provisions for elderly persons and those with physical disabilities (Park, 1980).

State Legislation

It should be noted that nearly half of the states had passed legislation pertaining to accessibility of public buildings prior to the passage of PL 90-480. Application of state legislation usually covers publicly funded buildings. Acts ensure that buildings financed with state monies are constructed accessible to and usable by elderly persons and those with physical disabilities. As stated earlier, *all* states have legislation comparable to PL 90-480. Table 3.2 on page 46 outlines some aspects of the legislation for three states: Indiana, Maryland, and Pennsylvania.

REHABILITATION ACTS AND AMENDMENTS

The original Vocational Rehabilitation Act was passed in 1954. The primary purpose of this act was to rehabilitate veterans with disabilities. Programs included direct medical assistance and vocational training. Nine years later, in 1963, the Rehabilitation Act Amendments included the phrase "recreation for ill and handicapped." Soon after this addition, several colleges and universities received federal monies from the Rehabilitation Services Administration (RSA) to initiate and/or develop master's degree programs to prepare recreators to work with persons with disabilities. Sessoms (1970) has stated that during the first five years of RSA support, 217 traineeships were awarded to 11 universities and colleges. Park (1980) suggested that more than 140 colleges and universities had received financial support by the end of the 1970s. Thus, hundreds of students received financial assistance through the RSA program. It is difficult to judge accurately the impact that the RSA traineeship program in recreation has had on either the profession of recreation or the number and quality of leisure services rendered to individuals with disabling conditions. However, it may be surmised that the impact has been significant. In addition, these academic programs laid the framework for the eventual development of therapeutic recreation options and emphases within recreation and parks curricula.

Table 3.2 Examples of State Legislation Relating to Architectural Barriers[a]

State	Legislation Date Effective	Application of Act	Compliance Adopts ANSI Standards	Covers Remodeling	Covers Leased Buildings	Enforcement			Inspection of New Buildings
						State	School	Local	
Indiana	Leg. Act Chap. # 49 (10/24/69)	Publ. owned bldg.	Yes	Yes	Yes	Admin. Bldg. Council			Yes
Maryland	Leg. Act Senate Bill # 404 added new Section # 51 to Article # 78, A (7/1/68)	Publ. funded bldgs.	Yes	Yes	Yes	Gen. Ser. Adm. State Dept. Ed. Pol. Subdiv.			Yes
Pennsylvania	Leg. Act # 348 Act of Gen. Assem. # 235 (9/1/65)	Publ. funded bldgs.	Yes	Yes	Yes	Dept. of Labor and Industry			Yes

[a]Taken from U.S. Dept. of HUD, Barrier Free Site Design, Appendix C, pp. 71–75, 1975.

Rehabilitation Act of 1973, PL 93-112

The 1973 amendments (PL 93-112) added new directions to recreation services. The "Vocational Rehabilitation Act" was changed to the "Rehabilitation Act." Thus, the concept of rehabilitation was broadened. This act continued the authorization of recreation services in both training and research but added new sections that have affected recreation services for persons with disabilities. Selected segments of the Rehabilitation Act follow.

1. Title II—*Research and Training.* This title continued to authorize funds for training recreation personnel to work with persons who have disabilities and for research monies for projects in recreation.

2. Title III, Section 304—*Special Projects and Demonstrations.* This section made monies available for grants for "operating programs to demonstrate methods of making recreational activities fully accessible" to individuals with disabilities. Several projects in recreation, such as the Parks and Recreation Commission in Wood County, West Virginia, which developed a recreation complex that is accessible to individuals with disabilities, have affected the delivery of recreation services.

3. Title V, Section 502—*Architectural and Transportation Barriers Compliance Board.* Section 502 created the Architectural and Transportation Barriers Compliance Board (A&TBCB) whose main function is to seek compliance with Public Law 90-480. Any citizen may file a complaint with this agency if a barrier is confronted in a public building or facility, particularly with respect to monuments, parks, and parklands covered by PL 90-480. Regulations entitled "Compliance with Standards for Access to and Use of Buildings by Handicapped Persons" were published by this agency in the Federal Register, Tuesday, November 25, 1980. Another function of the A&TBCB required by the Rehabilitation Act Amendments of 1978 (PL 95-602) was to establish minimum guidelines and requirements, which were published in the Federal Register on Friday, January 16, 1981, for the four federal standard-setting agencies. These four agencies designated by the Architectural Barriers Act are the General Services Administration, Department of Housing and Urban Development, Department of Defense, and the United States Postal Service. These agencies had one year from the effective date of the regulations (January 6, 1981) to issue final revised standards that have as a minimum the guidelines that were published. Many of the A&TBCB provisions were adopted from ANSI (A 117.1-1980). The 1980 ANSI code was not adopted by the A&TBCB; therefore, each federal agency will be issuing new accessibility codes; different design standards are issued by the many diverse federal agencies.

4. Title V, Section 504—*Nondiscrimination Under Federal Grants.* Section 504 is acknowledged to be landmark legislation for Americans with disabilities. The Department of Health and Human Services (formerly Department of Health, Education and Welfare) is the lead agency for Section 504 compliance. The Department of HHS published the first set of Section 504 regulations for recipients of HHS funds in the Federal Register, Wednesday, May 4, 1977, entitled "Nondiscrimination on Basis of Handicap: Programs and Activities Receiving or Benefiting from Federal Financial Assistance." This section states that "No otherwise qualified handicapped individual shall, solely by reason of his handicap, be excluded from the participation in, be denied the benefits of, or be subjected to discrimination under, any program or activity conducted by an executive agency or by the United States Postal Service." Failure to comply with the law can result in the withholding and/or withdrawal of federal financial assistance.

The impact of the Rehabilitation Act on public recreation services has not been determined. The issue of discrimination has been made unclear by attempts to soften legislation. For instance, the Architectural and Transportation Barriers Compliance Board adopted a softened plan on December 1, 1981, when members realized their original proposal faced certain rejection by the Administration and Congress. Dropped were rules requiring renovation of older transit stations and federally leased buildings, including thousands of postal offices. In the final analysis, such actions mean that fewer elevators, rails, ramps, and other special requirements will be built in either old or new buildings constructed with federal monies.

Rehabilitation Act Amendment of 1974, PL 93-516

The Rehabilitation Act Amendment of 1974 authorized the planning and implementation of the White House Conference on Handicapped Individuals, which was convened in May of 1977. Recreation was 1 of 16 major areas of concern at the White House Conference. The final report[1] noted the importance of recreation for individuals with disabilities and called for the expansion of recreation services, as well as an increase in the number of professionally trained individuals employed in the field of recreation.

Recreation and leisure services, outdoor recreation for persons with disabilities, and recreational programs and facilities are mentioned in the report. Generally, the main points of the report included funding incentives, accessibility, community-based recreation

---

1. The White House Conference on Handicapped Individuals, Volume Two: Final Report, Part C. Washington, D.C.: Superintendent of Documents, U.S. Government Printing Office, 1977.

programs, and employment and training of recreation professionals. In addition, under the heading of "Social Concerns," recreation was listed. The following is an abbreviated list of concerns dealing with the design of recreational services:

- accessibility
- program variety
- leisure skill development
- handicapped lobby

- transportation
- program integration
- funding for recreation
- public awareness

Rehabilitation Act of 1978, PL 95-602

As with many federal programs, the 1973 Rehabilitation Act and the programs it authorized expired at the end of five years. In 1978 legislation was introduced to extend and amend the 1973 act. The 1978 act contained six separate sections that called for recreation and leisure services as part of the rehabilitation process. PL 95-602 authorized the continuation of training programs, although training funds for recreation were curtailed in several regions of the country. The act included recreation as a service to be provided in rehabilitation facilities as well as in special public projects and demonstration programs such as the Regional Activities and Recreation Center for the Handicapped in Wood County, West Virginia.

The Senate Committee on Human Resources, in introducing the Senate bill to amend and extend the 1973 Rehabilitation Act, stated:

- In recognition of the recreational and social needs of handicapped individuals, the committee bill amends section 304 to authorize the secretary to make grants to states and public non-profit agencies and organizations for the purpose of initiating recreational programs for handicapped individuals.

- Recreational programs for handicapped individuals are greatly needed in order to assist them in developing their capacity for mobility and socialization. Unfortunately, existing programming for this purpose is limited; therefore, it is the committee's intent that this authority stimulate the development of and utilization of more community-based recreation programs.

- It is the committee's intent that handicapped individuals participate in existing regularly scheduled recreation programs to the maximum extent feasible; the committee realizes, however, that the specialized needs of handicapped individuals may necessitate adaptive equipment and programming and specially trained personnel. The committee therefore expects that such adaptive equipment and programming as well as specialized personnel attuned to the needs of handicapped persons will be an integral part of any recreation program initiated under this authority. It is further expected that such recreation programs should be coordinated with other recreational activities offered in the community. (Senate Report, 1978)

From a legislative funding perspective, recreation services to persons with disabilities have fared quite well. As a result of the amendments to the Rehabilitation Act of 1978 (PL 95-602), with reference to Sections 311 and 316, approximately $9 million have been allocated through the two sections to various agencies to make recreation facilities and programs accessible to persons with disabilities.

Section 311 provides grants to public or nonprofit agencies and organizations to pay part or all of the costs of special projects and demonstrations for operating programs and, where appropriate, renovating and constructing facilities to demonstrate methods of making *recreational* activities fully accessible to individuals who have disabilities.

Any project or demonstration assisted by a grant under this section that provides services to individuals with spinal cord injuries shall demonstrate and evaluate methods of community outreach for individuals with spinal cord injuries and community education in connection with the problems of such individuals in areas such as housing, transportation, *recreation,* employment, and community activities.

Section 316 provides grants to state and public nonprofit agencies and organizations for paying part or all of the cost of initiation of *recreation* programs to provide individuals with disabilities with *recreational* activities to aid in the mobility and socialization of such individuals. The activities authorized to be assisted under this section may include, but are not limited to, scouting and camping, 4-H activities, sports, music, dancing, handicrafts, art, and homemaking.

Two million dollars were allocated in 1984 through Section 316. In 1985, the National Recreation and Park Association urged the House Subcommittee on Labor, Health and Human Services, and Education to support supplemental appropriations for Section 316. This type of legislative support, along with support from the Special Education Program (Office of Special Education and Rehabilitation Services) in personnel preparation and research will continue to contribute to the growth and development of the profession (Reynolds & O'Morrow, 1985).

Finally, a major new section added to the 1978 act expanded the number of persons with disabilities eligible to receive services and "recreational and leisure time activities." Title VII, entitled Comprehensive Services for Independent Living, made funds available for the development of comprehensive services to persons with disabilities.

EDUCATION LEGISLATION

Education for Handicapped Children Act of 1967, PL 90-170

Legislation having great influence on recreation services for children with disabilities has been the Education for Handicapped Children Act of 1967, PL 90-170, amended by PL 93-380 and by PL 94-142. PL 90-170 provided a considerable amount of federal funds for the professional preparation of recreation personnel working with children with disabilities. In 1967, Senator Edward Kennedy (D-Mass.) introduced an amendment that created specific authorization for funds in the areas of physical education and recreation. More specifically, Title V, Section 501(a) stated:

> It is authorized to make grants to public and other non-profit institutions of higher learning to assist them in providing professional or advanced training for personnel engaged or preparing to engage in employment as physical educators or recreation personnel for mentally retarded and other handicapped children . . . or engaged or preparing to engage in research or teaching in fields relative to the physical education or recreation of such children.

This legislation enabled many colleges and universities to educate hundreds of students to work with children with disabling conditions in a variety of recreational settings.

Education for All Handicapped Children Act of 1975, PL 94-142 (Now Individuals with Disabilities Education Act, IDEA)

The Education for Handicapped Children Act was amended by PL 94-142 (1975). The amended act was titled the "Education for All Handicapped Children Act." It read, in part:

> It is the purpose of this act to assure that all handicapped children have available to them, within the time periods specified in Section 612 (2) (B), *a free appropriate public education* (FAPE) which emphasizes special education and related services designed to meet their unique needs, to assure that the rights of handicapped children and their parents or guardians are protected, to assist states and localities to provide for the education of all handicapped children, and to assess and assure the effectiveness of efforts to educate handicapped children.
>
> The term "related services" means transportation, and such development, corrective and other supportive services (including . . . *recreation* . . .) as may be required to assist a handicapped child to benefit from special education.

The regulations governing implementation of the law define recreation as including

1. assessment of leisure functioning
2. therapeutic recreation
3. recreation in schools and communities
4. leisure education

The inclusion of recreation as a related service provided a rationale for the inclusion of recreation as part of the individualized education plan (IEP) and suggested a framework for the delivery of recreation services. This particular point is highlighted in a hearing in Massachusetts involving a female student, Sandra T. In this court hearing, provisions on access to, and equal opportunity to participate in, extracurricular activities in after-school hours that were offered to students without disabilities was a major issue. Dispute between the parties centered on whether Sandra's special needs indicated that an after-school therapeutic recreation/leisure education component should be included in her IEP.

In short, a decision (BSEA # 3231)[2] ordered Old Rochester Regional School District to provide an after-school program of related services for Sandra T., incorporating socialization, recreation, physical development, and leisure education objectives for a minimum of six hours per week. Additionally, it was stated: "An aide shall be designated to carry out the program and a therapeutic recreation specialist shall provide a consulting and in-service program to interested teachers, etc., as well as provide direct service to Sandra individually or in a small group for a minimum of one hour per week."

In 1990, PL 101-476 amended the Education of the Handicapped Act to revise and extend the programs and purposes of PL 94-142. For example, under Related Services, the term "therapeutic" was added to the existing word "recreation."

Under Title IX, Section 601(a), the short title "Education of the Handicapped Act" was replaced by the title "Individuals with Disabilities Education Act" (IDEA). This change in wording as well as other changes, including replacing "disabilities" for "handicaps" and striking "handicapped children" and inserting "children with disabilities," updates the language of the law to reflect current terminology.

OTHER LEGISLATION

This section contains two other pieces of legislation that have had an impact on community recreation services for persons with disabilities.

Developmental Disabilities and Facilities Construction Act of 1970, PL 91-517

This act provided services to children and adults with developmental disabilities attributable to mental retardation, cerebral palsy, epilepsy, or other neurological conditions. This law was amended by PL 94-103, entitled "The Developmentally Disabled Assistance Bill of Rights Act of 1975," which added autism to the list of disabilities.

The developmental disabilities program does not provide direct services to individuals. Instead, it is oriented toward the provision of grant funds to a grantee who, in turn, provides the direct service to a population as a result of the acquired funds. Monies are awarded according to priorities established in the annual state plan.

These grants are for planning, administration, services, and construction of facilities and are awarded through Titles I and II of the Developmental Disabilities (DD) Act. Title I provides funding under a formula grant, which is money allocated to the states on a formula basis to be distributed by state agencies. "Recreation" as a fundable activity is mentioned in

---

2. This decision was issued pursuant to the requirements of M.G.L.C. 15, 31A, C. 718, The Education of All Handicapped Children Act (20 V.S.C. 1401–1461), The Rehabilitation Act of 1973, Section 502 (20 V.S.C. 794), . . . 1980.

The National Center on Accessibility, located at Bradford Woods in Indiana, provides information and assistance regarding legal mandates to ensure access for all. (Photo courtesy of Bradford Woods, Indiana University)

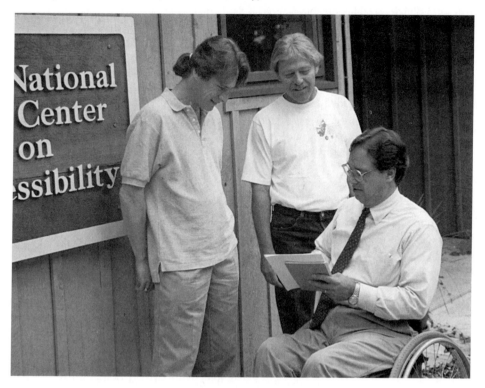

the law as one of the specific supportive services under the formula grants. Recreation services are aimed at providing opportunities for recreation, physical education, and open space acquisition and development.

Title II of the law is allocated for "interdisciplinary training programs in institutions of higher learning and for University Affiliated Facilities to house these programs." These facilities offer out-patient and in-patient services, provide training for service personnel, and improve the move toward integration and appropriate community services to individuals with developmental disabilities.

In 1978, the DD Act was amended through passage of the Rehabilitation Comprehensive Services and Developmental Disabilities Amendments. This had an impact on the expansion of services for individuals with disabilities. It affected the Rehabilitation Act of 1973, the Developmental Disabilities Services and Facilities Construction Act, and the Developmentally-Disabled Bill of Rights Act of 1975.

The overall purposes of the act were:

1. To assist in the provision of comprehensive services to persons with developmental disabilities, with priority to those persons whose needs cannot be covered or otherwise met under the Education for All Handicapped Children Act, the Rehabilitation Act of 1973, or other health, education, or welfare programs;
2. To assist states in appropriate planning activities;
3. To make grants to states and public and private nonprofit agencies to establish model programs, to demonstrate innovative habilitation techniques, and to train professional and paraprofessional personnel with respect to providing services to persons with developmental disabilities;
4. To make grants to university-affiliated facilities to assist them in administering and operating demonstration facilities for the provision of services to persons with developmental disabilities, and interdisciplinary training programs for personnel needed to provide specialized services for these persons; and
5. To make grants to support a system in each state to protect the legal and human rights of all persons with developmental disabilities.

The implications of these amendments to the recreation field are numerous. They allow recreation professionals opportunities to develop and implement special services, training, and research projects in the area of developmental disabilities. Some of the possibilities include (1) services necessary for community adjustment, such as counseling and educating the individual regarding leisure habits and resources for involvement in the community; (2) public awareness and educational programs to assist in the integration of individuals with disabilities into the mainstream of society; (3) coordination of all available community resources; (4) training of specialized personnel needed to service delivery or for research related to developmental disabilities; (5) development of demonstration techniques or projects to serve as a pilot for the expansion and continuation of innovative and successful programs; and (6) gathering and dissemination of information related to developmental disabilities.

The qualified recreation professional can actively involve himself or herself in the provision of quality services following acquisition of federal monies through grant writing. This law addresses the areas of facilities, research and training, demonstration projects, and special recreation programs.

Illinois Special Recreation Associations

In 1967, professionals in northern Illinois were aware that the leisure and recreational needs of persons with disabilities were not being met. As a result of two years of study and demonstration programs, members of the Illinois Senate and House pledged support of permissive legislation that allowed park districts and municipal recreation departments to join together to operate recreation programs for citizens with mental and physical disabilities. The legal base for all special recreation cooperatives is the result of Senate Bill 745 of the 1969 Illinois General Assembly. This bill made it possible for two or more park districts or municipal recreation departments to join together to provide recreation for the members of their communities who had disabilities. Funding for these special recreation cooperatives was made possible through legislation passed in 1972, which allowed park districts and municipalities to levy up to $.02 of $100 assessed valuation for recreation services for individuals with disabilities. Later, in 1975, Senate Bills 220 and 221 were passed; these allow park districts or municipal recreation departments, which are members of a cooperative of two or more such agencies, by the use of a referendum-by-petition, to tax their local citizens up to, but not to exceed, $.02 per $100 of assessed valuation. Currently districts are allowed to levy up to $.04 of $100 assessed valuation.

The first cooperative was the Northern Suburban Special Recreation Association (NSSRA), formed in 1970, and included eight local park districts in the northern Chicago metropolitan area. By 1973, there were a total of 10 member agencies of NSSRA serving portions of a two-county area (Keay, 1976).

SUMMARY

This chapter presented and discussed legislative acts aimed at equal rights for persons with disabilities. In particular, the Americans With Disabilities Act (ADA) was highlighted. This legislation has the goal of eliminating discrimination against persons with disabilities. It is intended to enhance the employment and social opportunities for millions of Americans with disabilities to participate more fully in everyday life. Aspects of the law cover nondiscrimination in employment activities, require state and local government programs and transportation to be made accessible to and usable by persons with disabilities, and cover the accessibility by private entities such as restaurants and movie theaters. ADA has implications for the operation of recreation programs and services and should be thoroughly understood by recreation professionals so that an inclusive position is adopted.

Both federal and state legislation dealing with accessibility have made the public more aware of architectural barriers. Legislation has also made new and remodeled federal and state buildings more accessible to and usable by persons who have physical disabilities as well as individuals who are elderly with mobility problems. Specifications for making buildings and facilities accessible to and usable by persons with disabilities are part of the legislative acts and are becoming common knowledge among professionals in a variety of fields. The Rehabilitation Acts have provided monies and opportunities to hundreds of recreation students to become professionally prepared to work in a variety of leisure settings with persons who have disabilities. In addition, the Individuals with Disabilities Education Act (1990) has provided a considerable amount of federal funding for the professional preparation of recreation personnel working with children with disabilities. The Developmental Disabilities Act (PL 91-517) has provided grants to recreation agencies so leisure services can be provided in community-based programs. The State of Illinois has passed legislation to allow park districts and municipal recreation departments to join together to operate recreation programs for individuals with disabilities.

All in all, legislation has had a profound impact on the delivery of recreational services to children and adults with disabilities. Acts have made buildings and other facilities accessible to and usable by people with disabilities. Appropriated monies have helped prepare professionals and paraprofessionals and have made direct services available via demonstration programs and construction projects.

SUGGESTED LEARNING ACTIVITIES

1. Discuss the implications of the various Rehabilitation Acts and Amendments on the field of recreation.
2. Go to the library or another source and outline all of the aspects pertaining to the Architectural Barriers Act in your state. Bring the information to class for discussion.
3. Review Public Law 94-142 and indicate the possible implications to community-based recreation programs for school-aged children with disabilities.
4. You are in charge of running an art program and there are several persons with disabilities who have signed up for the program. One person is in a wheelchair, another person has a hearing impairment, and a third individual is blind. Based on making reasonable accommodations as referenced in the Americans with Disabilities Act, what accommodations might you make so these individuals could participate in your art program?

REFERENCES

Keay, S. *Community Operated and Funded Recreation Programs for the Handicapped.* Report prepared on federally sponsored project under the direction of the Department of HEW. Highland Park, IL, 1976.

McGovern, J. N. *The ADA Self-Evaluation: A Handbook for Compliance with the Americans with Disabilities Act by Parks and Recreation Agencies.* Arlington, VA: National Recreation and Park Association, 1992.

Park, D. C. *Legislation Affecting Park Services and Recreation for Handicapped Individuals.* Published and distributed in part by the U.S. Department of Education, Office of Special Education, Washington, DC, and Hawkins and Associates, Washington, DC, 1980.

Reynolds, R. P., & G. S. O'Morrow. *Problems, Issues and Concepts in Therapeutic Recreation.* Englewood Cliffs, NJ: Prentice-Hall, 1985.

Schleien, S. J., & M. T. Ray. *Community Recreation and Persons with Disabilities: Strategies for Integration.* Baltimore: Brookes, 1988.

Senate Report on the Rehabilitation Act of 1978, PL 95-602.

Sessoms, H. D. The impact of the RSA Recreation Trainee Program, 1963–1968. *Therapeutic Recreation Journal, 14*(1), 23–29, 1970.

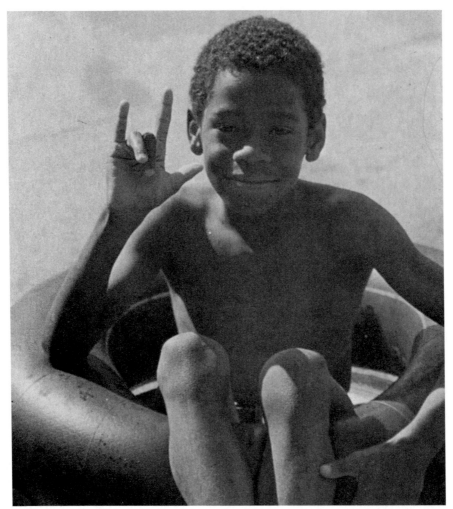

(Courtesy of The League: Serving People with Physical Disabilities, Inc., Baltimore, MD)

4

Disabling Conditions

. . .

Beginning at a very young age, people are capable of observing different objects and recognizing properties that make these objects similar. Tables, for example, are recognized as large, flat surfaces usually supported by four legs. Doors have handles and open to provide access to the outside or another room. This ability to categorize objects based on common characteristics is essential to human functioning. It not only enables us to recognize things that are essentially the same, but it also allows us to distinguish between items that have different qualities and/or functions. Failing to make such judgments could be catastrophic; i.e., it is essential to recognize that a chair is for sitting and a stove is for cooking, rather than vice versa.

LABELING

Categorizing, therefore, is a useful and necessary process in everyday life. However, it also presents problems. Categorizing can result in overlooking the uniqueness of each item within a category or class of objects. This is particularly troublesome when people, rather than objects, are categorized. Each human being desires to be recognized for his or her own talents and assets. However, placing a categorical label on people with similar disabilities, a process known as labeling, interferes with recognizing the unique qualities of each individual with a disability. Furthermore, stereotypes may be formed, and these generalizations accentuate the differences (real or imagined) from people without disabilities.

Rosenthal and Jacobson (1968) demonstrated that labeling not only creates expectations that a member of a group will behave in a predictable way, but also can result in a self-fulfilling prophecy. In other words, a person, once labeled, may actually behave in a certain way *solely* because such behavior is expected of him or her. As a consequence of a self-fulfilling prophecy, a child labeled as mentally retarded may fail to achieve according to his or her cognitive capabilities because others *expect* failure. An adult with a disability may remain physically dependent on others because he or she *expects* such behavior.

Figure 4.1. Self-fulfilling prophecy.

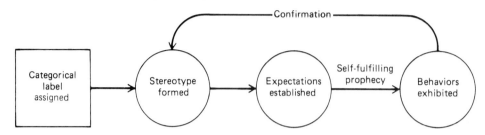

Figure 4.1 summarizes the sequence just described. Placing a categorical *label* on an individual results in the formation of a *stereotype*. This stereotype results in *expectations* regarding the individual's behavior. Because of these expectations, the labeled individual actually behaves as predicted. Thus, a *self-fulfilling prophecy* has occurred that appears to confirm the stereotype. It is a vicious cycle that many authorities feel precludes the use of labels for people with disabilities. Hutchison and Lord (1979) noted,

> The problems with a label are: 1) we tend to focus upon the person's disabilities rather than abilities, and 2) we make generalizations about the whole person based upon misconceptions regarding that label; in other words, a disability tends to have a spread effect in the minds of others. (p. 18)

Perhaps the self-fulfilling prophecy results because the *individual* focuses on the disability and makes generalizations about himself or herself. Consequently, it is sometimes difficult for a person with a disability to develop a positive self-concept. He or she may view himself or herself as different from and somehow less worthwhile than others who do not have disabilities. His or her concept of *self,* and perhaps perceptions of the entire world, are distorted by an overemphasis on the disabling condition. This overemphasis is exaggerated, if not caused, by the labeling process.

In addition to the possible consequences previously discussed, labeling someone has conceptual problems. The following questions clarify that identifying members of disability groups is not as easy as one might expect:

1. How severe does a disability or behavioral disorder have to be for a person to be classified as belonging to a disability group? For example, do people have to be legally blind before they are considered visually impaired?
2. Is it the degree of disability or the functional limitation that qualifies a person to be a member of a disability group? For example, should a person be categorized as "mentally retarded" even if he or she functions as well as most people who are not retarded?
3. Should the situation or task be taken into account in categorizing a person? For example, is a wheelchair user considered to have a disability when playing basketball, but not while eating or playing cards?

4. Does the generic term *disability* imply that people with different disabilities have common needs or problems? Should people with multiple sclerosis (who need cooler water to swim effectively) be classified under the same general term as people with cerebral palsy (who function best in warmer pool temperatures)?

The answers to these questions are by no means clear-cut. Rosenhan (1973) provided evidence that a person may be classified as belonging to a disability group *even if he or she has no disability or functional limitation.* In Rosenhan's study, eight nondisabled subjects admitted themselves to psychiatric hospitals and, once on the wards, behaved normally. Despite exhibiting no signs of psychological disorders, these "pseudo patients" were not detected as imposters by medical personnel. To the staff members of these institutions, Rosenhan's subjects were disabled. Ironically, a few "real" patients were the only ones to recognize that Rosenhan's subjects did not truly belong in a psychiatric facility. It is often said that beauty is in the eye of the beholder. Whether someone is classified as having a disability may likewise depend on the beholder.

The Paradox of Labels

We recognize the many shortcomings and problems of labeling individuals with disabilities. It seems paradoxical, therefore, that we find it necessary to discuss people in terms of their disabilities. When used in this textbook, the term *people with disabilities* is *not* meant to imply that all people who have disabilities are alike. On the contrary, the uniqueness of each person, whether disabled or not, is a concept that recurs throughout this text. For example, people who are classified as deaf (or hearing impaired) have similar, but not identical, limitations that may result in some common problems and needs. These same individuals, however, will have widely varied personalities, attitudes, functional behaviors, and so on. As with all other human beings, people with disabilities are alike in some ways, but in other ways they are quite dissimilar.

If emphasis is placed on individual differences within categories, many authorities contend that labels may prove useful. Labanowich and Hoessli (1979), for example, have pointed out that categorizing people with similar disabilities may serve as a "starting point for a deeper understanding" by the rest of society. Mandell and Fiscus (1981) gave two additional advantages of labeling according to disability characteristics: (1) Professionals can recognize and dispel any negative stereotypes they may have regarding specific disabling conditions, and (2) individuals with special needs can be referred to appropriate alternative services. It seems clear, therefore, that recreators must have some understanding of the nature of disabilities if they are to work effectively with *all* of their constituents. Although we fully recognize the potential problems of labeling, we do believe it is necessary to include selected information on a number of disabling conditions.

CONDITIONS AND CHARACTERISTICS

The next portion of this chapter provides selected factual statements about a variety of disabling conditions, including visual impairments, hearing impairments, learning impairments, motor impairments, psychological and behavioral disorders, brain injury, and AIDS. Although not disabling conditions per se, aging and at-risk youth have been included in this chapter because of the increasing importance of providing recreational opportunities for these persons.

It must be emphasized that the list in the prior paragraph does not include all possible categories of disability, nor are the statements that follow comprehensive in their content. The intent of each set of statements is to provide introductory applied information that may enhance the general understanding of recreators. Medical definitions, as well as etiologies (causes), prognoses (expected outcomes), and so on are *not* provided. The limited scope of this chapter does not allow for such depth; nor do most recreators who work in nonclinical settings require such detailed knowledge. Those desiring more depth on one or more disabling conditions are encouraged to refer to the references cited or to seek assistance from local volunteer health organizations, therapeutic recreation professionals, consumer groups, or information and referral sources.

Visual Impairments

Selected Facts

- Legal blindness is defined as having measured vision of 20/200 or less in the better eye with corrective lenses. In other words, a legally blind person is able to see at 20 feet or less what a person with average vision can see at 200 feet. A person with a visual field of less than an angle of 20 degrees is also legally blind.

- Most people with visual impairments have some vision. Only about 5 percent of people classified as legally blind have no vision or light perception (total blindness).

- Visual impairments are often present at birth, but people who have adventitious (after-birth) visual impairments will generally be able to create mental images of unseen objects based on prior sight.

- Language, motor, and cognitive skills are not significantly impaired by visual deficits, provided the person's environment has been structured to enhance development of these skills.

- Most people with visual impairments are not able to read Braille; those who do generally read much more slowly than a person with sight. Few Braille readers exceed 150 words per minute.

- Some people with visual impairments, particularly children, exhibit mannerisms known as "blindisms." These may be small or large body movements including head shaking, eye pressing, or body rocking.

Tips and Techniques for Recreation Professionals

- Try to involve *all* senses in recreational activities; using sounds, tastes, smells, and textures of materials can be enjoyed by everyone.

- Glare and other lighting conditions may create difficulties for some people with visual impairments. Because optimal conditions for vision vary from person to person, consult participants with visual impairments to determine the correct type and amount of lighting to provide.

- Placing information on audiotapes is generally preferable to Braille. Some commercial tapes offer compressed speech, which results from electronically cropping speech signals; thus, the speed of a recording is increased without distorting the sound.

- Bulletin boards and other visual displays (e.g., activity calendars) should use high-contrast (black-and-white), enlarged lettering.

- When walking with a person who has a visual impairment and needs assistance, ask how he or she wishes to be guided. One preferred method is for the person with the visual impairment to hold on to your elbow and walk to your side and slightly behind. Verbal cues can help to avoid obstacles.

- Be sure all directions are clear and concise, and demonstrate physical tasks. Allow individuals with visual impairments to be close enough to see or touch demonstrations. Use verbal instructions to create mental images for people with adventitious visual impairments.

- Orientation to play and recreational areas is important. Prior to participation, encourage individuals to walk around the area with a guide so they become comfortable with their surroundings. Tactile maps and signs may also allow individuals with visual impairments to orient themselves to unfamiliar surroundings.

- When approaching a person with a visual impairment, announce your presence using a calm, clear voice, and be sure to state your name. If you need to walk away, let him or her know you are leaving. If the person uses a guide dog, do not touch or speak to the dog, unless you first ask permission from the dog's owner.

Hearing Impairments

Selected Facts

- Only a small percentage of people with hearing impairments have extreme hearing loss (greater than 90 decibels in the better ear). Those who do, however, are unable to understand amplified speech; they experience sound through vibrations from loud noise.

- Hearing impairments occurring at birth or shortly afterward often result in delayed language development and difficulty with conceptual thinking. This is probably the greatest limitation experienced by people with hearing impairments.

- Many people with hearing impairments communicate by use of sign language and fingerspelling. Not all people with hearing impairments know and understand such communication methods, however, particularly those who developed hearing loss after early childhood.

Figure 4.2. Fingerspelling alphabet.

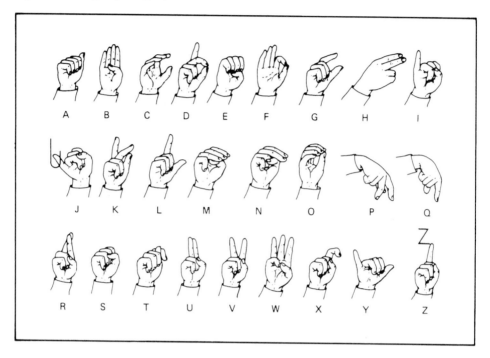

- Children with hearing impairments often appear to be hyperactive, but their behavior frequently results from difficulty communicating with the hearing world.
- Some people with hearing impairments have damage to their semicircular canals, which help control balance. Activities requiring balance, therefore, may prove difficult for these individuals.

Tips and Techniques for Recreation Professionals

- Whenever an individual who is deaf attends a recreational event, an interpreter should be provided to facilitate communication. Sign language and fingerspelling skills (see Fig. 4.2) would also prove useful for community recreational professionals. As a last resort, write messages on a pad of paper.
- When using sign language or fingerspelling, wear solid, dark-colored clothing to serve as a suitable background. Also, ensure that adequate lighting is provided.

- To gain the attention of a person with a severe hearing impairment, tap the person on the arm or wave your hand (not arm) near his or her visual field. You may also substitute visual cues, such as flashing lights, for auditory cues.

- When using speech to communicate with a person who has a hearing impairment, always face him or her and do not slow or exaggerate your speech.

- Written instructions should be expressed in short, clear sentences, and difficult vocabulary words should be avoided.

- When working with children who have hearing impairments, have several alternative activities prepared. To maintain their interest, it is sometimes necessary to redirect attention to a new activity.

- Because many participants with hearing impairments are unable to hear audible warnings of danger (e.g., traffic noise, verbal warnings), a high degree of structure and supervision is required with some activities and environments.

Mental Retardation and Other Learning Impairments

Selected Facts

- People with mental retardation have subaverage cognitive functioning, but they are able to learn. Their rate of learning is generally slower than that of nondisabled people, however. Deficits in decision making and problem solving may also accompany this delayed learning pattern.

- Mental retardation and other learning impairments encompass a wide range of cognitive and behavioral functioning. Most people with mental retardation are capable of obtaining jobs and functioning independently in the community. The greater the retardation, however, the greater the chance that a person will need some form of assistance with requirements of daily living.

- The majority of people with mental retardation do not differ in physical appearance from their nonretarded peers. In general, the higher the cognitive functioning of a person with a learning impairment, the less likely he or she is to have accompanying disabilities, motor deficits, or physical abnormalities.

- Socioeconomic conditions have been found to be associated with some learning impairments; for example, lower socioeconomic environments generally produce a higher-than-average percentage of people with mild mental retardation.

- Children with mental retardation and other learning impairments usually experience delays in their physical, cognitive, and social development; they exhibit behavior that is characteristic of children considerably younger in chronological age.

- People with learning disabilities, unlike individuals who have mental retardation, have average to above-average intelligence but do not function up to their cognitive potential. Sometimes learning disabilities affect specific types of information processing, like math or spelling skills.

- The signs of a learning disability vary widely. Problems in following directions, retaining information, performing paper-and-pencil tasks, and paying attention to appropriate cues are a few characteristics that may indicate the presence of a learning disability. Persons with learning disabilities sometimes also exhibit behavioral problems, such as hyperactivity, perceptual-motor deficits, emotional unpredictability, or aggression toward others (see the section on psychological and behavioral disorders).

Tips and Techniques for Recreation Professionals

- The wide range of behaviors and functional abilities of people with learning impairments necessitates careful consideration of each person's abilities. Assumptions about the individual based on a categorical designation must be avoided.

- Activities should be divided into manageable parts and carefully sequenced to offer a progression of skills. Repetition of important tasks may also facilitate learning. Whenever possible, it is helpful to provide a demonstration so participants with learning impairments can model the desired behavior. Also, avoid "multistep" commands when giving directions.

- Assist participants with mental retardation in selecting activities that are age appropriate and require skills that are useful in community living. Some people with learning impairments have inaccurate perceptions of their own capabilities; try to ensure that the challenges of an activity correspond with the skills of the participants.

- Small group and cooperative activities may facilitate social development for those with deficiencies in adaptive behavior.

- Use verbal instructions that are clear and easy to understand. Provide careful supervision of all activities, especially those in which accidents or injuries are possible. Be careful not to overprotect participants, however.

- Start an activity at the participant's current skill level rather than at the lowest possible level.

- With individuals who have learning disabilities, it is especially important to reduce extraneous stimuli; the leader should limit the quantity of materials, directions, verbal suggestions, and so on. Care should be taken *not* to eliminate choices or limit opportunities for creativity.

- For most children with learning impairments, especially those with learning disabilities, activities should involve as many of the senses as possible. Abstractions are often difficult for such children to grasp, so visible evidence of success, such as certificates of achievement, should be used.

Motor Impairments

Selected Facts

- The diversity of motor impairments makes the use of generalizations exceedingly difficult, if not impossible. Some are easily identified and have reasonably predictable physical effects (e.g., amputations). Others, however, manifest themselves in many ways and result in a wide range of functional limitations (e.g., cerebral palsy).

- Some motor impairments are present at birth (congenital), and others occur after birth (adventitious). Most remain stable or improve, but a few are progressive. As a result, the person's functional abilities may decrease across time (e.g., muscular dystrophy).

- Motor impairments may affect practically the entire body or may affect one specific area, such as the lower extremities. Common terminology for partial or full loss of function in a part of the body includes *monoplegia* (one extremity), *hemiplegia* (extremities on one side of the body), *paraplegia* (both lower extremities), and *quadriplegia* (all four extremities, perhaps including head involvement).

- Some people with motor impairments may have accompanying disabling conditions such as learning impairments, speech difficulties, or seizure disorders. Most people with motor impairments do not have multiple disabilities, however.

- Some children and young adults who have motor impairments experience an overly protective home environment, which places additional limits on their physical or social functioning.

Tips and Techniques for Recreation Professionals

- Most people with motor impairments can fully integrate into community recreational activities if an accessible environment is provided (see Chapters 5 and 6).

- The wide variety of functional abilities of people with motor impairments dictates careful attention to the needs of individual participants. Generalized programming tips for people with such diverse abilities are impossible, so seek advice from the participants who have disabilities.

- Ask participants with motor impairments if there are any specific conditions to avoid during recreational activities. For example, people with spastic cerebral palsy may have an exaggerated jerking response (stretch reflex) to a loud or unexpected noise. It would be unfortunate for the participant to ruin an art project, for example, because the instructor was unaware of this reaction.

- Because some people with motor impairments have been overprotected at home, encourage challenging, but safe, activities. Emphasize independent functioning, allowing the person to exert control over his or her environment. During activities, keep in mind that balance difficulties are common among people with mobility limitations.

- Participation in specific activities or exposure to certain weather conditions may be inadvisable for some people with motor impairments. Try to discuss the demands of an activity with participants in advance, and consult a therapeutic recreation specialist (or another knowledgeable professional) if there are any doubts about the advisability of participation.

Aging

Selected Facts

- It is generally accepted that old age begins at 65 years of age, but the physical, cognitive, psychological, and social functioning of people who are older varies considerably. People can be chronologically old yet exhibit few signs of advanced age. Conversely, some people display physical attributes associated with advanced age well before their 65th birthday.

- Most individuals who are older are self-sufficient in all aspects of their lives. Some, however, do experience a role-reversal situation. This happens when their offspring begin (or attempt) to make important life decisions for the person who is older. Such situations are extremely frustrating and may lead to feelings of futility and personal ineffectiveness.

- Approximately 95 percent of people who are older in the United States live and function within the community rather than in hospitals or nursing homes.

- Advanced age is usually accompanied by decreased visual acuity, some hearing loss (especially of higher-pitched sounds), and decreased motor performances. Generally, however, these declines do not place limits on most activities until a person is well into his or her 70s or beyond.

- In metropolitan areas, fear of crime and lack of financial resources are two major factors that may limit recreation and leisure participation among individuals who are elderly. Other factors include health considerations, lack of companionship, and transportation difficulties.

- Contrary to stereotypes held by many, people who are older *are* interested in sex. They can, and frequently do, engage in satisfying sexual relationships.

Tips and Techniques for Recreation Professionals

- It is essential that people who are older be given opportunities to maintain personal control over their own life activities. Citizens' councils and other organizations should be used to provide direction for community programs with participants who are elderly.

- Put to good use the skills that people who are older possess. Provide opportunities for individuals to serve as activity leaders, and try to offer a chance for them to share their life experiences with children as well as with people of all ages.

- Opportunities to socialize with age cohorts (those in the same stage of life) are important; flexible programs in a relaxed atmosphere should facilitate social interaction. Activities must be age-appropriate and should encourage older participants to proceed at their own pace and desired level of involvement.

- People who are older are very capable of learning new information and skills. Many welcome the chance to participate in adult education classes; identify topics, subjects, and skills of interest and provide opportunities for learning.

- Because visual, hearing, or motor impairments may accompany the aging process, the recreation leader should be prepared to integrate tips and techniques related to these impairments, as needed.

Psychological and Behavioral Disorders

Selected Facts

- Disruptive or abnormal behavior is manifested in a wide variety of ways and may result from one or more factors. Heredity, learning, physiological malfunctions, and environmental (situational) factors are often identified as contributing to problem behavior.

- For an individual to be considered to have a psychological or behavioral disorder, his or her behavior must be viewed in terms of degree, duration, or both. Extreme outbursts or withdrawal or consistently inappropriate behavior over time may indicate that professional intervention is necessary.

- Some prescription drugs may result in behaviors that appear to be signs of psychological or behavioral disorders. Many illegal drugs also have this effect on users.

- Of primary concern to most group leaders is the person whose actions distract other group members or disrupt group processes. Some behaviors, however, are not disruptive but may warrant similar attention, including extreme withdrawal, excessive shyness, submissiveness, frequent and prolonged daydreaming, fearfulness, and lack of interest in or response to environmental surroundings.

- The context in which abnormal behavior occurs, as well as the life situation of the individual, must be considered. Behavioral deviance is based on culturally defined norms and values. Much behavior that appears abnormal can be explained rationally by the heritage or life circumstances of the individual.

Tips and Techniques for Recreation Professionals

- Group leaders should become familiar with behavior management techniques and use them when necessary. Some specific techniques for dealing with problem behavior are included at the end of this chapter.

- No single technique of behavior management has been found effective with all people. Regardless of the technique used, consistency and empathy are essential. Be specific and firm about expected behavior, and express expectations in a clear and calm manner. Refrain from expressing negative emotions (e.g., blaming, threatening). If it becomes necessary to express displeasure, do so calmly and clarify that the *behavior*, not the person, is the concern.

- The presence of appropriate behavioral models in a warm and understanding environment may do a great deal to reduce or eliminate inappropriate behavior. Patience and acceptance of individual differences are also important.

- Learn to identify the physiological and psychological effects of popular drugs.

- If an individual's behavior appears to warrant outside intervention, seek the assistance of a qualified mental health professional.

Brain Injury

Selected Facts

- Brain injury (also referred to as head injury or closed head injury) is caused by trauma to the brain, usually resulting from an external blow to the head (e.g., auto accident, fall) or internal injury (e.g., embolism). The effects may be temporary or long term.

- The extent of impairment resulting from brain injury varies according to the severity of the injury and the specific portion of the brain most affected by the injury. For example, a person whose injury is greatest to the frontal portion of the brain may have significant difficulty with planning and initiating actions. Injury that is primarily to the back portion of the brain, however, is more likely to cause difficulty with visual perception and memory.

- The effects of brain injury vary greatly from person to person and often involve more than cognitive functioning. Ineffective social skills and limitations in motor functioning may also be associated with brain injury.

- Persons with brain injury often display one or more of the following characteristics: excessive talkativeness, impulsiveness, lack of inhibition, deficits in memory, inability to interpret situations accurately, and difficulty with time management.

- Depending on the nature and variety of the injury, a person with brain injury may be unaware of his or her limitations. In addition, the person may be unaware of the effects his or her behaviors have on others.

Tips and Techniques for Recreation Professionals

- Recreation leaders should become familiar with effective behavior management techniques. Many people who have brain injury need guidance with appropriate behavior in social situations. Such guidance should reinforce appropriate behaviors and, without being punitive, emphasize the consequences of inappropriate behaviors.

- When memory deficits are associated with brain injury, repetition of information, skills, and so on is helpful. It is important to keep in mind that the individual with a brain injury often does not realize that he or she has recently made a statement, asked a question, or performed a task. Try to respond to each repetition as if it were the first time.

- Initially, recreational activities should be *highly* structured for participants who have brain injury. Start with relatively simple (but age-appropriate) tasks that are sequenced in small, manageable steps. Doing so will facilitate success and encourage advancement to more complex tasks.

- Leadership of most activities that include participants with brain injury requires highly attentive supervision. Because the participant with brain injury may not recognize appropriate actions or his or her own limitations, the leader must be ready to intervene in any situation that has the potential for accidents or injuries.

Acquired Immunodeficiency Syndrome (AIDS)

Selected Facts

- More than one million people in the United States are believed to be infected with HIV, the virus that causes AIDS (Grossman, 1993). Statistics indicate that the incidence of AIDS is increasing in North America, and it is not confined to a few high-risk groups. Projections indicate that before the disease is eliminated, everyone in North America will know at least one person with AIDS.
- HIV is *not* transmitted by casual contact, nor can one get HIV from sweat, saliva, or tears. HIV is generally transmitted through bodily fluids such as semen and blood. Unprotected sexual contact and sharing needles or syringes with an infected person are the most common methods of transmission. Also, a baby may be born with HIV if the mother is infected.
- At present, AIDS is a chronic disease that cannot be cured. The average length of time between being infected with HIV and the onset of AIDS is more than 10 years. A person infected with HIV is capable of transmitting the virus even though he or she does not show any symptoms of being ill.
- Despite being protected by the Americans with Disabilities Act, people with HIV and AIDS often experience prejudice, discrimination, and social stigma. As a result, feelings of alienation, social isolation, and despair are frequently experienced by persons with HIV and AIDS.
- There is evidence that many recreation professionals have misconceptions about HIV and AIDS; moreover, they also have limited knowledge about high-risk behaviors and steps to reduce the risks of infection (Glenn & Dattilo, 1993; Grossman & Caroleo, 1992).
- Physical problems associated with AIDS may include loss of energy, loss of weight, bladder/bowel incontinence, and problems with coordination. Persons with AIDS also experience a wide variety of nutritional problems associated with their illness or medication (Caroleo, 1988). In addition to physical problems, most persons with AIDS will experience dementia during the latter stages of their illness. Symptoms may include impaired memory and concentration, confusion, and slowing of mental processes.

Tips and Techniques for Recreation Professionals

- Become knowledgeable about HIV and AIDS. Use that knowledge to provide appropriate environments and activities for participants with HIV or AIDS.
- Provide an atmosphere that enables participants with AIDS to feel relaxed, welcome, and supported by staff members. Friends and family members of participants with HIV or AIDS should be encouraged to attend.

- If refreshments are provided, be sure to provide choices that are consistent with dietary requirements of persons with AIDS. For example, foods high in yeast, fat, or lactose may be prohibited for some participants with AIDS.

- Include individuals with HIV or AIDS in activities and programs, *and* in the program planning process. Coping with AIDS requires discipline and necessitates adherence to physician directives; therefore, it is important to provide ample opportunities for choice and personal control during leisure.

- All recreation providers should include prevention education in conjunction with programs and activities. To date, prevention (e.g., safer sex practices) is the only method of controlling the spread of HIV infection and AIDS.

Youth At-Risk

Selected Facts

- The term *youth at-risk* means different things to different people. As used in this textbook, it refers to children and adolescents who, for a variety of reasons, are at risk of becoming juvenile offenders.

- Youth at-risk often come from socially disadvantaged backgrounds, lack basic academic skills, experience feelings of alienation and futility, and have limited support from family members. Most of these young persons do not succeed in school and many fail to complete their secondary education. The number of school dropouts is particularly high among minorities and those with low socioeconomic status.

- Most youth at-risk have low self-esteem; they experience, or have experienced, extremely stressful home environments. Family-related stressors include parental separation or divorce, physical and/or sexual abuse, alcoholism, and frequent residential moves. For many, peers (e.g., gangs) replace the family as the primary source of support, affiliation, and behavioral guidance.

- Delinquent and other behaviors that deviate from society's norms (e.g., physical aggression, disorderly conduct, destruction of property) usually occur during free time. Moreover, they may provide youth at-risk with fun and other feelings associated with leisure experiences (Aguilar, 1991; Reimer, 1981).

Tips and Techniques for Recreation Professionals

- Recreation leaders need to provide stimulating activities that can provide youth at-risk with high degrees of personal challenge. Outdoor-adventure programs and ropes courses are two commonly used activities that offer a progression of challenges to participants. Such activities also foster important interpersonal skills, such as acceptance of others and cooperation with group members. In addition, outdoor-adventure programs assist participants to develop a more realistic view of self (Gillis, 1992).

- Programs and activities should emphasize autonomy and choice making. Youth at-risk should be active contributors to the program planning process, and activities should be structured to optimize decision making and personal control among participants.

- Education regarding socially acceptable leisure participation should be incorporated into recreation programs. Educational activities that promote small group interaction and interdependence among group members may be particularly helpful since acceptance of peers is very important to many youth who are at-risk.

- Create a positive, caring, and accepting environment for youthful participants by displaying genuine interest in them and their experiences. Also, encourage their family members to become actively involved in recreation programs and activities. Since financial constraints are significant for many youth at-risk, fees for services should be kept to a minimum.

- Peers who are appropriate role models for youth at-risk should be encouraged to attend programs and share how they successfully adjusted to the demands of society. Recreation leaders and adults in the community may also serve as mentors to youth at-risk, offering guidance, support, and understanding.

- Early intervention is vitally important; therefore, recreation programs should be available to preschool and preteen youth who are considered to be at-risk. The most effective way of dealing with socially deviant behavior is to prevent it before it begins.

MANAGING PROBLEM BEHAVIOR

From time to time, most recreation leaders must deal with problem behavior exhibited by one or more participants. Managing such problem behavior is a difficult and frustrating task that requires patience and skill. Some of the disabilities discussed in this chapter (e.g., learning disabilities, brain injury, psychological disorders) may result in above-average incidents of problem behavior; however, behavior management techniques that are effective for the general population are also effective for persons who have disabilities. The following list of simple strategies,[1] although far from a cure-all, may help to increase appropriate behavior among participants whose behavior is difficult to manage.

1. *Reinforce desirable behavior.* It is usually much easier to establish desirable behavior patterns than to alter problem behavior after it has started. A smile, gesture, or brief word of support is frequently all that is necessary to encourage a participant to maintain or to increase acceptable behavior.

2. *Clearly state privileges as well as rules.* Tell participants what they may do; too many "don'ts" violate strategy 1. If participants clearly understand what is permitted, they will not need to test to determine acceptable limits. Participant involvement in establishing rules may help as well.

---

1. Modified from "A Camp Director's 10: A List of Strategies for Managing Problem Behavior of Young Campers" by Ralph W. Smith, in *Camping Magazine*, June 1980, Vol. 52, No. 7, p. 7. Reprinted with permission from the American Camping Association, Inc. Copyright © 1980 American Camping Association, Inc.

3. *Tolerate some annoying behavior.* Too much attention to annoying behavior may not only interfere with an activity's effectiveness, but may serve to reinforce undesirable actions. Also, certain annoying behaviors may be typical for a young person's developmental stage.

4. *Use nonverbal cues.* Eye contact, accompanied by a frown or gesture, may control undesirable behavior without the possibility of embarrassing the participant in front of his or her peers.

5. *Consider redirection to a different task or activity.* The challenges of any activity should be consistent with the participant's skill development, so plan for varying levels of skill and try to individualize tasks to each person's abilities. Many behavior problems result from activity dissatisfaction or boredom and may be eliminated by redirecting the person to another task or activity.

   NOTE: Despite careful attention to the above strategies, problem behaviors may occur that require immediate intervention. Any disciplinary action should be fair, consistent, and administered in an understanding manner. The next strategies may be helpful when intervention is required.

6. *Clarify consequences of unacceptable behavior.* A participant should clearly understand the personal impact of his or her behavior, such as anticipated disciplinary action. It also may be advisable to encourage young participants to clarify the consequences of his or her own actions by asking, "What things do you think will happen if you continue to act this way?" When clarifying consequences, it is important to avoid using a threatening tone of voice and, above all, the recreation professional must be prepared to follow through if the undesirable behavior continues.

7. *Clarify benefits of acceptable behavior.* This is the corollary to strategy 6, and may be useful in concert with it. Pointing out the benefits of acceptable behavior will be most effective if it occurs immediately after desirable behavior (strategy 1).

8. *Use time-out procedures.* It may be necessary to temporarily remove a disruptive person from the situation in which problem behavior is occurring and place him or her in a location where little or no enjoyable stimulation is received. Once removed, the person should be allowed to return after a short period of time, but it is important that this return be contingent on appropriate behavior.

9. *Punishment, if used, should be a last resort.* Punishment of any kind does not allow the person to avoid the consequences by exhibiting acceptable behavior. Thus, attention is directed to the punishment itself, rather than to the problem and alternative forms of behavior. Any form of punishment should be appropriate to the situation and, of course, must conform to agency policies.

10. *If in doubt, seek help.* This strategy should be used whenever the recreation leader feels incapable of coping with a particular situation or behavioral problem. It should be stressed that seeking help is not a sign of defeat or inadequacy. No one, regardless of experience, has all the answers to handling behavior problems.

One source of help, especially with severe behavior problems, is the Specialized Training Program, 1235, University of Oregon, Eugene, OR 97403-1235. This program, supported by the National Institute for Rehabilitation Research, has the mission of developing, evaluating, and disseminating practical behavior management technology that is effective with severe behavior problems. Techniques developed by the program are consistent with community standards for nonaversiveness, and can be used by staff in typical community settings and families.

SUMMARY

The traditional approach to recreation with persons who have disabilities is to focus extensively on characteristics that distinguish people with special needs from the general population. Medical terminology, facts and figures, and therapeutic interventions are often stressed. We feel, however, that this traditional approach overlooks the uniqueness of each person with a disability. Rather than give detailed characteristics and data for all disabling conditions, we have presented selected information that should be useful to any recreational professional. Readers interested in additional information regarding data, characteristics, techniques, and terminology associated with specific disabling conditions are encouraged to consult the following resources:

Adams, R., A. Daniel, & L. Rullman. *Games, Sports and Exercises for the Physically Handicapped* (4th ed.). Philadelphia: Lea and Febiger, 1991.

Austin, D. R., & M. E. Crawford, Eds. *Therapeutic Recreation: An Introduction.* Englewood Cliffs, NJ: Prentice-Hall, 1991.

Basmajian, J. V., Ed. *Therapeutic Exercise.* Baltimore: Williams & Wilkins, 1984.

Batshaw, M. L., & Y. M. Perret. *Children with Handicaps: A Medical Primer* (3rd ed.). Baltimore: Paul H. Brookes, 1992.

Botwinick, J. *Aging and Behavior.* New York: Springer, 1984.

Caplan, B., Ed. *Rehabilitation Psychology Desk Reference.* Rockville, MD: Aspen, 1987.

Carmi, A., S. Chigier, & S. Schneider. *Disability.* New York: Springer-Verlag, 1984.

Chilman, C. S., Ed. *Chronic Illness and Disability.* London: Sage, 1988.

Donmoyer, R., & R. Kos, Eds. *At-Risk Students: Portraits, Policies, Programs, and Practices.* Albany, NY: State University of New York Press, 1993.

Erickson, M. T. *Behavior Disorders of Children and Adolescents: Assessment, Etiology and Intervention.* (2nd ed). Englewood Cliffs, NJ: Prentice-Hall, 1992.

Garrison, W. T., & S. McQuiston. *Chronic Illness During Childhood and Adolescence.* London: Sage, 1989.

Kelley, J. D., Ed. *Recreation Programming for Visually Impaired Children and Youth.* New York: American Foundation for the Blind, 1981.

Mandell, C. J., & E. Fiscus. *Understanding Exceptional People.* St. Paul, MN: West Publishing, 1981.

National Rehabilitation Information Center, 8455 Colesville Road, Suite 935, Silver Spring, MD 20910-3319 (Provides information, data-based computer searches, and copies of available articles on a wide range of disability-related topics).

Rehab Briefs: Bringing Research into Effective Focus. (Periodic summaries of research or disability topics; available through National Institute on Disability and Rehabilitation Research, Office of Special Education and Rehabilitative Services, U.S. Department of Education, Washington, DC 20202).

Stolov, W., & M. Clowers. *Handbook of Severe Disability.* Washington, DC: U.S. Department of Education, Rehabilitation Services Administration, 1981.

Treischmann, R. B. *Spinal Cord Injuries: Physiological, Social, and Vocational Rehabilitation* (2nd ed.). New York: Demos, 1988.

SUGGESTED LEARNING ACTIVITIES

1. Explain the concept of a self-fulfilling prophecy. How do you think expectations could cause behavior?
2. Write a two-page paper that gives your personal opinion on the topic "Should Labels Be Used to Identify People with Disabilities?"
3. Learn the fingerspelling alphabet pictured in Figure 4.2. Practice this alphabet by fingerspelling a message to friends (they can use Figure 4.2 to interpret your message).
4. Research one disabling condition and
   (a) add two facts to the "Selected Facts" listed in the chapter;
   (b) add two suggestions to the "Tips and Techniques" provided in the chapter.

REFERENCES

Aguilar, T. E. Social deviancy. In D. Austin & M. E. Crawford, Eds. *Therapeutic Recreation: An Introduction.* Englewood Cliffs, NJ: Prentice-Hall, 1991, pp. 100–118.

Caroleo, O. O. AIDS: Meeting the needs through therapeutic recreation. *Therapeutic Recreation Journal, 22*(4), 71–78, 1988.

Gillis, H. L. Therapeutic uses of adventure-challenge-outdoor-wilderness theory and research. Paper presented at the Coalition for Education in the Outdoors, 1992.

Glenn, C., & J. Dattilo. TR professionals' attitudes toward and knowledge of AIDS. *Therapeutic Recreation Journal, 27,* 253–261, 1993.

Grossman, A. H. The faces of HIV/AIDS. *Parks and Recreation, 28*(3), 44–46, 1993.

Grossman, A. H., & O. Caroleo. A study of AIDS risk-behavior knowledge among therapeutic recreation specialists in New York State. *Therapeutic Recreation Journal, 26*(4), 55–60, 1992.

Hutchison, P., & J. Lord. *Recreation Integration.* Ontario, Canada: Leisurability Publications, 1979.

Labanowich, S., & P. Hoessli. Module 2: Knowing the campers. In D. A. Vinton & E. M. Farley, Eds. *Camp Staff Training Series.* Lexington, KY: University of Kentucky, 1979.

Mandell, C. J., & E. Fiscus. *Understanding Exceptional People.* St. Paul, MN: West Publishing, 1981.

Reimer, J. W. Deviance as fun. *Adolescence, 16*(61), 39–43, 1981.

Rosenhan, D. L. On being sane in insane places. *Science, 179*(4070) 250–253, 1973.

Rosenthal, R., & L. Jacobson. *Pygmalion in the Classroom: Teacher Expectations and Pupil's Intellectual Development.* New York: Holt, Rinehart & Winston, 1968.

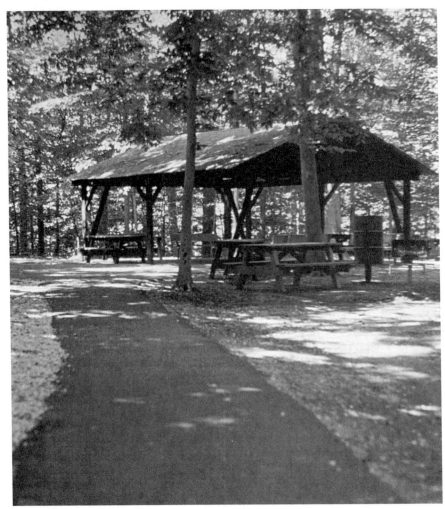

(Photo by Ralph W. Smith)

PART TWO

PROGRAM AND FACILITY PLANNING

Equal access to recreation programs and facilities is the thrust of Chapter 5, Barriers to Recreation Participation. This chapter discusses intrinsic, environmental, and communication barriers that prevent leisure participation by individuals with disabilities, along with means to overcome these barriers.

Chapter 6, Design of Accessible and Usable Recreation Environments, concerns designing appropriate recreation environments for all people, including persons with disabilities. A major portion of the chapter is devoted to guidelines and recommendations for creating accessible and usable public park and recreation facilities. A special section on playground design concludes Chapter 6.

Featured in Chapter 7, Program Planning and Evaluation Process, is a discussion of how to create recreation programs that facilitate inclusion of persons with disabilities. Needs assessment, selection and modification of activities, and implementation of inclusive recreational activities are highlighted. In addition, an overview of program evaluation is presented, including a detailed discussion of Importance-Performance Evaluation.

The final chapter in this section is Chapter 8, Special Recreation Programs—Exemplaries and Standards. This chapter presents information on several outstanding community-based inclusive and special recreation programs. Each program is highlighted, and the philosophy and goals of each are outlined.

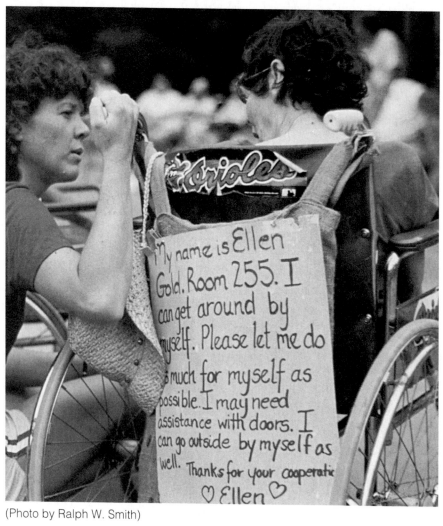

(Photo by Ralph W. Smith)

5

When a disability makes an individual physically dependent on others, the limits imposed are obvious. In some cases, an attendant or aide may be necessary to enable a person to participate in activities. It is not always easy for the person with a disability to ask for physical assistance, however. Szychowski (1993) wrote that asking for assistance "in some ways requires greater strength of spirit than it takes to face a monster [whitewater] rapid, for in those moments we risk intimacy and vulnerability" (pp. 20–21).

Psychological dependency is not always as obvious as physical dependency, but it can be even more limiting. Moore and Dattilo (1993), for example, theorized that differences in nature-related trail preferences between persons with and without disabilities may have resulted from "a willingness on the part of people with disabilities to accept limited accommodations as a result of 'internalized oppression'" (p. 28). Family members, friends, and rehabilitation professionals are all capable of fostering an atmosphere of psychological dependency (i.e., internalized oppression) for people with disabilities. Sometimes this situation is reciprocal, meaning that the person with a disability receives feelings of satisfaction from being protected and patronized, while the nondisabled person enjoys being needed by someone viewed as "less fortunate." Thus, both have their needs met by the other.

When psychological dependency occurs, the person's capacity for personal growth and self-development is severely limited (Wright, 1983). Many of the barriers that are faced by people with disabilities require personal initiative, creative thought, risk taking, and perseverance in action. These qualities do not develop fully in an atmosphere of psychological dependency. The fact that some rehabilitation professionals encourage their clients to be dependent also compounds this problem. As noted by Illich, Zola, McKnight, Caplan, and Shaiken (1977), "Life is paralyzed in permanent intensive care" (p. 27).

Skill/Challenge Gap. Csikszentmihalyi (1975) has studied enjoyment of activities for many years. In his book *Beyond Boredom and Anxiety*, he proposed that enjoyment of an activity is most often possible if the participant perceives that the challenges of an activity are in balance with his or her skills. If the challenges are thought to be too great, worry or anxiety may limit the chance for enjoyment. If the challenge is considered too easily achieved, boredom often results. Many individuals with disabilities do not possess skill levels appropriate for enjoying a number of leisure pursuits. Moreover, the presence of a skill/challenge gap may interfere with efforts to integrate individuals with disabilities into mainstream society (Miller, 1989). Sometimes the nature of their disabilities limits skill development, but often they do not get the opportunity to develop skills that could enhance participation. As a result, they correctly perceive that many activities are too challenging for their present skills. The result is usually nonparticipation.

This skill/challenge gap has many implications for recreation professionals. Proper progression in teaching specific skills may enable a person with a disability to gain the expertise necessary for participation. Also, an activity may be modified to accommodate the current skills of a participant with a disability (see Chapter 7). It is very important to keep in mind that the participant's *perception* of his or her skill level is a critical factor. Underestimating one's own skill may result in withdrawal from participation, whereas overestimating one's own skill may prove embarrassing or even dangerous. Many overconfident

Figure 5.2. Environmental barriers.

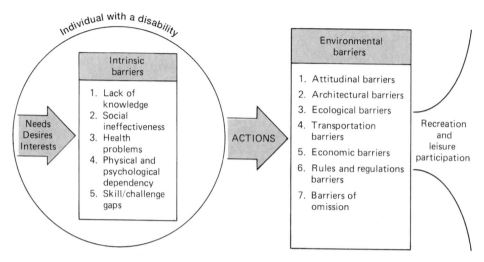

skiers, for example, have ended up in the hospital because they thought they were ready for the advanced slopes. As Bregha (1980) observed, the ability to select appropriate leisure pursuits requires more than knowledge of what is available or permissible. "Something deeper is required: the knowledge of oneself as well as one's milieu" (p. 31).

Environmental Barriers

No matter how successfully a person with a disability copes with intrinsic barriers to recreation participation, he or she will also be faced with external forces that limit participation. Figure 5.2 illustrates the idea that these external forces, known as environmental barriers, may block the actions that a person takes toward participation in recreation and leisure activities. Unlike intrinsic barriers, environmental barriers are imposed on the individual by societal or ecological conditions. Thus, the person is less likely to feel that he or she can overcome such barriers through individual action. Many intrinsic barriers can be partially or completely overcome through personal efforts such as physical rehabilitation, educational programs, and counseling. The solution to environmental barriers is much more complex and, therefore, more frustrating for individuals with disabilities. The following environmental barriers limit recreation and leisure participation for many persons with disabilities.

Attitudinal Barriers. Of all the barriers to participation faced by individuals with disabilities, attitudinal barriers are probably the most limiting. They are also the most difficult to overcome. The attitude concept is discussed in depth in Chapter 2, but it is important here to examine the types of behaviors that reflect barrier-producing attitudes. These behaviors, which may be exhibited by family and friends or by strangers, can be divided into three categories: (1) *negative* behaviors; (2) *paternalistic* behaviors; and (3) *apathetic* behaviors. To give readers a better understanding of these behaviors, we have provided the following information:

1. *Negative Behaviors.* From time to time, every person with a disability is subjected to behaviors that arise from negative attitudes toward people who are "different." Some of these behaviors are obvious, but others are subtle. However, they all clearly inform the individual that he or she has less value than a person who does not have a disability. One obvious sample of negative behavior is ridiculing or mocking the person with a visible disability. Less obvious, though, is avoidance of people with disabilities. Whether from fear, dislike, or discomfort, many nondisabled people avoid eye contact and maintain exaggerated social distance when in the presence of people with visible disabilities (Langer et al., 1976). Obsolete and derogatory labels, such as "cripple," "deaf and dumb," and "crazy," are also examples of negative behaviors. Such terms are not only demeaning, but their use encourages others to behave negatively toward people with disabilities.

2. *Paternalistic Behaviors.* Many people without disabilities treat adolescents or adults who have disabilities like children. (Often they treat children with disabilities like infants!) Unlike negative behaviors, paternalistic actions frequently arise from a desire to show a "favorable" view of people who have disabilities. Unfortunately, the message conveyed by paternalistic behavior is that people with disabilities lack competence, maturity, and the capacity for independence. Head patting, giving undue or excessive praise, and providing help when it is not needed are all examples of paternalistic behavior. The importance of *not* overhelping individuals with disabilities was highlighted by Karol Davenport, a wheelchair athlete from Pennsylvania. Upon returning from her first wheelchair track-and-field competition, Karol was glowing from her success and the camaraderie she shared with others. Finally, she said, "But you know what I liked best of all? People *didn't* help me when I said I didn't need help!" (K. Davenport, personal communication, 1981).

3. *Apathetic Behaviors.* People who are apathetic toward individuals with disabilities express no feelings of sympathy, understanding, or caring toward people who have disabilities. Rather than being negative or paternalistic, such people totally ignore the needs and concerns of people with disabilities. They behave as if such people did not exist. Doug Wakefield, who is blind, talked about one personal experience with public apathy. Doug and his guide dog were using Washington's subway system. They got off the train at an unfamiliar station, and Doug did not know the direction of his exit. His guide dog, which is trained to keep him from dangerous situations, preceded Doug as he paced back and forth on the landing trying to determine the appropriate direction. Despite the fact that it was obvious Doug and his dog were pacing aimlessly, none of the passengers and bystanders offered assistance. Some people may have failed to help because of negative feelings, but Doug felt that most were simply apathetic toward his dilemma. Ironically, public apathy prevented him from climbing out of a Washington subway station, but in 1981, Doug Wakefield was part of a team of individuals with and without disabilities who scaled Mt. Rainier (D. Wakefield, personal communication, 1981).

The effects of attitudinal barriers on persons with disabilities are overwhelming. Heyne, Schleien, and McAvoy (1993), for example, found that "fearful and negative attitudes about people with disabilities" was one of the most frequently reported obstacles to friendship development between persons with and without disabilities. In his poignant and eloquent book *The Body Silent*, Robert Murphy (1987) described the effects of a progressive disability on his daily activities and social relationships. He wrote, "The greatest impediment to a person's taking full part in his society are not his physical flaws, but rather the issue of myths, fears, and misunderstandings that society attaches to them" (p. 113).

Architectural Barriers. Structures such as buildings, walkways, and so on, that are usable by nondisabled people but present obstacles for people with disabilities, are known as architectural barriers. These barriers limit mobility and often deprive individuals with disabilities access to worthwhile leisure activities. David Park (1977), the National Park Service's Chief of Special Programs and Populations, noted, "A major reason many persons with disabilities do not participate in existing recreation programs is simply that facilities are not physically accessible and barrier-free" (p. 129).

Despite legislation (e.g., ADA) and the U.S. Access Board's efforts to increase accessibility in the United States, architectural barriers continue to be a significant problem for persons with disabilities. Although not all people with disabilities are inconvenienced by architectural barriers, it has been estimated that at least 21 million Americans are so affected (Socio-Technological Instrumental Modules Project, 1978). Architectural barriers give an unspoken message to these 21 million people: Society is not concerned with the needs of individuals who have disabilities. In effect, they are second-class citizens. The result is often frustration, anger, and alienation. As one person expressed, "I am not a shut in, I am a shut out" (Bruck, 1978, p. 21).

Progress toward eliminating architectural barriers has been made during the past decade, but there is still much work to be done. Freedom of mobility and access to programs are rights that should be extended to *every* citizen. (See Chapter 6 for an in-depth examination of architectural barriers.)

Ecological Barriers. Physical obstacles that occur in the natural environment may be termed ecological barriers. Hills, trees, sand, rain, snow, and wind are some examples. The physical impact of such barriers is roughly the same as that of architectural barriers, but there are two important differences. First, ecological barriers are much less frustrating for individuals who have disabilities, because they are not intentionally constructed by human beings. Therefore, they are not reminders of societal insensitivity toward people with disabilities. "I have to accept the fact that I will never backpack unassisted through the wilderness," commented one wheelchair user, "but I deserve the right to go to the store independently!"

The second difference between ecological and architectural barriers is that legislation cannot be used to counteract ecological barriers. Rather than eliminating ecological barriers, the main emphasis must be on minimizing their impact on people with disabilities. Careful advance planning may help minimize or avoid ecological barriers. For example, prior to participating in a nature walk, the individual with a disability can ensure that the program leader selects an access route that avoids ecological barriers such as gullies or large tree roots. Sometimes, however, overcoming rather than avoiding an ecological barrier may offer a greater reward. Satisfaction and pride are feelings that we *all* receive when we face and overcome nature's obstacles.

Transportation Barriers. The lack of usable and affordable methods of transportation often prevents individuals who have disabilities from benefiting from available community resources, including recreation services. As Goldman (1987) noted, "Transportation links the diverse facets of our lives . . . making each of them, and in turn, each of us, nondisabled and disabled, more accessible" (p. 106). Yet, automobile or van modifications are expensive, mass transportation is often inaccessible or inconvenient, and specially arranged (dial-a-ride) programs are few and often have many restrictions. Even when accessible public transportation is available, it usually requires considerable advance planning and constricts the lives of persons with disabilities. Murphy (1987) wrote:

> The inability to drive was more than a retreat from mobility, for it was one more step away from spontaneity and the free exercise of will. Whereas I could once act on whim and fancy, I now had to exercise planning and foresight. . . . This loss of spontaneity invaded my entire assessment of time. It rigidified my short-range perspectives and introduced a calculating quality into an existence that formerly had been pleasantly disordered. (p. 76)

Although some recreational programs do offer transportation services, these are usually segregated programs that do not meet the needs of all people who have disabilities. Too often, the person with a disability faces the choice of either staying home or imposing on family and friends by requesting transportation to recreational activities.

The American Bar Association (1979) has observed that an accessible transportation system would "increase significantly" the number of trips taken by people with disabilities. Nevertheless, the U.S. government has no national policy on transportation for individuals who have disabilities. Until such a policy is formulated and accompanied by a commitment to fund it, many people with disabilities in the United States will continue to face difficulties in finding and affording transportation to recreational programs.

Canada, unlike the United States, has had a national policy on transportation of persons with disabilities since 1983. The Coalition of Provincial Organizations of the Handicapped (COPOH, 1987) stated that the Canadian national policy guarantees for persons with disabilities "reasonable, reliable, and equitable transportation services and facilities; dignified travel; no unreasonable terms and conditions of travel; and self-determination" (p. 6). In addition, a Canadian Transportation Commission ruling known as the Kelly Decision has profound implications for the traveler who has a disability. This decision, an outcome of Clarris Kelly being denied transport because she was traveling without an attendant, established four significant principles: (1) self-determination (the traveler with a disability decides whether he or she requires an attendant); (2) one person/one fare (an attendant travels without charge); (3) equality of access (architectural barriers must not prevent travel); and (4) dignity of risk (travelers with disabilities are entitled to take the same risks as everyone else) (COPOH, 1987). As part of Canada's National Strategy for the Integration of Persons with Disabilities, Transport Canada is investing $24.6 million over a five-year period to make its transportation network more accessible. "Since the transportation network consists of many systems joined together, Transport Canada is working closely with all levels of government and the private sector to achieve equal access" ("Flying High," 1993, p. 17).

Such steps to improve transportation for persons with disabilities are of vital importance because, as Bowe (1979) noted, the availability of transportation "expands the alternatives from which a [person with a disability] can design his or her life" (p. 484).

Economic Barriers. Even in times of low unemployment, job opportunities are more limited for people who have disabilities. Furthermore, when they are able to find employment, individuals with disabilities frequently find themselves in low-paying positions with limited opportunity for advancement. These difficulties are compounded by higher-than-average expenses, such as for special transportation arrangements. Studies in the United States and Canada (International Center for the Disabled, 1986; Roeher Institute, 1988), have emphasized the economic plight of many people who have disabilities. Generally, people with disabilities have considerably less disposable income than people without disabilities; thus, their leisure activity choices and life experiences are constrained by their economic circumstances (Bridge & Gold, 1989). Ferris (1987), for example, found that 44 percent of the respondents in his study cited the home as their primary location for physical activity. Moreover, even when enough money is available to participate in activities outside the home, there may not be sufficient funds to fully enjoy the experience. Ferrel (1989) provided a poignant illustration of this point:

> Finally, I saved enough to pay for a week-end retreat and to go home each night by taxi. I enjoyed meeting new people and discovering new feelings of relaxation. The opportunity to go out for dinner afterwards with the group was important to me, but I felt peculiar when I could only afford to order an appetizer. My lack of income, rather than my disability, made me feel different from the others. (p. 15)

Interestingly, some studies have found that people with disabilities do not perceive lack of money to be a significant barrier to leisure participation (Caldwell & Adolph, 1989; Ferris, 1987). Nevertheless, these and other investigations have noted that people with disabilities often report recreational pursuits that are home based and require minimal expenditure of money. It is entirely possible that financial limitations, rather than personal preferences, determine the nature of leisure participation for many people who have disabilities. As Crawford (1989) stated, "For most, the economics of disability determine what life at the sidelines is like" (p. 8).

Rules and Regulations Barriers. Historically, people with disabilities have faced many rules and regulations that limited their ability to participate in all aspects of our society. Educational opportunities were systematically denied to people with severe disabilities; literacy tests prevented many capable people with disabilities from

In general, people with disabilities have less income than people without disabilities. Unfortunately, many have greater expenses as well. (Reprinted with permission from "There's Lint in Your Bellybutton! A Disabled Fable" by Audry King, © 1987 Canadian Rehabilitation Council for the Disabled [CRCD])

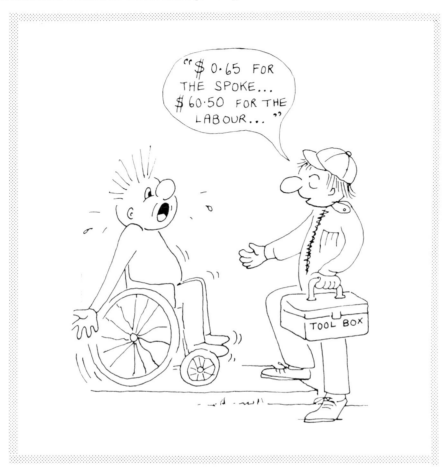

voting; and employers overtly discriminated against people with disabilities by establishing requirements that were unrelated to job performance.

Fortunately, legislation (e.g., ADA) has reduced or eliminated many discriminatory policies. Rules and regulations often die hard, however. In 1978, for example, the New York City Marathon Committee turned down the applications of two wheelchair users. The decision was eventually overturned, but not without controversy. Barbara Kelves, who has published many articles on running, supported the original decision. Kelves wrote to

The New York Times, "I believe the disabled racers lack the basic qualifications for the sport. . . . As race director, let [Fred Lebow] exercise his right mandated by the A.A.U. to protect the safety of all participants. Since Lebow wants to bar wheelchair racers from the New York Marathon they should be kept out" (October 7, 1979, Section 5, Page 2).

Rules and regulations are necessary if society is to function effectively. At the same time, they must not be used as an excuse to exclude people with disabilities from participation in leisure activities. Susan Sygall (1985), a highly independent wheelchair user, described the excellent accessibility at the National Theatre in England, but then stated, "Would you believe they refused to sell us two 'wheelchair seats' because we didn't have an able-bodied chaperone?" (p. 50). Such incidents provide evidence that fair rules and regulations, plus sensible enforcement, are needed if individuals with disabilities are to have equal access to recreational activities.

Barriers of Omission. Most environmental barriers to participation are actions or obstacles that limit people who have disabilities. Sometimes, however, what is *not* done creates barriers as well. The failure of society to provide for the needs of individuals who have disabilities results in barriers of omission. The following are examples of such barriers:

- Lack of appropriate education opportunities, including education for leisure.
- Lack of available recreation services that provide for people who have disabilities. Specifically, individualized services are needed to allow a person with a disability to function at his or her maximum level.
- Failure to publicize adequately those programs that could offer appropriate services to people who have disabilities.
- Failure to include participants with disabilities in the planning and implementation of leisure services.
- Lack of appropriate technology to maximize the leisure functioning of individuals with disabilities.
- Failure to enforce existing legislation that would reduce other barriers to participation.
- Lack of adequate leisure role models for youngsters with disabilities and adults with recent disabilities.

Communication Barriers

The locus of intrinsic barriers is primarily within the individual. Environmental barriers are external forces. Communication barriers, however, cannot be thought of as either primarily intrinsic or extrinsic to the individual with a disability. Communication barriers result from a reciprocal interaction between individuals with disabilities and their social environment. There is the old expression "It takes two to tango." It also takes two to establish effective communication; a message needs to be sent, but it must be received as well.

If communication is to occur, the sender *and* the receiver must be active participants in the process. This is true whether the message is spoken or written. If the message sender

Effective communication requires *active* participation by both the sender and receiver of a message. For physically disabled people with speech difficulties, pointing to letters on a "letter board" may facilitate this two-way interaction process. (Courtesy of The League: Serving People with Disabilities, Inc., Baltimore, MD)

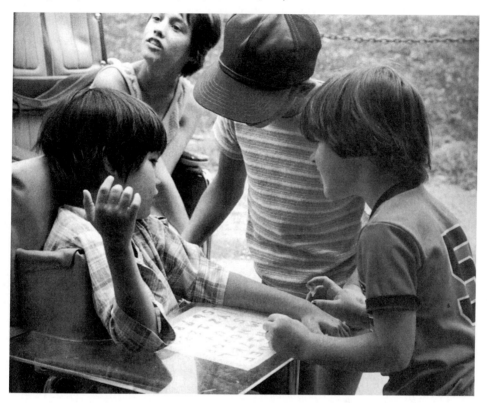

is not able to make the message clear enough to be understood by others, an *expressive* block limits communication. On the other hand, if a clearly expressed message is not received correctly, a *receptive* block interferes with the communication process.

Communication barriers are rarely caused exclusively by expressive blocks or receptive blocks, however. An individual with speech difficulties may find it impossible to pronounce words clearly. This difficulty could be an expressive block to communication. The listener, however, may not concentrate on what is said or take the time to ask for unclear words to be repeated. Thus, the listener could be responsible for a receptive block. Most communication barriers between people with and without disabilities result from a combination of expressive blocks and receptive blocks. If effective communication is to occur, *both* individuals with disabilities and society at large must make an effort to overcome expressive and receptive blocks to communication.

People with hearing impairments are probably the most familiar individuals affected by communication barriers. To varying degrees, however, most people with disabilities experience communication barriers. Many youth with behavioral disorders feel that their parents don't listen to them. Their parents, in turn, may complain that they don't even speak the same language. Some people with physical disabilities claim that politicians do not listen to their complaints. At the same time, these politicians express frustration because they feel that activists with physical disabilities do not want to discuss the problems of funding social programs.

The importance of communication barriers such as those just discussed cannot be overemphasized. Communication links the individual who has a disability with his or her environment. A two-way dialogue needs to exist between persons with disabilities and the rest of society, including individuals and societal institutions. If blocks are allowed to interfere with this communication, there is little hope of overcoming the many barriers to participation.

OVERCOMING BARRIERS

It is important to recognize that individuals with and without disabilities regularly overcome their personal barriers to recreation participation. Recent research on constraints to recreation participation for persons both with and without disabilities confirms that the presence of barriers (i.e., constraints) does not necessarily limit participation in activities (Henderson, Bedini, Hecht, & Schuler, 1993; Jackson & Rucks, in press; Kay & Jackson, 1991). Rather, people who are faced with barriers often "negotiate" their way through or around these barriers. People with disabilities are *not* powerless against the many barriers listed previously; however, they may require assistance to negotiate some barriers they face. As a result, recreation professionals have the *obligation* to work for the reduction or elimination of these barriers. Witt (1977) emphasized this obligation in the following statement:

> The group of individuals who we need to deal with when we consider overcoming attitudinal barriers often also includes "ourselves" as well, i.e., those of us who feel committed to "helping" but may place limits on how much help we are willing to give; how far rights really extend; and how much we are prepared to go beyond what is easy and obvious. (p. 17)

Despite this obligation, there are so many barriers to participation that working for their removal may seem like an overwhelming task. Most recreators rightfully feel that their jobs are so time-consuming that they have little time for additional efforts. Much of what needs to be done to remove barriers, however, can be accomplished within the scope of a recreator's job. The following concepts may help recreation professionals to provide the proper atmosphere for reducing or eliminating barriers to participation.

Accessible and inclusive programs encourage cooperative interaction between persons with and without disabilities. (Courtesy of Maryland—National Capital Park and Planning Commission, Special Populations Division; Photo by Steve Abramowitz)

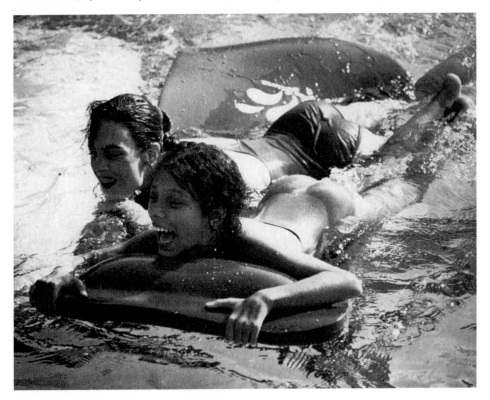

Provide Accessible Programs

It is essential that recreation professionals respond to the intent of the ADA (see Chapter 3) by planning and implementing programs that are accessible to persons with disabilities. This means more than simply providing ramps into buildings; it involves planning programs that avoid as many barriers to participation as possible. The following suggestions may assist with this process:

- Offer activities that (a) include a range of cognitive and physical skill requirements, (b) allow for proper skill progression, (c) give opportunities for both formal and informal involvement, and (d) encourage cooperative interaction between participants with and without disabilities.

- Coordinate activities offered with public transportation schedules, and consider establishing car or van pools to activities.

- Ensure that buildings and facilities, including parking lots, comply with Americans with Disabilities Act Architectural Guidelines for accessibility.

- Develop ways for economically disadvantaged individuals to "pay" for services that require fees; for example, in-kind services such as volunteer work could be used.

- Coordinate programs with agencies and organizations that specialize in services to people with special needs, thus ensuring that a continuum of services is available within the community.

- Publicize programs thoroughly and advertise that they are accessible to people with disabilities (including interpreters for participants with hearing impairments).

Establish Priorities for Action

The traditional approach to overcoming barriers to participation has been for the recreation professional to concentrate on intrinsic barriers. This approach involves using recreation participation to improve the person's social, physical, or cognitive functioning. Emphasis may be on improving a person's disability or "problem," or it may be on strengthening the person's abilities. Regardless, this traditional approach means that the recreation professional focuses on changing the participant.

A number of authorities (Bowe, 1978; Howe-Murphy & Charboneau, 1987; Schleien & Ray, 1988; Wright, 1980) have challenged this traditional approach, however. They contend that professionals should not focus solely on changing individuals with disabilities, but should work toward reducing or eliminating environmental barriers. In 1980, Hutchison developed and used a Barriers to Community Involvement scale to determine the impact of 13 intrinsic and environmental barriers. Her results "suggest that disabled persons largely see barriers to community involvement as lying beyond themselves" (p. 10). She stated that this was a "noteworthy finding and should be analyzed further, since much of the focus in rehabilitation, education, and vocational services is upon changing disabled persons rather than the community" (pp. 10–11). The individual with a disability does not live in a vacuum. If people with disabilities are to become fully integrated into society, most authorities agree that *both* intrinsic and environmental barriers must receive everyone's attention.

Although recreational professionals can and should help to reduce or eliminate intrinsic and environmental barriers, the *unique* contribution that recreators can make is with the third type of barrier—communication barriers. By eliminating communication barriers as their first priority, recreators can help provide a vital link between individuals with disabilities and their social environments. Once this is accomplished, the job of overcoming other barriers will become much easier.

Facilitate Communication

Providing accessible programs is one way to facilitate communication between individuals with and without disabilities. Such programs bring people together and offer an opportunity for interpersonal communication. Recreation professionals must do more than just bring people together, however. Recreators should set an example for their constituents without disabilities by interacting appropriately with people who have disabilities. Additionally, recreators should aid the communication process between people who have disabilities and society's policymakers.

People who lack experience interacting with individuals with visible disabilities sometimes feel uncomfortable initiating conversation. Hesitancy and some discomfort are normal reactions to any unfamiliar situation, so recreators should expect to feel uneasy at first. It is essential to overcome these initial feelings, however. Before long, the person's disability will become less noticeable, and his or her "normalcy" will become apparent. The following tips for interacting with an individual who has a disability are modified from "When You Meet a Handicapped Person," by an unknown author. They provide an excellent guideline for community recreators.

- Remember, a person with a disability is a person *first*. He or she is like anyone else, except for specific physical or mental limitations.
- Just be yourself, and show friendly personal interest in him or her.
- Learn basic signs and fingerspelling for talking with individuals who are hearing impaired.
- Talk about the same things you would with anyone else.
- Give physical assistance only if requested by the individual.
- Independence is important to everyone. If the situation dictates, perhaps ask, "Do you need assistance?"
- Be patient and let the person with a disability set the pace in walking or talking.
- Don't be afraid to laugh with him or her.
- Don't be overprotective or shower the individual with kindness. Don't offer pity or charity.
- Avoid making up your mind in advance about the capabilities of the person. You may be surprised how wrong you can be in making judgments about the individual's interests and abilities.

Facilitating interpersonal communication is extremely important. It is equally important, however, for recreators to facilitate communication between individuals with disabilities and leaders in the community. Hopkins, Tilley, and Salisbury (1988), Hutchison and Lord (1979), Owen (1981), and many others have stressed the necessity for people with disabilities to express their own needs to policymakers. Hutchison (1980) noted, "As with many other change movements, greatest progress will be made when those oppressed by negative attitudes and poor services take an active role in changing attitudes and practices which block community involvement" (p. 7). Recreation professionals should search for ways to assist with this process. The following are some possibilities:

- Assist in the development of consumer groups, which bring together people with disabilities who have similar needs, interests, and goals.

- Analyze the community's power structure (Jewell, 1983), identify decision makers, and assist efforts to increase their awareness of barriers to participation.

- Keep abreast of meetings, hearings, and so on, that offer opportunities for people with disabilities to express their views.

- Provide consumers with information and resources that may be useful in discussions with policymakers.

- Offer seminars on interpersonal communication for people with disabilities to include ways to improve both expressive and receptive communication.

- If necessary, serve as an advocate to speak for people with disabilities who are unable to articulate their own needs.

Recreation professionals are in a unique position. Their jobs offer the chance to provide an ideal atmosphere for eliminating communication barriers, and effective communication between individuals with disabilities and the rest of society is the key to reducing or eliminating most barriers to participation. Careful planning and a great deal of energy are required, but it is well worth the effort. As Bowe (1978) emphasized, "We are talking about retrofitting an entire society, renovating buildings and subways, altering entrenched bureaucracies, and, perhaps most difficult of all, changing people themselves. But it must be done" (p. 225).

SUMMARY

Barriers to participation in recreation and leisure activities are experienced by everyone, but people who have disabilities face more and greater barriers than their nondisabled peers. Some of these barriers are *intrinsic;* they result from the individual's own limitations. Other barriers are *environmental;* they are caused by external forces that impose limits on the individual. Finally, some are *communication* barriers, which block interaction between the individual and his or her social environment. Although recreation professionals can assist with overcoming all types of barriers, they should establish the elimination of communication barriers as their first priority. By reducing or eliminating communication barriers, recreators can help create a vital link between people with disabilities and their social environments. Once this is accomplished, the task of overcoming other barriers becomes much easier.

SUGGESTED LEARNING ACTIVITIES

1. Make a list of 10 items regarding elimination of barriers to recreation participation that you would address if asked to testify before your city council.
2. Explain how an individual's perception of his or her own skill can act as a barrier to recreation participation.
3. Simulate a disability (blindness, paraplegia, etc.) and attend an organized recreational program. Identify each barrier encountered according to the types listed in the chapter.
4. Interview the director of a community recreation program and determine what actions are being taken to eliminate barriers to participation in that program. Discuss the strengths and weaknesses of these actions.
5. Of the three types of barriers outlined in the chapter, which is the key to reducing or eliminating most other barriers to participation? Explain why.
6. Interview an individual with a disability and determine (a) his or her recreational needs, interests, and desires, and (b) intrinsic, environmental, and communication barriers that limit his or her participation.

REFERENCES

American Bar Association. *Eliminating Environmental Barriers.* Washington, DC: ABA Commission on the Mentally Disabled, 1979.

Bedini, L. A. Transition and integration in leisure for people with disabilities. *Parks & Recreation, 28*(11), 20–24, 1993.

Bowe, F. *Handicapping America: Barriers to Disabled People.* New York: Harper and Row, 1978.

Bowe, F. Transportation: Key to independent living. *Archives of Physical Medicine and Rehabilitation, 60*(10), 484, 1979.

Bregha, F. J. Leisure and freedom re-examined. In T. L. Goodale & P. A. Witt, Eds. *Recreation and Leisure and Issues in an Era of Change.* State College, PA: Venture Publishing, 1980, pp. 30–37.

Bridge, N. J., & D. Gold. An analysis of the relationship between leisure and economics. *Journal of Leisurability, 16*(2), 10–14, 1989.

Bruck L. *Access: The Guide to a Better Life for Disabled Americans.* New York: Random House, 1978.

Caldwell, L., & S. Adolph. Economic issues associated with disability: And then there is leisure. *Journal of Leisurability, 16*(2), 19–24, 1989.

COPOH. Transportation and disabled citizens: Policies on eligibility and reciprocity. *Journal of Leisurability, 14*(1), 4–12, 1987.

Crawford, C. A view from the sidelines: Disability, poverty, and recreation in Canada. *Journal of Leisurability, 16*(2), 3–9, 1989.

Crawford, D. W., E. L. Jackson, & G. Godbey. A hierarchical model of leisure constraints. *Leisure Sciences, 13,* 309–320, 1991.

Csikszentmihalyi, M. *Beyond Boredom and Anxiety.* San Francisco: Jossey-Bass, 1975.

Ferrel, M. No income: No leisure. *Journal of Leisurability, 16*(2), 15–16, 1989.

Ferris, B. F. Reflection on the physical activity patterns of disabled Canadians: Challenges for practitioners. *Journal of Leisurability, 14*(2), 18–23, 1987.

Flying high. *Abilities,* 17, Spring, 1993.

Goldman, C. D. *Disability Rights Guide: Practical Solutions to Problems Affecting People with Disabilities.* Lincoln, NE: Media, 1987.

Henderson, K. A., L. A. Bedini, L. Hecht, & R. Schuler. *Women With Physical Disabilities and the Negotiation of Leisure Constraints.* Paper presented at the Canadian Congress on Leisure Research, Winnipeg, Manitoba, Canada, May, 1993.

Heyne, L. A., S. J. Schleien, & L. H. McAvoy. *Friendship Development Between Children With and Without Developmental Disabilities in Recreational Activities.* Paper presented at the 1993 Symposium on Leisure Research, San Jose, CA, October, 1993.

Hopkins, J., A. Tilley, & T. Salisbury. Thoughts and reflections from British Columbia. *Journal of Leisurability, 15*(2), 20–23, 1988.

Howe-Murphy, R., & B. G. Charboneau. *Therapeutic Recreation Intervention: An Ecological Perspective.* Englewood Cliffs, NJ: Prentice-Hall, 1987.

Hutchison, P. Perceptions of disabled persons regarding barriers to community involvement. *Journal of Leisurability, 7*(3), 4–16, 1980.

Hutchison, P., & J. Lord. *Recreation Integration.* Ontario, Canada: Leisurability Publications, 1979.

Illich, I., I. K. Zola, J. McKnight, J. Caplan, & H. Shaiken. *Disabling Professions.* London: Marion Boyers, 1977.

International Center for the Disabled. *The ICD Survey of Disabled Americans: Bringing Disabled Americans into the Mainstream.* New York: Louis Harris and Associates, 1986.

Jackson, E. L. Special issue introduction: Leisure constraints/constrained leisure. *Leisure Sciences, 13,* 203–215. 1991.

Jackson, E. L., D. W. Crawford, & G. Godbey. Negotiation of leisure constraints. *Leisure Sciences, 15,* 1–11, 1993.

Jackson, E. L., & V. C. Rucks. Reasons for ceasing participation and barriers to participation: Further examination of constrained leisure as an internally homogeneous concept. *Leisure Sciences, 15,* 217–230, 1993.

Jackson. E. L., & V. C. Rucks. Negotiation of leisure constraints by junior-high and high-school students: An exploratory study. *Journal of Leisure Research,* in press.

Jewell, D. C. Comprehending concepts of community power structure: Prerequisite for recreation-integration. *Journal of Leisurability, 10*(1), 24–30, 1983.

Kay, T., & G. Jackson. Leisure despite constraint: The impact of leisure constraints on leisure participation. *Journal of Leisure Research, 23,* 301–313, 1991.

Langer, E. J., S. Fiske, S. E. Taylor, & B. Chanowitz. Stigma, staring, and discomfort: A novel-stimulus hypothesis. *Journal of Experimental Social Psychology, 12*(5), 451–463, 1976.

Matthews, P. R. Why the mentally retarded do not participate in certain types of recreational activities. *Therapeutic Recreation Journal, 14*(1), 44–50, 1980.

Miller, H. L. Integration of disabled people in mainstream sports: Case study of a partially sighted child. *Adapted Physical Activity Quarterly, 6,* 17–31, 1989.

Moore, R. L., & J. Dattilo. Greenway preferences: A comparison between people with and without disabilities. In *Abstracts from the 1993 Symposium on Leisure Research* (p. 28). Arlington, VA: National Recreation and Park Association, 1993.

Murphy, J. F. An enabling approach to leisure service delivery. In T. L. Goodale and P. A. Witt, Eds. *Recreation and Leisure: Issues in an Era of Change.* State College, PA: Venture Publishing, 1980, pp. 197–210.

Murphy, R. *The body silent.* New York: Holt, 1987.

National Organization on Disability. New survey shows people with disabilities not well informed on ADA. *National Organization on Disability Report,* 1–3, Summer, 1993.

Owen, J. Advocacy 'with' instead of 'for' consumers. *Journal of Leisurability, 8*(3), 19–20, 1981.

Park, D. Recreation. In the White House Conference on Handicapped Individuals, *Volume One: Awareness Papers* pp. 119–131. Washington, DC: The White House Conference on Handicapped Individuals, 1977.

Roeher Institute. *Income Insecurity: The Disability Income System in Canada.* Downsview, Ontario: The G. Allan Roeher Institute, 1988.

Schleien, S., & M. T. Ray. *Community Recreation and Persons with Disabilities: Strategies for Integration.* Baltimore, MD: Paul H. Brookes, 1988.

Sneegas, J. J. Social skills: An integral component of leisure participation and the therapeutic recreation services. *Therapeutic Recreation Journal, 23*(2), 30–40, 1989.

Socio-Technological Instrumental Modules Project. *Accessibility for the Handicapped.* Stony Brook, NY: State University of New York at Stony Brook, 1978.

Sygall, S. Travelling tips. *The Exceptional Parent, 15*(8), 50–51, 1985.

Szychowski, E. River of dreams. *Sports 'n Spokes, 18*(1), 19–22, 1993.

Witt, P. *Community Leisure Services and Disabled Individuals.* Washington, DC: Hawkins and Associates, 1977.

Wright, B. A. Developing constructive views of life with a disability. *Rehabilitation Literature, 41*(11–12), 274–279, 1980.

Wright, B. A. *Physical Disability—A Psychosocial Approach.* New York: Harper and Row, 1983.

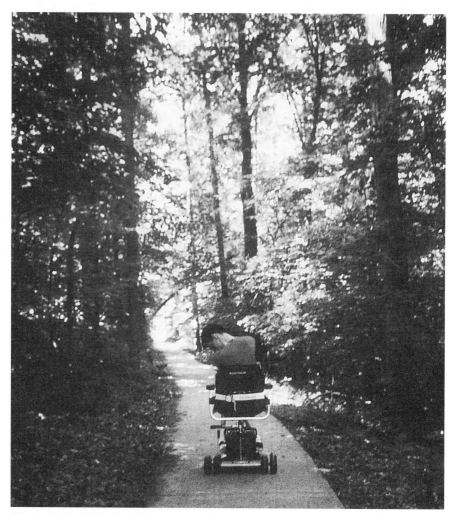

(Photo by David R. Austin)

6

Design of Accessible and Usable Recreation Environments

. . .

In the past, a vast number of recreation facilities in the United States have been usable only by persons who do not have visual, audile, mental, or mobility impairments. Today, however, there is a growing public consciousness regarding environmental design for persons with disabilities. This consciousness is manifested by the Americans with Disabilities Act of 1990.

This chapter deals with the design of appropriate recreation environments for all people, including persons with disabilities. Initial coverage is given to common terms and pertinent legislation. The major portion of the chapter is devoted to a discussion of guidelines and recommendations for creating usable public recreation facilities, with special attention directed to playgrounds.

TERMINOLOGY

For the purpose of this chapter, it is necessary to define two important terms often found in the literature concerning recreation environments designed to meet the needs of persons with disabilities. These terms are *accessibility* and *usability,* and each is defined as follows:

- *Accessibility* refers to the elements in the constructed environment (site or building) that allow approach, entrance, and use of facilities by persons with disabling conditions. The term is often used to indicate that a facility complies with specified standards to permit use by those whose sensory or physical impairments might otherwise limit their use of the facility.
- *Usability* refers to a constructed environment providing the opportunity for maximum use by those with sensory or mobility impairments. Occasionally, the word is used with the term *accessibility* to indicate that a facility not only meets minimum accessibility standards but is actually usable by individuals with disabling conditions.

LEGISLATION

Growing public awareness of the problems of persons with disabilities has led to several pieces of federal legislation that have an effect on the design of recreation facilities. Chief among these are the Architectural Barriers Act of 1968 (PL 90-480), Section 504 of the Rehabilitation Act of 1973 (PL 93-112), and the Americans with Disabilities Act of 1990 (PL 101-336).

The language of PL 90-480 and PL 93-112 dictates that the needs of persons with disabilities be considered by those recreation agencies that utilize federal funds. The Architectural Barriers Act specifies that "Any building, or facility, constructed in whole or in part by federal funds must be made accessible to and usable by the physically handicapped." Section 504 of the Rehabilitation Act states, "no otherwise qualified handicapped individual in the U.S. . . . shall solely, by reason of his handicap, be excluded from participation in, be denied the benefits of, or be subjected to discrimination under any program or activity receiving federal assistance." The Americans with Disabilities Act (ADA) prohibits discrimination against people with disabilities. The ADA extends the Architectural Barriers Act to all public facilities regardless of funding. Thus, it is clearly the mandate of the government of the United States that recreational facilities open to the public be accessible to all people. In addition, many state and local laws stipulate barrier-free architectural design for public facilities. For more detailed information on legislation, see Chapter 3.

GENERAL GUIDELINES FOR PLANNING RECREATION FACILITIES

Dimensions—Space Requirements

A basic point of departure in thinking about design components for persons with disabilities is to deal with dimensional requirements. To do this, space requirements for an average adult wheelchair user are considered since designs to accommodate this individual should ensure spaces large enough for other persons.

Wheelchair Dimensions. Dimensions for an average, manual, adult-sized wheelchair (Fig. 6.1) are as follows:

- The length of the chair itself will be 42 in. to 48 in. With another 6 in. required for toe space, the total length required for wheelchair users is 48 in. to 54 in.
- The width of the average wheelchair is 24 in. to 26 in. When collapsed, the most commonly used wheelchairs are 11 in. wide.
- The height of the seat from the floor is approximately 19 in.

Figure 6.1. Dimensions of adult-sized wheelchairs.

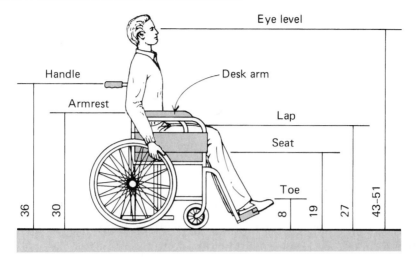

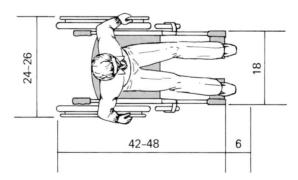

- It is 27 in. from the floor to the user's lap and 30 in. from the floor to the armrests.
- The height of the pusher handles is 36 in. from the floor.

Some specially equipped adult-sized wheelchairs may exceed these dimensions. Of course, children's wheelchairs will be smaller than those designed for adults. The junior-sized chair has a seat 16 in. wide and 18 in. from the floor. Thus, space requirements such as the turning radius will necessarily be reduced for children.

Space Requirements for Maneuvering Wheelchairs. The following are space requirements for those using standard, adult-sized wheelchairs:

- A turning radius of 64 in. × 64 in. is required to make a full 360° turn.

- A minimum width for a corridor or path that allows a pedestrian and a wheelchair user to pass is 48 in., although a wider width to accommodate two wheelchairs to pass is recommended.

- The minimum width for a corridor or path that allows two wheelchairs to pass is 60 in., although a space of 72 in. would be recommended.

- A minimum door opening width of 32 in. is needed by a person in a wheelchair.

- The width of a corridor or path with a door or gate should exceed the width of the door or gate by 18 in. to 24 in. to allow the space needed to maneuver the chair while opening the door or gate.

Reaching from a Wheelchair. Each wheelchair user is unique in his or her range of reach because of differences in size, strength, range of motion, and degree of involvement. The reach dimensions presented here are averages. Devices should therefore be placed well within the figures presented so they may be accessible to all.

- The reach for a wheelchair user facing a wall and reaching diagonally is approximately 48 in. from the floor. Thus, switches, telephones, and other such devices should be placed less than 48 in. from the floor. Minimum height is 15 in. from the floor.

- An upward side reach can be made to the height of 54 in. from the floor. A downward side reach can be made down to 9 in. from the floor. Thus, shelves and cabinets should be placed within the range of 9 in. to 54 in. from the floor.

- An average person in a wheelchair can reach a maximum of 25 in. across a table when seated at the table. A comfortable reach would, of course, be less. Thus, relatively narrow shelves and work spaces are dictated.

Special Considerations for Other Persons

General concepts to consider when planning areas and facilities for other populations are as follows:

- Some persons experience difficulty in operating devices that call for grasping or twisting because of chronic impairments that affect the skills required to manipulate objects (such as doorknobs). Therefore, devices should be chosen that make it possible to manipulate the objects without the need to grasp or twist.

- Persons may lack the strength and stamina needed to be successful in completing tasks such as opening heavy doors or using revolving doors. Decreased strength and stamina may particularly be a problem for older people. Doors should not be heavy to open, and rest areas should be considered in all recreation facilities, especially along paths.

- For those with visual impairments, raised letters should be used on signs.

- The use of different textures on walks or paths may be used to provide location cues to persons who have visual impairments. Textured borders on the edge of paths are an example of such a cueing aid.

- Audible cues may be provided, such as bells signaling once for an up elevator, twice for a down elevator, or verbal announcements of each floor on the elevator.

- For those with severe auditory impairments, signage is particularly important. Signs with precise and clear messages should be placed at a height within the range of vision of both children and adults.

- Simplicity should be a keynote in design for persons possessing mental impairments. For example, signs should be as simple as possible (i.e., use short words or easily understood symbols). In the design of buildings and other facilities, ambiguity should be avoided so as to minimize uncertainty and confusion.

PARKS AND OUTDOOR RECREATION AREAS

Numerous design elements are found within park and outdoor recreation areas. Although in the section that follows, a number of these elements will be treated as separate entities, it is critical to remember the importance of the physical relationship among these design elements. Unless it is possible to get from one area to another, the value of making a specific area accessible is minimized.

Gilbert (1987) has noted an interrelationship among design and other elements critical to accessibility of parks and outdoor recreation areas. Citing the results of a Canadian survey, Gilbert identified four key issues related to park access:

1. Transportation—Both to get to the [parks and historic] areas and within the park itself.
2. Accessibility—The need to remove all barriers to enable participation by all.
3. The need to consider disabilities other than physical disabilities.
4. The need for more education programs to impact on society's attitudes toward disabled persons. (p. 27)

The emphasis in this chapter is on design elements. However, it is important to keep in mind that the design characteristics discussed are interrelated and have important psychosocial implications for park and recreation facility users, particularly those who have disabilities.

Signage. Identification, directional, and information signs are helpful to all users of park and recreation facilities. Proper signage is particularly beneficial for persons with hearing and speech impairments, because they may not be able to communicate with others to obtain information.

The international symbol of accessibility (see Fig. 6.2) should be displayed at the entrance and at various points within the park or recreation area to inform people that it provides access for persons with disabilities. Facilities within the park or recreation area that should be appropriately marked with the symbol include rest rooms, entrances to

Figure 6.2. International symbol of accessibility.

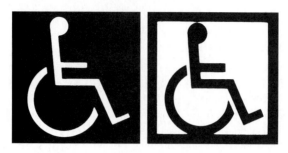

buildings, trails, and picnic areas. In addition, all parking spaces designated for use by individuals with disabilities should be clearly marked with the symbol of accessibility, and where diagrams or maps are provided, the symbol should be used to indicate accessible buildings or areas.

Signs should be placed at a height within the range of vision and reach for both children and adults. Preferably, signs should be located at eye level (between 43 in. and 51 in.) for wheelchair users. Consistency should be employed in height and location when mounting signs so that they may be found easily.

For ease in reading, signs should be made with light-colored characters or symbols on a dark background and have a nonglare surface. Identification signs for rooms (including rest rooms) should have raised characters, using the standard alphabet and Arabic numbers, since the vast majority of persons with severe visual impairments do no read Braille. The characters should be at least 5/8 in. in height but no higher than 2 in. They should be raised a minimum of 1/32 in. and have clearly defined edges. Signs with raised letters can also be used to identify and interpret points of interest. Most authorities would probably agree, however, that sighted guides or audiotape devices are more effective means of presenting information.

Parking. Special parking accommodations are required for persons with disabilities. These spaces allow drivers with disabilities who need extra space to transfer safely. Those with stamina limitations and individuals with visual impairments who must have safe access to and from parking areas may also use accessible spaces. Because of this, parking spaces need to be located as close as possible to the shortest accessible route to the building or area being utilized. Accessible paths (with a minimum 48 in. width) adjacent to parking areas must be wide enough to allow for the possibility of parked cars overhanging the walkway. Accessible parking stalls must be at least 96 in. wide. Passenger access aisles (at least 60 in. wide) next to the stalls for cars permit persons who have disabilities to gain access to automobiles. The overall dimensions of the area should be approximately 14 ft wide (including the 60 in. zone for the access aisle) and 18 ft long.

Figure 6.3. Returned curb.

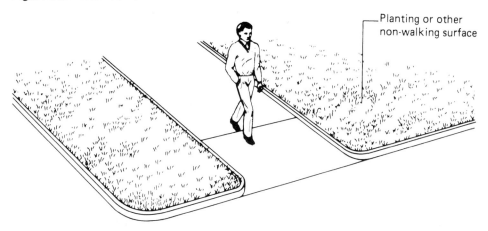

Planting or other
non-walking surface

One accessible space must be provided per 25 spaces in lots that hold 100 cars or less. In lots with more than 100 spaces, an additional accessible space must be added for each additional 50 spaces up to 400 spaces (i.e., 8 accessible spaces in a 400-space lot). Lots having 401 to 500 spaces must have 9 accessible spaces. In lots of 501 to 1,000 spaces, 2% of the spaces must be accessible. Finally, in lots of 1,001 spaces and more, the required number of accessible spaces is 20 plus 1 per 100 above 1,000. One out of every 8 accessible stalls needs to be designated as van accessible. Van stalls, like those for cars, are 9 ft wide, but the access aisle must be at least 96 in. (as compared to 60 in. for cars).

Both car and van accessible stalls must be painted solid blue with a white international symbol of accessibility, or must be outlined in blue with a 3-ft-square accessibility symbol. Finally, a sign at least 70 square in. in size, displaying the international symbol of accessibility, should be posted so the bottom edge is at least 80 in. above the surface.

Passenger Loading Zones. Passenger loading zones need to be designed for accessibility. The space for the vehicle must be at least 20 ft in length, with a 60 in. minimum aisle running along the entire length. The access aisle must be the same level as the pull-up space or a curb ramp needs to be provided. The slope of the curb ramp cannot exceed 1:12 (8.33%).

Two common types of curb ramps are the ramp with a returned curb (Fig. 6.3) and the flared ramp (Fig. 6.4). If there is a flare on the sides of the ramp, it should be no steeper than 1:8 (12.3%). No matter the type, curb ramps should be a minimum of 36 in. wide. Ramps should be constructed to blend at a common level with the street or parking lot and the walk. It is recommended that the entire curb ramp be made to contrast in color and texture with the walk surface so that it is not a hazard for those who have visual impairments.

Figure 6.4. Flared sides.

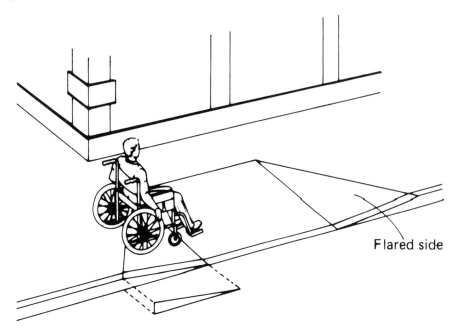

Flared side

Walks and Trails. Parks and outdoor recreation areas commonly provide walks to connect major buildings with other areas. Trails are also common features in parks and outdoor recreation areas.

When walks join parking lots and streets, they must be made to meet the level of the other surfaces. In many instances, curbs are not constructed in park and recreation areas so that there is a natural blending of walks with parking lots and streets. Illustrations presented in the previous section cover the design features when curb ramps are necessary in parking facilities. These same principles may be employed when a walk meets a street or driveway. Design features become far more complex, however, when walks meet the intersection of two curbed streets. It is recommended that information be sought from experts or illustrated literature on accessibility be reviewed to obtain alternatives for designing acceptable curb ramps at intersections.

Walks should be a minimum of 48 in. wide. However, a width of 60 in. to 72 in. is preferable so that wheelchairs can easily pass. Walk gradients should not exceed 1:20 (5%) and preferably should be less. If a walk does approach the maximum grade or is unusually long, rest areas with benches and room for wheelchairs should be provided. Surfaces in front of rest stops should be textured differently than the walk to provide location cues for persons with visual impairments. Nonslip surfaces such as brushed concrete or asphalt are recommended for the overall walk surface. Minimum use of expansion joints is also recommended, and where joints are used they should not exceed 1/2 in.

Ecological barriers, such as hills and rough terrains, may limit independent participation by wheelchair users. Accessible walks and trails enable most people with disabilities to enjoy nature without depending on others for assistance. (Courtesy of The League: Serving People with Physical Disabilities, Inc., Baltimore, MD)

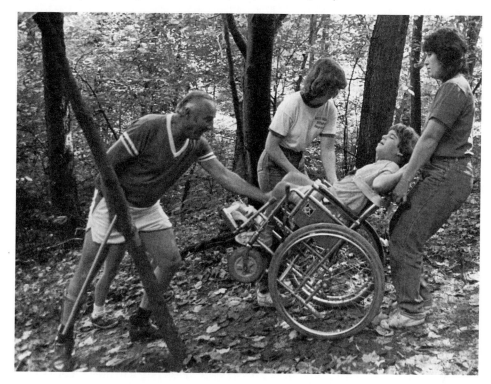

Most authorities object to the designation of "handicapped trails." An alternative to designating trails for the use of persons with disabilities is to provide several different types of recreational trails within a park or outdoor recreation area. The trail system can then reflect a wide range of user preferences and abilities. *A Guide to Designing Accessible Outdoor Recreation Facilities* (1980), published by the U.S. Department of Interior, suggests five classifications for trails. A brief description of each follows.

- Class I trails are short (0 ft to 1/4 mi), hard surface (concrete or asphalt) trails with very little grade (a maximum of 1:50 or 2% slope). The recommended width is 48 in. (one way) to 72 in. (two ways). Rest areas with benches, shelters, and interpretation stations are placed every 100 ft to 150 ft.

- Class II trails are 1/4 to 1 mi, surfaced with asphalt, wooden planking, or solidly packed crushed stone, and may have a slope of 1:20 (5%). The width for Class II trails is 36 in. to 48 in. (one way) to 48 in. to 60 in. (two ways). Rest areas with benches, shelters, and interpretation stations are placed every 200 ft to 300 ft.

- Class III trails are 1 to 3 mi long, are surfaced with a firm, well-compacted material (such as pea gravel), and may have a slope of 1:12 (8.33%). The width of the trail is 36 in. to 48 in. Rest areas consist of occasional natural benches and interpretation stations where needed (using 500 ft to 600 ft as a guideline.)

- Class IV trails are 3 to 10 mi in length, are surfaced with bound wood chips or class 5 gravel mixed coarse, and may have a slope of 1:8 (12.5%). The trail width is 24 in. to 36 in. A rest area or interpretation station is located every mile.

- Class V trails are more than 10 miles, have surfaces that are sandy or made of rocks or rough, unbound wood chips, and that follow the slope of the land or use steps. The width of the trail is not defined and rest areas are not developed unless there is a particularly unique feature that requires interpretation.

By employing this five-level classification system or a similar system, parks and recreation professionals can provide appropriate levels of experiences to suit persons with a variety of interests and abilities. Of course, proper signage is important to the successful utilization of such a trail system, since users must be informed of the length and difficulty of each trail.

An alternative means to the classification system is the mapping of trails using computerized mapping techniques in order to provide users objective data on the difficulty of each trail. Such maps offer much more specific and objective information than can a general classification system (Axelson & Chelini, 1993).

Before closing this segment on trails, we should mention that a particularly interesting approach to trail design is displayed by the "All People's Trail," located in the Shaker Lakes Regional Nature Center in Cleveland, Ohio. The "All People's Trail" is a completely accessible trail constructed of wood and concrete. The use of wood allowed the designers to elevate parts of the trail so that all can enjoy being in the middle of a marsh area, overlooking a small waterfall, looking down into a creek, and, in general, having a new perspective from which to view nature. The trail truly provides a unique outdoor experience in which all may participate.

Picnic Areas. Picnic tables need to be designed to accommodate wheelchair users. Usually this is accomplished by designing picnic tables so that a wheelchair user can sit comfortably at one end of the table. Paths should lead to at least some of the tables in any picnic area, and grills should be usable by all those in wheelchairs. Specific dimensions for tables and grills are provided in the following section on furnishings.

Furnishings. Site furniture includes tables, grills, benches, drinking fountains, and telephones. *Picnic tables* should be a minimum of 27 in. from the underside of the table to the ground and should allow 19 in. clearance in depth and 30 in. in width for knee space. *Grills* 30 in. in height and located adjacent to hard surfacing can be most easily utilized by wheelchair users. While not all grills in any picnic area need to accommodate persons in wheelchairs, a number should be provided adequate to the needs of the population using the facility. *Benches* with setting heights of 18 in. to 20 in. and widths of no more than 18 in. are most ideal. Backrests and arm supports should be included. Benches should be set back so that they do not obstruct walkways, and adequate space should be provided around them so that a wheelchair user can sit in his or her wheelchair beside someone seated on the bench. *Drinking fountains* should be surrounded with paved areas to provide easy access and avoid mud puddles. Hand-operated levers allow the greatest ease in turning in the water. For adults, the spout should preferably be 34 in. to 36 in. from the paved area. For children, the height should be approximately 30 in. A push-button public *telephone* should be located on a hard surface for use by persons with disabilities. The entrance to the phone should be at least 30 in. wide to allow wheelchair users access to the coin slot, receiver, and push buttons. Normally it is best to plan for the highest operable part of the telephone to be no more than 54 in. from the surface.

Water-Related Areas and Playfields

Some of the most popular recreational activities take place in water-related areas. The section that follows discusses swimming, fishing, and boating facilities.

Beaches. Sand—a highly desirable element at the beach—can create difficulties for wheelchair users and those who may have mobility problems. Designers must, therefore, make certain there are walks or pathways through the sand to the water. Concrete walks can be constructed. An alternative is to build a stabilized sand path to the water. No matter what method is used, the walk or path should not be steep (a maximum slope of 8.33% is recommended), and it should lead to the water's edge or to swimming platforms or docks. Where platforms or docks do not extend into the lake, a concrete pad can be constructed so that there is a hard surface under the water to aid the entry of persons with disabilities. Sometimes handrails (placed at about 32 in. in height) are constructed to follow the walk and entry into the water.

Pools. The best pool design is one that allows people who have disabilities to choose from several options to enter the water. One means to aid entry is to construct a ramp a minimum of 36 in. wide. Such a ramp should have a slip-resistant surface, handrails that are 34 in. to 38 in. high, and a slope of no more than 8.33%. A second means is to provide steps with treads at least 18 in. wide. Steps should be deep enough to allow adults to sit on them. Handrails (34 in. to 38 in. high) can be provided along the steps. It would also be helpful to have a second rail 6 in. above the nosings (the projecting edge of a step). A third means for people to enter the pool is for them to sit on the pool deck and swing their legs over the side into the water. A portable device with steps can be placed on the deck so that wheelchair users may transfer to it and then move down its steps to deck level. A final means of helping people with disabilities into a pool is a hydraulic lift. Such a lift will normally not be required. However, in instances when large persons must be assisted into the pool, the hydraulic lift can be very helpful.

Fishing Piers. Fishing piers can be constructed to meet the needs of persons with disabilities. Of course, fishing piers should be accessible by a walk or hard surface pathway.

Fishing piers, if properly constructed, can provide access to persons who use wheelchairs or other mobility aids. (Courtesy of Bradford Woods, Indiana University)

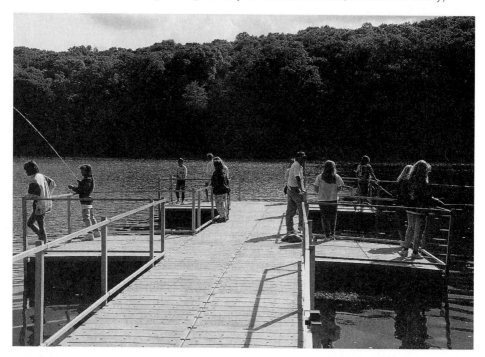

It is important that the walk or path blend with the pier so there is no difference in level between the two. The surface of the pier should have spaces of less than 1/2 in. between the planks. Around the bottom edge of the pier, there should be a kick plate to keep foot pedals of wheelchairs from slipping off the pier. Handrails or armrests and bait shelves should be provided. Probably the best design is to build an armrest about 36 in. high with a slope of approximately 30°. This board can be used by those fishing to rest their arms and fishing poles. An 8 in. to 12 in. bait shelf about 30 in. from the surface of the pier offers a place for fishing gear. If children are the principal users of the pier, then slightly reduced heights would be appropriate for the armrest and bait shelf. Benches and some type of shaded seating area are other features that may enhance fishing piers.

Boat Docks. As with fishing piers, access to boat docks should be over hard surface walks or paths, and there should be no difference in level between the dock and the walk or path. Again, as in the case of the fishing pier, spaces between planks should be no wider than 1/2 in. Handrails may be constructed around the edge of the dock where they do not restrict access to boats.

Playfields with Seating Areas

Ticket Booths. At least one ticket booth must be accessible although it is desirable to have more. The front of the booth needs to have a level surface area of 30 in. by 48 in. The ticket window or counter must not be higher than 36 in. above the surface in order to accommodate persons in wheelchairs. The counter should be 36 in. wide.

Seating Areas. The number of wheelchair spaces that need to be provided depends on the seating capacity of the facility. One space is required for a capacity of 4 to 25. Two spaces are required for 26 to 50, four for 51 to 300, six for 301 to 500, and six plus one per 100 additional seats for more than 500. Spaces provided for wheelchair users cannot be segregated and wheelchair seating must be provided at each seat pricing level. The size of the space depends on approachability. If the user can pull forward into the space, the space needs to be 33 in. by 48 in. If maneuvering from the side is necessary, then a space of 33 in. by 60 in. is required. A companion seat must be made available next to the wheelchair space.

Recreation Buildings

This section covers accessibility information about recreation buildings. Both exterior and interior design elements are discussed.

Exterior Circulation and Entrances. Designated parking spaces need to be located as near as is practical to the accessible entrance of each recreation facility. The guidelines on parking noted earlier in the chapter provide more exact information on design features for parking areas.

Ideally, the approach to the entrance of the building will not be on a slope, or any slope will be minimum. The suggested guidelines for walks presented earlier in this chapter may be applied when designing walks leading to buildings. Chief among design considerations for walks are their grade, width, and surface.

All major entrances to recreation buildings should be made accessible to avoid having persons with disabilities use the back door, service entrance, or other similar entrance. Involved in this principle is not only respect for individuals with disabilities but the need for all persons to have access to major exits in cases of emergency.

The surface directly in front of entrances should be level or have only a very slight slope (no more than 2%). When an automatic door is not provided, adequate space should be allowed on either side of the door to permit wheelchair users to easily open the door. Manual doors should be equipped with handles that do not require grasping or a twisting motion of the wrist. The door should have a width of at least 32 in. and should have a threshold of no more than 1/2 in. to allow wheelchair access. The pressure required to open the door should never exceed 15 lb for exterior doors and is preferably much less than this maximum. Revolving doors are not practical, because they cannot be used by people in wheelchairs.

Ramps. Both exterior and interior ramps may be used in recreation buildings. Any walk or path may be designated a ramp if it has a slope of 5% or more. While curb ramps may be slightly steeper, other ramps should not exceed a slope of 8.33% (1:12 ratio) with a slope of 5% preferred (1:20 ratio). Handrails on both sides are a necessity on practically all ramps (except curb ramps) to protect people or to provide support. Normally, handrails on ramps are placed around 34 in. to 38 in. in height. However, if the building is often used by children, a second set of handrails 24 in. in height should be added. Handrails should extend 12 in. beyond both ends of the ramp.

The minimum width for ramps is 36 in., with 60 in. needed for ramps over which wheelchairs often pass. A level space at least 5 ft in length and as wide as the ramp should be provided at the approach and at the top of the ramp. Long ramps or ramps with turns should have level platforms to allow users to rest or to negotiate the turn. On long, straight-run ramps, a rest platform of 3 ft in length is recommended. Turning platforms are larger. The platform for a ramp with one 90° turn should be 4 ft deep by 5 ft long. For a switchback type of ramp, the turning platform needs to be at least 8 ft deep and 5 ft wide.

Stairs. Stairs and elevators should be provided in addition to ramps because some persons have difficulty using ramps. Persons wearing leg braces and others may trip if the nosing of stair steps is squared; therefore, a smooth nosing on steps is recommended. As with ramps, handrails should be installed on both sides of the stairs. The handrails (between 1 1/4 in. and 1 1/2 in. in diameter) should be placed about 34 in. to 38 in. above the stair nosings and should extend 12 in. beyond both the top step and the bottom step. A second set of handrails should be provided in recreation facilities that serve children. These should be placed 24 in. above the surface of the steps.

Tactile warning devices can be used as cueing aids for persons with visual impairments to alert them of stairs. For example, in buildings with carpeting or vinyl tiles, rubber tiles can be laid at the top of stairs to offer a surface tactile warning signal. It is important that tactile warning signals remain consistent throughout the entire building. Finally, adequate lighting on stairs is necessary to allow users to detect the step nosing.

Elevators. Elevators should be placed in an area close to the main entrance of the building and in the normal path of travel of building users. The elevator call buttons should be located so wheelchair users can reach them. It is recommended that the center of the button panel be 40 in. from the floor. Raised numbers can be placed on the button panel to identify the floor. These numbers should be raised a minimum of 1/32 in. from the surface and be at least 1/2 in. high. They should have clearly defined edges. To be easily seen, the numbers should contrast in color with the background on which they are placed. Brailled characters should also identify buttons.

Visual and audible cueing devices should be used to indicate the direction of an approaching elevator car. Visual signals can be given by installing arrow-shaped direction indicators. The up indicator arrow should be white and the down arrow red. Audible cues can be given by signals that sound once for up cars and twice for down cars.

The inside of the elevator car must be large enough to accommodate at least one person in a wheelchair and allow this individual to move to a position from which he or she can operate the elevator controls. The controls need to be located so that the highest button is no more than 54 in. from the floor of the elevator. Emergency controls should be located below the standard controls so that they are accessible to wheelchair users. Also inside the car should be handrails mounted on the side walls (and preferably rear wall) at a height of 30 in. to 32 in. from the floor of the elevator.

It is of course necessary that all elevators be adjusted so that, when stopped, the floor of the car is level with the building floor. Elevator doors should have safety edges and door-opening sensing devices to prevent the door from closing and injuring someone entering or leaving the car.

Transient Lodging. Newly constructed or remodeled transient lodging units must provide for the needs of people with disabilities. Ideally, all resort, lodge, or cabin bedrooms will be made accessible to persons who have physical disabilities. If this is not possible, then a certain percentage of rooms should accommodate individuals who have disabilities. ADA standards call for one accessible room per 25 total rooms, up to 100 (e.g., three accessible rooms per 75 total rooms). Five accessible rooms are required for 101 to 150 rooms, six for 151 to 200, seven for 201 to 300, eight for 301 to 400 and nine for 401 to 500. For establishments with 501 to 1,000 rooms, 2% of the total number of rooms are required to be accessible, and in those with more than 1,001 rooms, there must be 20 accessible rooms, plus one for each 100 over 1,000.

Hallways and corridors should be a least 44 in. wide if occupancy exceeds 50 people and 36 in. wide if occupancy is 50 or fewer. All doors should have a minimum width of 32 in. Within the rooms, floor space should be large enough to permit furniture to be placed with adequate space (approximately 5 ft) for wheelchair users to move about. The floor should be unwaxed. If carpeting is used, it should be low-pile, wall-to-wall carpet so that wheelchairs can move easily on it.

It is important that essential elements are of the proper height. The top of the mattress on the beds should be approximately the same height as the seat of the wheelchair to allow for ease in transferring. Controls such as light switches and thermostats should be placed within reach of wheelchair users, at a maximum of 4 ft from the floor. Windows should be easy to open and close by persons in wheelchairs. Ideally, windows will be placed low enough so people who use wheelchairs may be able to see the out-of-doors from them.

Closets and other clothing-storage facilities should be designed with wheelchair users in mind. Closets should allow ease in entry and should have hanging rods within comfortable reach. Spring-close or self-closing drawers should be avoided.

Many of the suggestions in the next section on rest rooms can be applied to bathrooms for bedroom units. Of course, the floor space of individual bathrooms for bedroom units will be much smaller than for public rest rooms. Therefore it is important to design individual bathrooms so that those in wheelchairs can close the door for privacy and have sufficient room to move about.

Cabin at Bradford Woods, home of Camp Riley for campers with disabilities. (Photo courtesy of Bradford Woods, Indiana University)

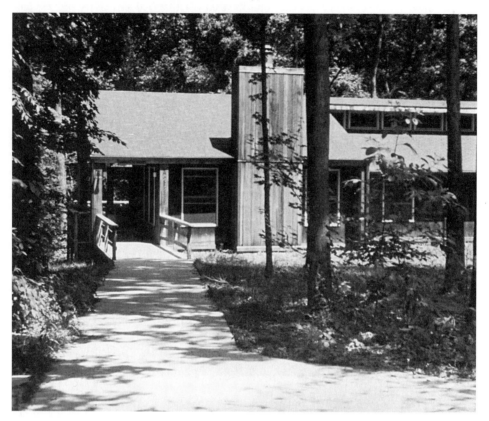

Rest Rooms. Within any given park and recreation area, it is important to have at least one public rest room for each sex that accommodates persons with disabilities. Accessible rest rooms should be identified by a 12 in. gender symbol centered 60 in. above the floor and raised 1/4 in. from the door surface. The international symbol of accessibility should also be displayed if not all rest rooms in a facility are accessible.

Rest room entry corridors must be 44 in. wide, or 48 in. wide if wheelchair users are required to turn around an obstruction to enter. Inside the rest room, a minimum of 5 ft by 5 ft of clear floor space must be provided so that wheelchair users can have sufficient turning space. There must be at least 44 in. between all fixed elements in the rest room to allow wheelchairs to move through the room.

At least one accessible toilet stall should exist in each rest room. There must be 48 in. of clear space outside the stall door. Doors must open outward and have an opening of

32 in. if the stall is entered from the front and 34 in. if the stall is entered from the side. In the stall, there must be 18 in. from one wall to the centerline of the toilet and 32 in. between the wall and the edge of the toilet on the other side. The overall width of the stall must be at least 60 in. There must be 48 in. between the front of the toilet and the door (or opposite wall for side-entry stalls). The toilet seat should be 17 in. to 19 in. from the floor to allow ease in transferring.

Grab bars must be placed 33 in. above the floor. On a tank-type toilet, they may be 36 in. above the floor. The rear grab bar needs to be at least 36 in. long, while the side grab bar must be at least 42 in. long. An outside diameter of 1 1/4 in. to 1 1/2 in. is required for grab bars, which should be exactly 1 1/2 in. from the wall. Grab bars should support at least 250 lb.

Men's rest rooms should have at least one wall-mounted urinal. Accessible urinals should be placed with the basin lip not more than 17 in. from the floor and the rim projecting at least 14 in. from the wall.

The lavatory should be mounted to provide a 29 in. clearance from the floor, with a maximum height to the top of the rim of 34 in. All pipes under the lavatory should be covered or insulated to protect wheelchair users from burning themselves. This is particularly important for protecting those without sensation in their legs.

Towel racks, towel dispensers, hand dryers, and other such devices should be placed so that they are easily accessible to wheelchair users. These should be placed no higher than 40 in. from the floor.

Showers are sometimes found in rest rooms or locker rooms in recreation facilities. If showers are provided, they should accommodate persons who have disabilities. Shower stalls equipped for individuals with disabilities should not have thresholds (or only slight thresholds) and should have nonslip surfaces. On each shower stall, a hinged seat should be mounted 33 in. to 36 in. from the floor so that it can be folded out during shower use. Grab rails are a necessity and should be placed at a height of approximately 18 in. Water control levers should allow for ease in gripping and, along with the soap tray, should be placed between 38 in. and 48 in. from the floor. The provision of a hand-held diversionary showerhead with a flexible hose allows those seated to shower more easily.

Concluding Statement on the Design of Parks and Outdoor Recreation Areas

Many sources of information on design considerations for people with disabilities are available to parks and recreation professionals. No matter what the source of information, it is important to consider *all* parts of the facility, since these must flow together to ensure that the area is truly accessible. Table 6.1 provides a checklist that may be used to determine the accessibility of park and recreation facilities.

Within this chapter and Table 6.1, an attempt has been made to stipulate ADA accessibility guidelines from the *Federal Register* (Vol. 56, No. 144, July 26, 1991). Readers

Table 6.1 Checklist for Accessibility of Park and Recreation Facilities

Signage

1. Is the international symbol of accessibility displayed at the entrance?
2. Is the international symbol of accessibility displayed at various points within the facility to inform persons of accessibility?
3. Are parking spaces designated for use by persons with disabilities marked with the symbol of accessibility?
4. Do diagrams or maps provide the symbol of accessibility to indicate accessible buildings or areas?
5. Are signs located at eye level (43 in. to 51 in.) for wheelchair users?
6. Are signs made with light-colored characters or symbols on dark backgrounds?
7. Do identification signs for rooms (including rest rooms) have raised characters at least 5/8 in. in height but no greater than 2 in.?
8. Are signs placed near the closest approach?
9. Are signs well lighted, if used at night?
10. If used, are exhibit labels large enough to read?

Parking

1. Is a loading zone 20 ft long available, with a 60 in. area parallel to the auto allowing the car door to open fully?
2. Is the loading zone separated from the walk by a curb, bollards, or similar objects?
3. Is there a curb ramp if a curb is next to the loading area?
4. Are accessible van spaces 9 ft wide and 18 ft long with 96 in. access aisles?
5. Are car spaces 8 ft wide and 18 ft long with 60 in. access aisles?
6. Do spaces have provisions to keep cars from overhanging walks?
7. If a curb exists, is there a curb ramp?
8. Are curb ramps no more than 8.33% grade?
9. Are curb ramps made to contrast both in color and texture with the walk surface?
10. Are adequate numbers of spaces provided for persons with disabilities?

Walks and Trails

1. Are walks that join parking lots and streets made to meet the level of the other surfaces?
2. Are walks at least 48 in. wide?
3. Are walk gradients 5% or less?
4. Do walks approaching the maximum grade, or those unusually long, have rest areas? Are surfaces in front of the rest areas textured differently than the walks?
5. Do walks have nonslip surfaces?
6. Do trails reflect a wide range of user preferences and abilities?
7. Are trails clearly marked for length and degree of difficulty?
8. Are overhanging tree branches on trails cut?
9. Are textural changes used on hard surface trails to indicate interpretations or rest areas?

Table 6.1 *(Continued)*

Picnic Areas

1. Are picnic tables designed to accommodate wheelchair users (with a minimum of 27 in. to the ground and 19 in. from the end of the table to the undersupport)?
2. Do paths lead to some of the picnic tables? Grills?
3. Are grills approximately 30 in. in height?
4. Do benches have sitting heights of 18 in. to 20 in. and widths of no more than 18 in.? Are backrests and arm supports included?
5. Is there adequate space around benches so that wheelchair users may sit beside someone seated on the bench?
6. Are drinking fountains set in paved areas? Do they stand 34 in. to 36 in. from the ground for adults? 30 in. for children?

Telephones

1. Is a push-button public telephone available? Is it located on a hard surface?
2. Is the entrance to the phone at least 30 in. wide?
3. Is the highest operable part of the telephone no more than 54 in. from the surface?
4. Are telephones equipped for persons with hearing impairments?

Water-Related Areas

1. Are pathways provided on beaches through the sand to the water?
2. Are paths sloped no more than 8.33%?
3. Is the pool designed to allow persons to enter the water by means of a ramp? Steps? Portable device with steps placed on the deck? Hydraulic lift?
4. Are fishing piers made accessible by providing a path to them?
5. Do the surfaces of docks and piers have spaces of less than 1/2 in. between planks?
6. Is there a kick plate at the bottom edge of fishing piers? Are handrails provided?

Buildings and Ramps

1. Are designated parking spaces for persons with disabilities located near the entrance?
2. Are all major entrances accessible?
3. Are surfaces in front of entrances level or have only a very small slope?
4. Are entry doors at least 32 in. wide with a threshold of no more than 1/2 in.?
5. Are manual doors equipped with proper handles?
6. Are doors relatively easy to pull open?
7. Are ramps on a slope of 8.33% or less?
8. Are there proper handrails on ramps?
9. Are ramps at least 36 in. wide? Do they have nonslip surfaces?
10. Are level spaces (5 ft in length or more) provided at the approach and at the top of the ramps?

Table 6.1 *(Continued)*

Stairs and Elevators

1. Are stairs and elevators provided in addition to ramps?
2. Do stair steps have smooth nosing?
3. Are handrails on both sides of the stairs?
4. Are handrails 34 in. to 38 in. from the surface of each step? Do they extend 12 in. beyond both the top step and the bottom step?
5. Are tactile warning cues provided to alert persons with visual impairments to stairs?
6. If the building serves children, are handrails provided 24 in. from the surface of each step?
7. Are stairs adequately lighted?
8. Are elevators placed near the main entrance?
9. Are elevator cars large enough to accommodate at least one person in a wheelchair and to allow that person to move to a position to operate the controls?
10. Are elevator buttons easily accessible to wheelchair users?
11. Are raised numbers placed on the button panel?
12. Are visual and auditory cueing devices used to indicate the direction of approaching elevator cars?

Transient Lodging

1. Do doors have a clear opening of at least 32 in.?
2. Are hallways and corridors at least 36 in. wide?
3. Does floor space in rooms permit wheelchair users to move freely around furniture?
4. Do floors have nonslip surfaces? If carpeting is used, is it low-pile, wall-to-wall carpet?
5. Are light switches and other controls within reach of wheelchair users (a maximum of 4 ft from the floor)?
6. Are bed mattresses approximately the same height as the seats of the wheelchair users who usually occupy the room (i.e., children or adults)?
7. Do closets allow use by wheelchair users?

Rest Rooms

1. Is there at least one rest room for each sex that accommodates persons with physical disabilities?
2. Can wheelchair users easily enter the rest rooms?
3. Is there a minimum of 5 ft × 5 ft of clear floor space to provide turning space for wheelchair users?
4. Are toilet stalls at least 60 in. wide? Equipped with doors at least 32 in. wide that open outward? Equipped with grab bars approximately 33 in. high and 42 in. long with an outside diameter of 1 1/4 in. to 1 1/2 in.?
5. Is the seat in toilet stalls 17 in. to 19 in. from the floor and designed for persons with disabilities?

Table 6.1 *(Continued)*

6. Does the men's rest room have at least one wall-mounted urinal with a basin lip of not more than 17 in. projecting at least 14 in. from the wall?

7. Is the lavatory mounted to provide 29 in. clearance from the floor with a maximum height to the top of the rim of 34 in.?

8. Are drain pipes and hot water pipes covered or insulated?

9. Are mirrors, towel racks, dispensers, hand dryers, and other such equipment placed so they are easily accessible to wheelchair users, no more than 40 in. from the floor?

10. Do showers, if provided, accommodate persons with physical disabilities by having no thresholds (or very slight thresholds)? Nonslip surfaces? A hinged seat, mounted 18 in. from the floor? Grab rails at 33 in. to 36 in.? Control levers between 38 in. and 48 in. from the floor?

---

may wish to refer to publications such as McGovern (1992) or Goltsman, Gilbert, and Wohlford (1993b) for further details on ADA standards. The U.S. Architectural and Transportation Barriers Compliance Board (Access Board) is to publish ADA guidelines specifically for amusement parks, boating and marine facilities, golf facilities, playgrounds, sports facilities, and outdoor developed facilities (such as ski areas and campgrounds). The Access Board may be contacted at 1331 F Street NW, Washington, DC 20004-1111 (Greenwell, 1993). The National Center on Accessibility (NCA) offers the latest information regarding accessibility. NCA is located at Bradford Woods, 5040 State Road 67 North, Martinsville, IN 46151.

Although the design of facilities to meet the needs of children has been mentioned several times, the central focus of this chapter has been on adults. If children are the primary users of a facility, their needs should be given a great amount of consideration. Those planning facilities for children should remain ever conscious of the need to accommodate children with disabling conditions. One of the primary play areas of children is the playground. The final portion of this chapter deals with the design of playgrounds to accommodate the child who has a disability.

PLAYGROUNDS

Through play, children develop intellectually, emotionally, and motorically. As stated in *The Universal Playground: A Planning Guide* (1990), "Play is an essential activity for all children. It is one way children explore their world" (p. 9). Stout (1988) has written this about playgrounds for children with disabilities: "A safe, accessible, and challenging playground encourages social interaction and physical and mental exercise. All children have the right of access to appropriate play opportunities" (p. 653).

Gordon (1972) has observed a tendency for many infants and children with disabling conditions to be passive and to display a superficiality in relating to people and objects.

Frost and Klein (1979) have suggested that children who have disabilities may have difficulties in the following skills: "Extent of exploration; initiation of activities; response and approach to others; attention to people, materials, and tasks; acceptance of limits and routines; respect for rights of others; seeing self as able to do and achieve" (p. 219). Obviously, infants and children displaying such behaviors have not had the experiences required to allow them to develop the competencies to interact with confidence with other persons or with the physical environment. Sadly, as Smith (1989) has noted:

> It appears that our nation's community playgrounds offer few architecturally barrier-free play opportunities to children with disabilities. Only 14 percent of the play equipment surveyed was designed for use by a child in a wheelchair, and only 16 percent of the play equipment provided for wheelchair accessibility up to the equipment. The latter is particularly disturbing because a child who uses a wheelchair might be able to transfer onto and use a conventional play structure, *providing* he or she could position the chair adjacent to the equipment. (p. 88)

As a result of this situation, it appears that most of the children with disabilities in the United States have been deprived of the opportunity to experience play environments that encourage the realization of natural developmental outcomes. This is not to say, however, that special playgrounds must be designed for the exclusive use of children with disabling conditions. One of the most important concepts to remember about children with disabilities is that they are, first and foremost, children. Most children with special needs have one or perhaps two disabilities and are average or above average in most areas of ability. Also, by constructing playgrounds to serve all children, children both with and without disabilities can gain experiences playing with children possessing different characteristics. Such exposures have the potential to broaden the understanding of all children regarding individual differences (Schleien, 1993). In addition, among the many positive outcomes of such integrated play experiences are appropriate responses to peer aggression, increased social and cognitive skills, and improved communication skills for children who have disabilities (Odom, Strain, Karger, & Smith, 1986). Finally, fundamental economic reasoning dictates that a single playground would be less expensive than two playgrounds. From all perspectives, it seems to make little sense to build community playgrounds for the use of any single group. Therefore, as a general principle, playgrounds should be designed so they are usable by *all* children.

The Inadequacy of Traditional American Playgrounds

Traditional American playgrounds were seemingly designed to serve two primary purposes. Apparently, the major reason for the establishment of playgrounds was to provide gross motor activities. The slides, swings, merry-go-rounds, seesaws, and monkey bars of the traditional playground certainly do not encourage types of play other than motor behaviors.

This playground design offers safety, novelty, challenge, and accessibility to users. (Preschool developmental play center designed by Dr. Louis Bowers, University of South Florida; Photo by David R. Austin)

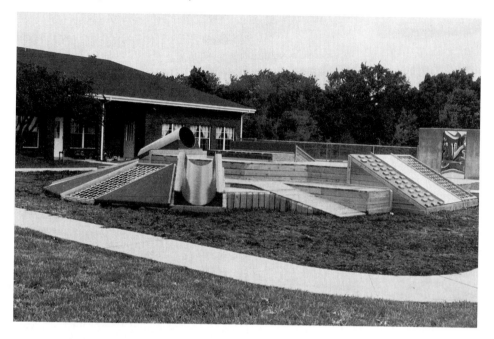

The second major purpose of the design was evidently to allow ease of maintenance. This was commonly done by having all apparatus made of steel and usually placing this equipment in a sea of asphalt. Traditional American playgrounds, to say the least, were unimaginative in design and built with the needs of the maintenance crews ever in mind.

What Should Playgrounds Be Like?

Unquestionably those responsible for traditional American playgrounds failed to provide well-designed play areas for our children. But what should playgrounds be like? A number of authors have attempted to answer this question (e.g., Bruya & Langendorfer, 1988; Harrison, 1993; Thompson & Bowers, 1989). Most of these authors have given consideration to the needs of children with disabilities in their writings. Still other authors (e.g., Austin, 1978; Beckwith, 1985; Grosse, 1980; and Stout, 1988) have published works that have focused specifically on designing playgrounds that meet the needs of children with disabilities.

In reviewing this body of literature, four broad areas of concern emerge. These are (1) accessibility, (2) health and safety considerations, (3) the provision of an interesting and challenging environment, and (4) the need for variety. The sections that follow review these four areas.

Accessibility

Children who use wheelchairs, children using crutches or other mobility aids, and children with braces are regularly denied play experiences because play areas have not been made accessible (Grosse, 1980). To be sure, accessibility is a primary issue in the design of community playgrounds.

A number of design features can be employed to make an outside play area accessible. The following recommendations for increasing accessibility have been primarily drawn from *The Accessibility Checklist* (Goltsman, Gilbert, & Wohlford, 1993a).

Hard Surface Paths. Hard surface paths should allow entry to the play area and then wind their way throughout the playground so that a child can reach any piece of apparatus by use of the path. Paths need to be slip-resistant surfaces (e.g., brushed concrete) free of level changes caused by tree roots, cracks, or expansion joints. Abrupt changes in level should not exceed 1/4 in., with gradual changes of 1/2 in. permissible if they are beveled with a slope of not more than 1:2. Paths should be wide enough to permit two wheelchairs to pass (88 in.). Gentle curves, not sharp angles, should be used in laying out the path system. Steep slopes should be avoided. Paths should not exceed a grade of 5% (1:20), with slopes of 3% or 4% preferred. Cross slopes should not exceed 1:50. Finally, space close to each piece of apparatus should be provided so that children can park their wheelchairs or leave crutches or walkers to give them the freedom to crawl or use the apparatus for support while exploring the play environment.

Ramps. Ramps (44 in. wide) can make playgrounds accessible by first permitting access to the play area and then allowing children access to play apparatus. A slope of not more than 1:16 is recommended for all ramps. The cross slope should not exceed 1:50. Ramps are well suited to replace stairs or ladders. For example, a ramp can provide access to a slide. Freestanding ramps need to be designed to prevent the child from accidentally slipping off the edge. This may be done by means of two railings—one at the bottom edge of the ramp and a second, higher one that may be used as a handrail. Or, walls may be constructed on the ramps and handrails attached to the walls. Two sets of handrails at two different heights will enable children of various sizes to negotiate the ramp. The highest handrail should be 24 in. from the floor of the ramp. In general, ramps should blend into the playground rather than being obtrusive signs that the site was developed for persons with mobility impairments (Harrison, 1993).

Railings. Railings can be used to enable children to move about the playground more easily. Children with balance problems can use the equipment by supporting themselves with the railings. Children who have visual impairments can employ the railings to guide their movements. The use of bright paint on the rails can serve as visual cues for children who are partially sighted. Of course, it is important to make the railings the proper height to accommodate the children using them. The diameter of the railing is also important. For children with mobility limitations, a railing of 3/4 in. to 1 1/2 in. has been recommended by *The Accessibility Checklist* (Goltsman et al., 1993a). Another source (*A Playground for all Children*, 1978) has suggested that handrails should have a diameter of no more than 3/4 in. to allow ease in use by amputees with hooks.

Elevated Areas. Elevated areas can be constructed to allow children in wheelchairs to engage in sand and water play or to complete gardening projects. Freestanding sand and water tables, which accommodate children who use wheelchairs, can be purchased or constructed. Their trays should not be more than 30 in. above the ground, with at least 24 in. between the underside of the table and the ground and 19 in. of knee space. For sand play, a mound can be covered with sand. A small wall can be constructed to surround the cutout area (an indentation cut into the mound). It is important that the cutout area be the correct height (approximately 30 in.) for allowing the child to easily reach the sand. Garden boxes can be built of railroad ties, which can be stacked to form boxes and filled with soil. Again, proper height is important. The child who uses a wheelchair should be able to reach the soil from his or her wheelchair or by transferring from the wheelchair to sit on the top rail. Most designers believe that children should be afforded the option to leave their wheelchairs whenever they desire. Therefore, it is probably best not to overdesign playgrounds by building too many elevated areas, because this may discourage children from leaving their wheelchairs.

Transfer Platforms and Handholds. Children in wheelchairs may access equipment by means of transfer platforms. There needs to be a clear space (60 in. × 60 in.) on one side of the platform to allow the child to transfer. The platform itself should be at least 24 in. × 24 in. in size at a height of approximately 15 in. to 17 in. from the ground. Handholds should be mounted on the apparatus approximately 25 in. to 27 in. from the ground to help the child transfer from the chair to the platform. Handholds or grab bars should also be provided at each level change on the play structure itself. Every piece of equipment does not have to have a platform and handholds but an effort should be made to allow access to each type of play apparatus on the playground.

Health and Safety Considerations

A recent nationwide survey of playground equipment in U.S. community parks (Thompson & Bowers, 1989) documented a myriad of health and safety problems. Analyzing the results of this survey, Smith (1989) has listed many *significant* problems that reveal that "our nation's playgrounds may simply be too unsafe for use by the people for whom they were built—children" (p. 85). A few common-sense measures, however, can help ensure a safe and healthy play environment that challenges children without posing undue risks. Several recommendations follow under the headings of general considerations, surfacing, and apparatus. Primary sources for this section are Gordon (1972), Frost and Klein (1979), *A Guide to Designing Accessible Outdoor Recreation Facilities* (1980) produced by the U.S. Department of Interior, and Thompson and Bowers (1989).

General Considerations. One often-neglected element on playgrounds is seating for adults who accompany children to the play area and who wish to have a comfortable vantage point from which to view the child at play (Thompson & Bowers, 1989). Benches should, if possible, be in a shaded area. Protection from the sun should also be provided for the children. Trees or shelters may be used for this purpose. For some, a shaded area is a desirable convenience. For others it is essential. Children taking certain medications may need to avoid exposure to the sun to prevent nausea, severe sunburns, or other harmful reactions. Those who do not perspire normally must have shade to avoid becoming overheated. Other children who lack skin sensitivity may be burned by contact with metal parts on apparatus that have become hot from exposure to the sun (Pittsburgh Architects Workshop, 1979). Another general consideration is to provide accessible rest rooms and drinking fountains a short distance from the playground. Easy access to water is imperative for some persons with physical disabilities who require regular fluid intake (R. W. Smith, personal communication, November 11, 1981). Finally, a fence with gates (32 in. to 48 in. wide) that can be locked should be provided around playgrounds adjacent to a street or those used primarily by young children.

Surfacing. Children occasionally fall from apparatus. Therefore, falls should be anticipated and prepared for when installing surfaces. While hard surfaces such as asphalt and cement are desirable from a maintenance perspective, these surfaces are not desirable from a safety standpoint. Grass is a most desirable surface for open areas of the playground, but resilient surfaces are needed under all equipment. A protective surface must be installed under equipment where falls would be anticipated. Materials such as rubber padding and astroturf can be used to form a protective surface (Goltsman et al., 1993a).

Apparatus. One basic playground safety principle is that all apparatus should have rounded edges. All rough or jagged edges need to be smoothed off when equipment is put in place, and regular maintenance checks need to be made to ensure that the edges remain safe.

Another basic principle is to avoid the use of hard, wooden seats on swings. Flexible rubber seats provide a better alternative for traditional swings. Safety belts may be installed for swings adapted for use by children with disabilities. For children with strength limitations, those who have amputations or paralysis, and others who can benefit from the stabilization provided, safety belts (along with back supports and leg supports) are useful additions to swings. In fact, safety belts can be used not only on swings but on seesaws and other pieces of apparatus where children are seated (Pittsburgh Architects Workshop, 1979).

Stabilization is a critical factor to consider in designing equipment for children with disabilities. There is a noticeable absence of support devices on many traditional pieces of playground equipment. Swings, seesaws, spring animals, and similar pieces require a

Play and exercise equipment often needs modification for safety and visibility. For example, a webbed traverse can be modified by placing a mat over the webbing. (Photo courtesy of Bradford Woods, Indiana University)

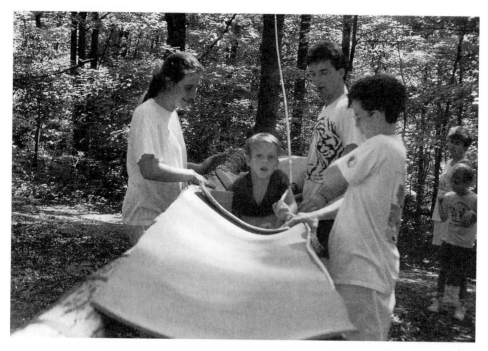

great deal of balance and control; the lack of some type of device to provide back and leg support makes their use quite difficult for many children who have conditions. Therefore, to allow these children safe access to this equipment, alterations need to be made (Pittsburgh Architects Workshop, 1979). Specific guidelines for making adaptations for swings, seesaws, and merry-go-rounds are provided later in this chapter.

It is important that *everyone* be able to move safely about the play area. Swings and other rapidly moving equipment should have barriers strategically placed to protect all passersby, but especially those with visual limitations. Currently, only 11% of community playgrounds in the United States have such barriers (Thompson & Bowers, 1989). To enable children with strength or mobility limitations to move safely, handholds and handrails should be installed where appropriate. Of course, handrails are essential to ramped areas and steps. Here it may be desirable to provide two sets of handrails to accommodate children of various sizes.

A final area of concern is that of height. A great deal of analysis should go into the selection of equipment and its installation to be sure it is a safe height for the user. Smaller children naturally need smaller apparatus. Other design concepts, such as building slides into hillsides or using climbing ropes or platforms set on one another to allow children access to a slide, not only eliminate the need for a ladder but reduce the danger of having a child fall from a high place.

The Provision of an Interesting and Challenging Environment

Besides being unsafe to varying degrees, most community parks in the United States feature play structures that are "dominated by traditional pieces of equipment that offer children limited opportunities for social interaction, creative expression, and fine motor development" (Smith, 1989, p. 85). There are, however, several concepts that could be used to provide interesting, challenging, and developmentally sound playgrounds for *all* children. The concepts that follow are based largely on the work of Frost and Klein (1979) and Moore and the University of Wisconsin-Milwaukee group (Moore, Cohen, Oerbel, & van Ryzin, 1979).

Multiple Skill Level. The play environment should provide for multiple levels of skill so that the child is challenged without unreasonable demands being made on his or her abilities. Ideally, there is just enough challenge to stimulate the child to try the next skill level. Therefore, it is important to provide graded levels of complexity on the playground. For example, there may be several ways to reach the top of a slide, each of which may be slightly more challenging to the child. These might range from a ramp to platforms to climbing a cargo net. Such alternatives also provide clear points of accomplishment so the child will realize he or she has succeeded at the task. All children, and particularly children with disabilities, need successes to build positive self-concepts.

Opportunities for Sensory Stimulation. Children need opportunities for all sorts of sensory stimulation. Playgrounds should offer a wide variety of sensory experiences including things to feel, smell, see, and hear (Hart, 1989). For example, surfaces can be made to have different textures so that children with visual impairments can learn to discriminate between types of surfaces. Flowers and other plants can be grown to offer visual beauty as well as pleasing aromas. A variety of colors can be used on the playground, and some equipment may be designed so that children can manipulate it to produce sounds.

Soft Playthings Offer Emotional Release and a Sense of Control. Not all equipment must be of steel or wood. A soft play environment made of foam rubber covered with a variety of colored fabrics can offer new experiences to children. In such an environment, children can release tensions and emotions without harming themselves. Designers of the New York University Medical Center playground (Gordon, 1972) used pits made of covered foam rubber so that children with severely limited mobility could express themselves through motion by moving their bodies on the soft, giving surface. An alternative to foam rubber is an air-filled apparatus.

Equipment Placement to Facilitate Continuous Play. Play should be allowed to flow naturally from one activity to another. In the placement of equipment, consideration should be given to possible alternative play behaviors once a particular activity ends. The

An interesting preschool playground at Flower Mound, New Town, in Texas. (Photo by David R. Austin)

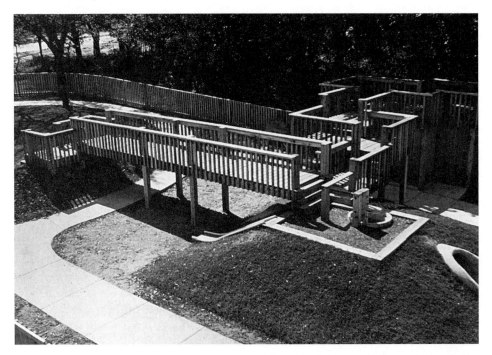

child should be given several alternatives from which to choose his or her next play activity. For example, are opportunities other than returning for more sliding available at the bottom of the slide? Play patterns can grow and expand if adequate environmental cues are provided to the child. On the other hand, overstimulation at decision points must be avoided for those children not yet ready to tolerate dealing with too many stimuli.

The Need for Variety

Closely related to the need for an interesting and challenging environment is the necessity for variety in play environments. The content for this section, like the one that preceded it, has been drawn primarily from the works of Frost and Klein (1979) and Moore and his colleagues (1979).

Broad Range of Areas and Equipment. The playground should provide for almost any imaginable type of play in which children normally engage. Children certainly need equipment that allows for gross motor activity. But children also require places for play involving organized games, drama, building things, growing plants, and other activities. Defined boundaries should set apart the more active areas from other areas of the playground.

One means of zoning the playground is by building waist-high railings throughout the play area. Such a railing system also serves as a guide for visually impaired children and enables children with braces, crutches, canes, and walkers to stabilize themselves as they move about the playground (Pittsburgh Architects Workshop, 1979).

Equipment Offering a Variety of Uses. Some equipment defines its own use, since it has a singular purpose. Swings are for swinging and slides are for sliding. This equipment is generally not as useful as equipment that serves multiple functions. The playground designer should analyze each piece of apparatus to see if it provides for a variety of uses. For example, many different spatial experiences might be gained by a piece of apparatus that allows the child to crawl or climb under it, on it, through it, beside it, across it, above it, and around it. Ambiguous objects such as wooden climbing structures or rocks allow children to be creative and to use their imaginations.

Manipulation of Loose Parts. Closely related to the principle of offering a variety of uses is the idea of providing loose parts that the child can manipulate in a number of ways. Moore and his colleagues (1979) classify loose parts into three categories: (1) manufactured objects that are to be made into a specific end product (e.g., a puzzle), (2) things that are manufactured but have a variable finished form (e.g., Tinker Toys), and (3) things found in the natural environment (e.g., old tires, boards, sand) that can be used in any variety of ways. The use of loose parts allows the child to have some control over his or her environment—to change it or to manipulate it. Adventure playgrounds are made up entirely of loose parts such as lumber, bricks, cardboard boxes, and old tires from which the children build whatever they desire. Moore and his colleagues (1979) state that the use of loose parts (including adventure playgrounds) has been successfully employed with children who have mental and physical disabilities. Furthermore, Roger Hart (1989), an internationally recognized expert on innovative design of children's play environments, has noted that *creating* playhouses and other play structures appears to be more important to children than playing in them once they are made.

Places and Spaces. Children need a variety of places to accommodate different types of play. Open spaces are required for group play and games. Other places should be provided for play by a single child or a small group of children. While children require opportunities for group play, they also need places where they can gain privacy on the playground. Some small spaces need to be provided for solitary play or for just escaping. Small group play may be facilitated by designing areas where two to four children can play together. Sand and water areas or playhouses may be designed for this purpose.

ADAPTING EXISTING EQUIPMENT

One means to begin ensuring adequate play areas for children with disabilities is to modify equipment on existing playgrounds. Specific suggestions have been offered by the Pittsburgh Architects Workshop (1979) on how to adapt traditional playground apparatus to make them usable by children with disabling conditions. The material that follows is based on the work of Pittsburgh Architects Workshop.

Slides

A soft ground surface may limit access to both conventional and timber slides. An initial improvement would be to provide a hard surface path to a surface pad (with a 6 ft diameter) at the base of the steps or ramp leading to the top of the slide.

Conventional Slides. Steps on conventional metal slides are too steep and too narrow for the use of children who are semiambulatory. The original steps may be replaced by ones adjusted to 45° or less. These new steps should be 2 ft 6 in. to 3 ft wide with a depth of 4 in. to 6 in. The space between steps should preferably be 4 in. and no more than 6 in. In replacing existing handrails on steps, ones approximately 3/4 in. in diameter should be used. At the top of the steps, a platform 2 ft long (from front to back) and approximately 3 ft wide should be constructed to allow space for the child to prepare to go down the slide. The sliding board should be 2 ft 6 in. to 3 ft 6 in. in width, rather than the standard 1 ft 6 in. to 2 ft 6 in. size, to accommodate children who have disabilities. A soft landing surface (6 ft in diameter) should be provided at the bottom of the sliding board. Outside this landing area, a hard surface circulation path should be located for the use of semi-ambulatory children. Within the landing area, a short railing extending from either side of the bottom of the sliding board may be constructed to aid children with physical disabilities in getting up after coming off the end of the slide into the landing area. Finally, trees may be planted near the slide to provide shade to keep the sliding surface relatively cool on hot summer days.

Timber Slides. Pipes are often placed on timber slides to be used as climbers to reach the platform. Since this access would be difficult for many children with disabilities, alternatives may need to be employed to allow access to this apparatus. One means is to use either telephone poles or railroad ties cut at various lengths and placed on end to form stairs up the platform. Handholds may be placed on the support posts of the apparatus for use by children in gaining stability and pulling themselves up the stairs. Another alternative is to construct a ramp at least 4 ft wide. As with any ramp, handrails should be placed on either side to facilitate movement by the children. Rubber coverings can be used on handrails and on the tops of support posts to cushion falls. On the platform, an elevated box can be constructed to allow children a gradual transfer to the surface of the sliding board. It is recommended that the box be 2 ft long, 3 ft wide, and 1 ft to 1 ft 6 in. high. As with a conventional metal slide, the sliding board and landing areas should be made to accommodate the needs of children with disabilities. (See the prior section on conventional slides for details).

Seesaws

Another piece of traditional apparatus discussed by the Pittsburgh Architects Workshop (1979) is the seesaw. A basic improvement, as with the slides, is to allow access to the seesaw by means of a hard surface path.

To provide stability when the child is mounting the seesaw, a pipe or post device can be constructed on which the end of the seesaw can rest. A permanent installation of this device would require a seesaw that could be swung to the side so it can be placed on the stationary post for mounting and then be returned to its original position. An alternative to having a seesaw that rotates is to build a stabilizer post that can be moved once the child had mounted the seesaw.

Two things can be done to lessen the impact of the seesaw when it hits the ground. One is to provide a soft surface beneath the seesaw. The second is to add shock-absorbent padding at the ends of the seesaw. Various types of rubber padding (e.g., a piece of auto tire) may be attached to the bottom of the seesaw to absorb the shock.

Several adaptations can be made to the seat to better accommodate children with disabilities. The first is to make the seat wider (10 in. to 12 in.) so it is easier to straddle. A second is to add a back support to provide stability for children with balance problems. Another is to attach leg supports 1 ft 6 in. to 2 ft from the front of the seat. These supports, which extend about 8 in. from each side, should be curved up on their ends to keep the legs from falling off. Finally, the addition of safety belts allows a margin of safety for those children who experience difficulty with balance and stability.

Handles on conventional seesaws are 1 in. to 1 1/2 in. in diameter. As indicated earlier, this size is too large for many children with disabilities. To accommodate these children, a 3/4 in. piece of pipe can be bolted into the existing handle.

Swings

A hard surface path leading to a 6-ft-diameter concrete pad directly under the swing offers the child who uses a wheelchair the opportunity to transfer to the seat of the swing. The path should come into the pad at a 45° angle so that there is a soft landing area directly in front of the swing. The placement of an inverted U-shaped metal pipe (1 in. to 1 1/2 in. in diameter and 2 ft to 2 ft 6 in. in height) in the concrete pad would enable users to stabilize themselves while getting seated. This railing should be set in the pad 10 in. to 12 in. from the path of the swing. (Even though this clearance is recommended by the Pittsburgh Architects Workshop, it seems highly important to make certain that the swing cannot strike the railing.)

Other modifications for an adapted swing include the addition of a back support, leg support, and safety belts. The back support should be at least 1 ft 6 in. in height. The leg support should fold back under the wooden or metal seat when it is not needed by the child who has the ability to operate the swing without the device. When extended, the leg support should clear the ground by at least 6 in. to 8 in. The safety belts help ensure that the child with balance limitations will not fall from the swing. They are easily attached to the seat.

It is recommended by the Pittsburgh Architects Workshop (1979) that in each set of four swings, one swing should be adapted in the fashion indicated in this section. For those agencies that do not wish to modify existing swings, commercial playground equipment manufacturers now offer molded plastic seats for purchase.

Merry-Go-Round

As with other adapted equipment, it is important that a hard surface path lead to the merry-go-round. It is not desirable, however, to have a hard surface surrounding the merry-go-round; a soft ground surface should be provided around the merry-go-round to minimize injuries from falls.

Handrails on merry-go-rounds are usually made of metal pipe 1 1/4 in. to 1 1/2 in. in diameter. At minimum, one set of handrails should be replaced with smaller pipe (i.e., 3/4 in. to 1 in.). Other adaptations that can be made are to stretch wire mesh or a rope net between the posts for the handrails to form a back support and to attach safety belts to the base of the pipes.

Railings Around Equipment

As noted earlier, a waist-high railing around an area such as the merry-go-round or seesaw will zone it off to protect children with visual or perceptual impairments from getting hurt by moving into the equipment when it is in use. Such railings also serve to guide visually impaired children around the playground. An optional refinement is the attachment of a sound-producing device to the merry-go-round, seesaws, or other apparatus to indicate to the visually impaired that it is in use.

The interested reader is referred to *Access to Play* by the Pittsburgh Architects Workshop (1979) for further details on the adaptations covered in this section. *Access to Play* contains many excellent diagrams that illustrate suggested adaptations.

A Final Word on Playgrounds

As previously stated, it is not normally necessary or desirable to provide separate playgrounds for children with disabilities. Playgrounds can be designed with all children in mind. If play environments are well designed, the great majority of children with disabilities can join their peers without disabilities in healthful play experiences in our community parks, on our school grounds, or wherever playgrounds are provided.

SUMMARY

This chapter dealt with concerns in designing appropriate recreation environments for all people, including those with disabilities. The chapter began with a discussion of terminology and legislation related to designing environments to meet the needs of individuals with disabilities. Following this introduction, the major portion of the chapter was devoted to guidelines and recommendations for creating usable recreation facilities. The final segment of the chapter covered the topic of designing playgrounds so that they will accommodate children who have disabilities.

SUGGESTED LEARNING ACTIVITIES

1. Using Table 6.1, assess a local park or campus recreation facility. Several students may join together to assess a state, regional, or national park.
2. Drawing on the information from the section on playgrounds, assess a local playground for design criteria.
3. Using an actual playground, report how you would adapt existing equipment to meet the needs of all children, including those with disabilities.
4. Prepare a slide show on the proper design of either parks or playgrounds.
5. Participate in a telephone lecture given by an authority on playground design for children with disabilities.
6. View an audiovisual presentation on facility or playground design for persons with disabilities. Several films and slide shows are available through Indiana University, the University of Missouri, and the University of South Florida. Local libraries and universities may also be of assistance.

REFERENCES

Austin, D. R. Playgrounds for the handicapped. In D. J. Bradamus, Ed. *New Thoughts on Leisure.* Champaign, IL: Office of Recreation and Park Resources, University of Illinois, 1978.

Axelson, P. W., & D. Chelini. *Inventory and Computerized Mapping of Trails: The First Step Towards Access.* Santa Cruz, CA: Beneficial Designs, 1993.

Beckwith, J. Play environments for all children. *Leisure Today.* In *Journal of Physical Education, Recreation and Dance, 56*(5), 32–35, 1985.

Bruya, L., & S. Langendorfer, Eds. *Where Our Children Play, Volume I: Elementary School Playground Equipment.* Reston, VA: American Alliance for Health, Physical Education, Recreation and Dance, 1988.

Frost, J. L., & B. L. Klein. *Children's Play and Playgrounds.* Boston: Allyn and Bacon, Inc., 1979.

Gilbert, A. Should a path be paved to the top of a mountain? Access to Heritage/parks areas. *Leisurability, 14*(1), 26–30, 1987.

Goltsman, S. M., T. A. Gilbert, & S. D. Wohlford. *The Accessibility Checklist: Vol. II Survey Form.* Berkeley, CA: MIG Communications, 1993a.

Goltsman, S. M., T. A. Gilbert, & S. D. Wohlford. *The Accessibility Checklist User's Guide* (2nd ed.). Berkeley, CA: MIG Communications, 1993b.

Gordon, R. *The Design of a Pre-School Therapeutic Playground: An Outdoor "Learning Laboratory."* New York: Institute of Rehabilitation Medicine, New York University Medical Centers, 1972.

Greenwell, P. H. Access board begins work on recreation guidelines. *Access Today, 2*(2), 1, 1993.

Grosse, S. J. Making outdoor play areas usable for all children. *Practical Pointers.* Reston, VA: American Alliance for Health, Physical Education, Recreation and Dance, 1980.

A Guide to Designing Accessible Outdoor Recreation Facilities. Ann Arbor, MI: Heritage Conservation and Recreation Service, U.S. Department of Interior, 1980.

Harrison, M. J. Customizing playgrounds. *Parks & Recreation 28*(4), 42–45, 91, 1993.

Hart, R. Child development and the design of preschool play environments. Presentation to the College of Health and Human Development, Penn State University, February 2, 1989.

McGovern, J. *The ADA Self-Evaluation: A Handbook for Compliance with the Americans with Disabilities Act by Parks and Recreation Agencies.* Arlington, VA: National Recreation and Park Association, 1992.

Moore, G. T., U. Cohen, J. Oerbel, & L. van Ryzin. *Designing Environments for Handicapped Children: A Design Guide and Case Study.* New York: Educational Facilities Laboratories, 1979.

Odom, S. L., P. S. Strain, M. A. Karger, & J. D. Smith. Using single and multiple peers to promote social interaction of preschool children with handicaps. *Journal of the Division of Early Childhood, 10*(1), 53–64, 1986.

Pittsburgh Architects Workshop. *Access to Play: Design Criteria for Adaptation of Existing Playground Equipment for Use by Handicapped Children.* Pittsburgh: Pittsburgh Architects Workshop, Inc., 1979.

A Playground for All Children: Resource Book. Washington, DC: U.S. Government Printing Office, 1978.

Schleien, S. J. Assess and inclusion in community leisure services. *Parks & Recreation 28*(4), 66–72, 1993.

Smith, R. W. Plan of action: Reflections and recommendations. In D. Thompson and L. Bowers, Eds. *Where Our Children Play: Community Park Playground Equipment.* Reston, VA: American Alliance for Health, Physical Education, Recreation and Dance, 1989, pp. 85–97.

Stout, J. Planning playgrounds for children with disabilities. *The American Journal of Occupational Therapy, 42*, 653–658, 1988.

Thompson, D., & L. Bowers, Eds. *Where Our Children Play: Community Park Playground Equipment.* Reston, VA: American Alliance for Health, Physical Education, Recreation and Dance, 1989.

The Universal Playground: A Planning Guide. Province of British Columbia: Ministry of Education, 1990.

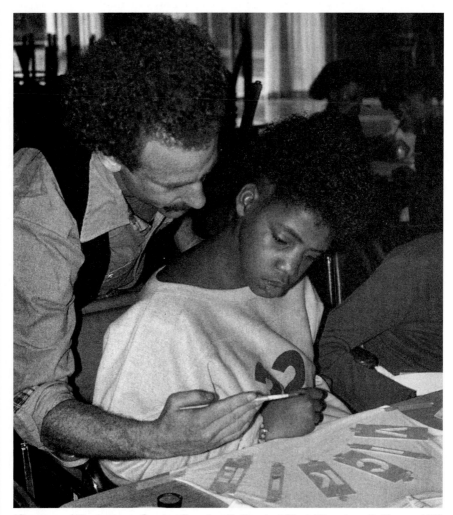

(Courtesy of The League: Serving People with Physical Disabilities, Inc., Baltimore, MD)

7

Program Planning and Evaluation Process

■ ■ ■

If you were asked to conduct a three-day camp program for children with and without disabilities, would you immediately begin planning activities such as arts and crafts, a campfire program, and cooperative games, or would you attempt to find out more information before beginning your planning? If you answered "yes" to finding out more information before planning, you would be correct. Regardless of the setting, it is important that recreation professionals follow an organized approach when planning and providing recreational activities. One example of a systematic approach involves a series of steps, including *assessment, planning, implementation,* and *evaluation.*

Throughout this program planning process, recreation professionals should be aware of the strategies and techniques used to integrate persons with disabilities into their programs. This is important because changes in legislation and shifts in philosophy have resulted in increasing inclusion of persons with disabilities into regular community recreation programs (see Chapters 2 and 3). All evidence points to this inclusionary trend continuing in the future. Recreation professionals should, therefore, consider the needs of this segment of the population when planning programs.

This chapter examines the *program planning and evaluation process,* and includes information that will assist recreation providers in ensuring that the needs of persons with disabilities are taken into account.

NEEDS ASSESSMENT

The number of persons with disabilities in the community or geographic area where programming is to take place should be identified. The fact that persons who have disabilities reside in the community will, in part, help justify leisure services. Some communities

The authors would like to thank Christine Camps for her extensive contributions to this chapter. Ms. Camps, from Toronto, has work experience integrating persons with developmental disabilities into community recreation programs, and has taught in the therapeutic recreation program at Georgian College. Ms. Camps assisted with this chapter during her graduate study at The Pennsylvania State University.

have conducted surveys to establish such information. The kind of information that might be useful includes age, sex, disabling condition, geographic location, and special considerations. Special considerations may include specific needs of the person related to transportation barriers, architectural barriers such as steps and curbs, the need for medication, and special kinds of assistance, such as transferring persons from their wheelchairs to the swimming pool.

The first step in the program planning process is to assess the needs of participants and potential participants. The goal of needs assessment is to facilitate effective program planning (Farrell & Lundegren, 1978). Assessment of needs in recreation can take many forms. Methods for establishing the needs of persons with disabilities are included in the following section.

Determining Needs Within a Community

According to a Harris poll, approximately 15% of the U.S. population has some sort of disability (International Center for the Disabled, 1986). It would be wise, therefore, for recreation providers to determine if their services and programs are meeting the needs of these individuals. Perrin, Wiele, Wilder, and Perrin (1992) suggested several methods for considering the recreational needs of persons with disabilities. Developing partnerships with persons with disabilities and their advocates is one method that may help determine how their needs can best be met. Often, individuals with disabilities are a good source of information about "what is not being done effectively," and they frequently can provide suggestions for change. The importance of including persons with disabilities in *all* aspects of the program planning process cannot be overemphasized. Bedini and Henderson (1994), for example, used interviews to explore the lives of 30 women with disabilities to determine implications for parks, recreation, and leisure providers. These women "reported feeling that they did not have opportunities or support to express their needs and interests concerning recreation and leisure" (p. 28). Moreover, many of these women emphasized that recreation providers need to be proactive in seeking the opinions of persons with disabilities. One woman advised:

> It would be very empowering for [persons with disabilities] to say what it is that they want as opposed to being told by a recreation department these are the things we have available for you. . . . I would probably pose a question, "What would you like to experiment with that you have not been able to do on your own? . . . and we'll brainstorm and come up with a way to make it possible. (pp. 28–29)

Heyne, McAvoy, and Schleien (1994) suggest that focus group techniques are an excellent way to encourage persons with disabilities to express their opinions and relate their personal experiences. Focus groups typically include 7 to 10 participants in "a carefully planned discussion designed to obtain perceptions on a defined area of interest in a permissive, nonthreatening environment" (Kruger, 1988, p. 18). Heyne et al. note that focus groups enable recreation service providers to "stay in touch with needs of individuals with

Activity analysis may clarify the need to modify an activity in order to meet the needs of participants with disabilities. (Courtesy of Courage Center, Golden Valley, MN)

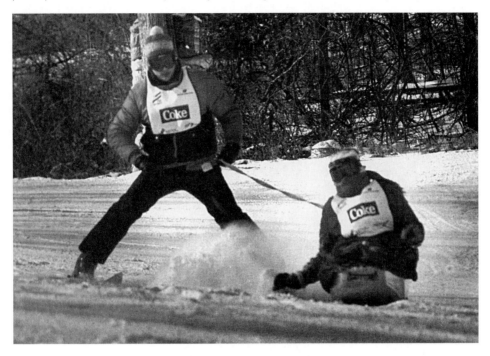

use of an outrigger (a ski-like attachment to a pole). Both of these adaptations allow individuals with disabilities to take part in a sport that would otherwise be difficult for them to participate in.

A second reason for adapting an activity may be to enhance achievement of the program's goals and objectives. For example, if one of the goals of the program was to "provide opportunities for social interaction," the leader might modify an activity like T-shirt painting, which is traditionally done alone, by requesting that all projects be done in pairs. This way, individuals with and without disabilities would have to work together to complete the task.

A third reason for adapting activities is to accommodate any operational concerns that the leader may have. Insufficient staff, facilities, participants, or equipment may make it difficult or dangerous to perform an activity the way it was meant to be performed. For example, if a woodworking program were being offered but there were not enough staff to supervise the machinery, the activity may need to be modified so that the participants only do the sanding and finishing on their projects; thus, their safety is not put in jeopardy.

A fourth and final reason for adapting activities is to provide novelty, or a variation from routine. Participants may become bored with always taking part in the same activities the same way. If bingo is a popular activity with participants, occasionally varying the way the game is played can add excitement. With children, for example, letters or symbols could be called out in place of numbers (this could also help develop their reading and sign recognition skills). Alternatively, "Barnyard Bingo" could be played: each time their card has the number that is called out, the children make a farm animal noise. Variations of activities for the sake of novelty are limited only by the creativity of leaders and participants!

Guidelines for Modification

The rationale for the adaptations cited here is not meant to give the impression that activities should be altered with little thought to the implications of the modifications. A point that Labanowich (1978) made about wheelchair sports is that we need to be careful not to slant recreational activities toward an air of "temporariness," particularly for children and youth. According to Labanowich, such activities may "fail to convey a sense of realism for the participant projected against their utility as later life pastimes" (p. 12). Keeping in mind that activities should be beneficial or meaningful to the individual, the leader should ask the question: "Will modifying or adapting the activity be unfair and/or detract from the meaningfulness of the activity for the individual?" The following are some guidelines that should be considered when selecting and modifying activities for persons who have disabilities.

1. Change as little as necessary. For example, try to keep the structure and the rules of a game as close as possible to the existing game. It is better to undermodify so as to challenge the individual and to provide normalized experiences.

2. Where possible, involve the person in the selection and activity modification process. Many times, the user is a good source of information. The rules for wheelchair basketball are based on this phenomenon. All rule modifications of the National Wheelchair Basketball Association need the approval of participants.

3. Don't make assumptions about an individual based on his or her disability. No two persons with the same disability have the exact same modification needs. Get to know the person before deciding on any needed modifications.

4. There may be elements of competition to consider when working with groups of children and adults. In the Special Olympics, for instance, past performance, age, and sex of the participant are usually taken into consideration when pitting one person against another.

5. Try to offer activities that are characteristic of individuals who are in the mainstream of society. That is, offer to persons with disabilities the same leisure opportunities that exist in society. The normalization principle should be emphasized and the idea of inventing activities should be deemphasized.

6. Where possible, activities should have common denominators, especially if they are modified. For example, in wheelchair basketball, everyone plays in a wheelchair and follows the same rules. The wheelchair and the fact that everyone follows the same rules are the common denominators for equality in participation.

7. In many instances, the person with a disability is cast in the role of spectator. The authors of this text strongly feel that individuals should be provided opportunities to participate in, and be encouraged to join, participant-based programs. If full and active participation is not possible, then the person with the disability should be provided with opportunities for partial participation.

8. Start at the level where the participants are currently functioning. This does *not* mean starting at the lowest level.

9. Individuals should be given opportunities for free choice. This may enhance the feeling of control and reduce feelings of "learned helplessness."

Categories of Modification

Keeping the aforementioned guidelines for modification in mind, there are several types of adaptations that could be utilized, if needed, to facilitate the inclusion of persons with disabilities. These modifications fall into one of the following four categories:

1. *Procedural/operational adaptations:* These are changes or alterations in the actual operation of play that achieve the same purpose as the original activity. This may involve modifications to the rules (e.g., shortening the length of time a game is played to accommodate short attention spans), changes in the procedures for action (e.g., having participants walk instead of run during an activity), changes in the roles of the participants (e.g., using the buddy system in the outfield in baseball if a participant with a disability needs assistance), or changes in the social interaction requirements of an activity (e.g., allowing two people to answer questions together in a trivia quiz).

2. *Environmental adaptations:* This involves adaptations that are directly related to the environment in which the activity is taking place. For example, if a participant has a mobility impairment, the leader could use barriers around the group to decrease the distance that the ball rolls. Or, if a participant has a visual impairment, arrangements could be made to ensure that the lighting does not hamper that person's ability to track objects.

3. *Equipment adaptations:* There are two types of equipment adaptations. The first type, aids to existing equipment, allows individuals to use standard equipment. Examples of such aids include card holders for people unable to hold playing cards and vises to hold craft projects for people who have use of one hand. The second type of equipment modification, specialized equipment, involves changes to standard equipment or the creation of new equipment to allow activity participation. Examples of specialized equipment include four-holed scissors, with which an instructor can physically help a person cut something, talking books for people unable to read regular books, and sledges, used in an adapted form of ice hockey played by persons with and without a physical impairment. Many sources of adaptive and specialized equipment can be found in Appendix C.

4. *Human intervention:* This involves a leader, volunteer, or peer assisting with an individual's participation in an activity. This may take the form of passive assistance (providing verbal prompting, encouragement, or praise), or more active assistance (providing physical prompts, hand-over-hand assistance, or actually moving with the individual). In either case, the individual with the disability should be allowed to do as much for him- or herself as possible.

Recreation professionals should be encouraged to utilize creativity and flexibility in trying to accommodate all individuals in programs. The use of innovative adaptations allows participation in a particular activity by many people who would otherwise find it difficult or impossible.

SAMM Model

Peterson (1976) presented what she termed a "Selection of Activity and Modification Model" (SAMM). The important feature stressed in the SAMM is answering questions and making the appropriate decision. If the answer is *no* for the question "Do clients have the physical skills necessary for participation?" then another question is posed: "Can the activity be modified for the existing skill level?" If *yes,* then follow the guidelines for selecting and modifying activities. Figure 7.2 is a modified version of the Selection of Activity and Modification Model (Peterson & Gunn, 1984).

IMPLEMENTATION

Having assessed the needs of the participants in the program, selected appropriate activities, and decided how these activities may need to be modified to allow the successful participation of a person or persons with disabilities, the recreation professional then takes the next step, implementing these activities. One important facet during this phase of the program planning process is to provide appropriate awareness, education, and support to all persons involved, including staff, volunteers, and program participants with and without disabilities.

Staff Education, Awareness, and Support

People who work in recreation settings generally take part in some type of orientation or preservice training designed to help them carry out the functions of their job more effectively. Part of this training should be devoted to developing the skills and positive attitudes that will assist persons with disabilities to participate successfully in the recreation programs offered. McGill (1984) makes the case that inadequate staff training decreases the likelihood of successful inclusion of persons with disabilities. A variety of topics should be covered in such a training program. First and foremost, the agency must make its commitment to inclusion well known to the staff, and must attempt to foster a welcoming attitude toward persons with disabilities. This may be done by using preprepared training packages that focus on dispelling myths about persons with disabilities, and by making staff feel more at ease in including these individuals in their programs. Examples of these training packages include "All Ways Welcome," from the Ontario Ministry of Tourism and Recreation, and "Disability Awareness Training," developed by the Canadian Rehabilitation Council for the Disabled. Information on obtaining these and other

Figure 7.2. Modified version of the Selection of Activity and Modification Model (Peterson, 1976). (Used with permission of the National Recreation and Park Association)

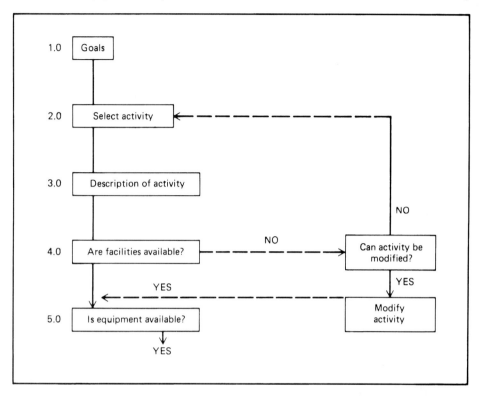

training packages is included at the end of this chapter. Regardless of what type of training is given, it should include an overview of the methods used by the agency to support individuals with disabilities (see Methods of Support following). The agency's training program may also include some leadership hints and tips for working with people with particular disabilities, such as persons with visual impairments or brain injuries (see Chapter 4). Methods of analyzing and adapting activities, as outlined in this chapter, could also be a useful part of the training process.

To be most effective, the training program should involve a variety of training methods, such as videos, printed material, discussions, problem solving, hands-on experiences, and presentations. The training itself can be implemented using a number of sources. Someone within the agency who has the appropriate background may initiate the training program, or departments may wish to hire a therapeutic recreation specialist as a consultant to conduct this training (Schleien & Ray, 1988). Professionals from agencies that serve persons with disabilities can also be a good source of information, and could be active participants in the education process (Burt Perrin Associates, 1989). If possible, staff training should include the involvement of persons with disabilities. They have firsthand experience with what works and what doesn't (Hutchison & McGill, 1992).

Training and education should not be limited to a formal program conducted upon hiring. Staff should have open access to printed resources that may be of assistance, to further training programs as they are made available, and to ongoing support that may be needed to help solve problems as they arise. Sable (1992), for example, described using biweekly group sessions and individual supervision meetings with staff to facilitate integration in a residential camp. Timely and effective staff training will go a long way toward ensuring the successful inclusion of persons with disabilities.

METHODS OF SUPPORT

Many persons with disabilities may be able to participate independently in community recreation programs if consideration is given to their needs during the assessment and planning phases. For some individuals with disabilities, however, additional supports may be required during the program to allow them to take part. Many recreation departments and agencies have implemented one or a number of such support services. The following section briefly highlights some methods of support that are currently used throughout the United States and Canada.

Paid Support

Some agencies or parks and recreation departments hire an individual to act as a Special Needs Coordinator or Integration Specialist. This person is generally responsible for ensuring that the needs of persons with disabilities are being met by the programs offered, and he or she also oversees any additional support services that are provided. Some agencies that serve persons with disabilities employ what Dattilo and St. Peter (1991) term a Leisure Coach. The Leisure Coach is available to teach persons with disabilities those skills necessary for participation in recreational activities, to provide inclusion information and support to the recreation staff, and to offer assistance to the participant with a disability during the activity, if needed. Recreation providers can assist in this process by allowing the person with a disability and the Coach to observe or try a number of different activities to gain exposure, and by providing tours and information about programs and facilities, as requested.

Volunteers

Volunteers are used in many agencies and recreation departments to assist in the inclusion of persons with disabilities. Names such as Leisure Buddy, Leisure Link, or Volunteer Advocate denote programs where an individual without a disability is matched with an individual with a disability, and the two of them participate in a community recreation program together. The Montgomery County (Maryland) Mainstreaming Initiative, for example, uses this approach to ensure that programs are open to all county residents (see Chapter 8).

It is important that volunteers who assist in recreation programs also receive appropriate training so that both the participant with a disability and the volunteer have the best possible experience. Volunteers should be made aware of what type of assistance may be needed (information that is best provided by the person with the disability), and should encourage the participant to do as much for him- or herself as possible.

Group Support

One idea that is increasing in popularity is the notion of a group in which the participants without disabilities form a natural support system for the person with a disability. Sometimes referred to as a Circle of Friends (Schleien, 1993), the participants without disabilities work with the person who has a disability to develop strategies for overcoming barriers that might prevent group acceptance and participation. This type of approach provides opportunities for developing friendships and interactions among people with and without disabilities (Bedini, 1993).

Climate of Cooperation

Leaders of recreation programs can structure activities so as to encourage positive interaction as well as the development of skills and friendships among participants. One of the best ways to do this is to offer activities that create a climate of cooperation. Although persons with disabilities should be given the opportunity to participate in competitive activities if desired, competition can create situations where the person with a disability does not succeed. By eliminating the focus on winning and dominance, cooperative activities create an atmosphere that allows participants to express themselves more freely and support one another (LeFevre, 1988). Removing anxiety about performance creates an atmosphere of interdependence, and the result will most likely be positive social interactions among persons with and without disabilities (Rynders & Schleien, 1991).

If a competitive structure is selected, leaders should still facilitate a climate of cooperation. One way to do this is to be aware of the abilities of participants and consider altering the activity to facilitate inclusion. If an activity is by nature one in which individuals compete against each other, the activity could be altered so that people compete against themselves by trying to improve their own performance. In bowling, for example, rather than competing for the highest score, individuals could try to beat their own average, with the person scoring the most pins over average being declared the winner. This structure gives all participants an equal opportunity to succeed.

Another way to structure competitive activities that allow individuals with disabilities equal opportunities for succeeding and developing peer friendships is to structure activities that create an interdependence among team members. With this structure, every

Creating a climate of cooperation encourages positive interaction among persons with and without disabilities. (Courtesy of Maryland-National Capital Park and Planning Commission, Special Populations Division; Photo by Steve Abramowitz)

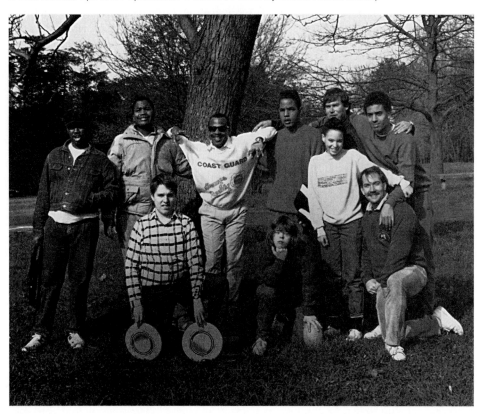

member's contribution to the task at hand is what determines "winning" (Rynders & Schleien, 1991). For example, in a group chili-making contest, the rules could state that each member of the group must perform a given number of tasks in the preparation of the chili. Moreover, the rules could state that each participant must do "blind taste tests" to help determine the winners. In this way, persons with and without disabilities are equal partners in influencing the outcome of their group's efforts.

When planning group activities, leaders should give consideration to the most appropriate size for the group. Johnson and Johnson (1980) have indicated that, to best facilitate integration, the decision for group size should be based on several factors. Generally speaking, the younger the group, the more complex the task, the weaker the cooperative skills of the group members, and the shorter the time available to complete the task, the smaller the group should be. Also, offering a progression from small-group to large-group activities may facilitate social integration.

Recreation leaders should make every effort to allow persons with disabilities to participate to the best of their abilities. By following some of the strategies for educating staff and providing the necessary support outlined in this section of the chapter, recreation providers will be well on their way to inclusive programming.

EVALUATION

According to Kennedy and Lundegren (1981), "Evaluation is the key to successful program planning, since inherent in it are suggestions for increasing effectiveness" (p. 24). Recreation boards and commissions, administrators, the public, and clients like to see hard evidence that recreation programs are effective. How do you get this evidence? Program evaluation is the only reliable method of obtaining the information needed to justify recreation programs and the corresponding financial needs.

Reasons for Program Evaluation

Why should professional recreators evaluate their programs? There are a multitude of reasons. The following are just a few examples.

- To determine if program objectives have been accomplished
- To discover the impact the program had on the participants
- To decide if the program was cost effective
- To provide information for future program planning and modification
- To obtain key information necessary to justify future financial support for the program
- To obtain information for formal reports to the board, planning committees, and other target audiences
- To provide information necessary to market the program to potential clients, decision makers, and program sponsors

What Are We Trying to Evaluate?

It is important to clarify what we mean by success in your programming efforts. As one example, quantitative information helps track the number of participants in a recreation program. Over time, comparisons can be made to determine whether the number of participants with disabilities increased, decreased, or stayed about the same. Knowing information about the number of people may reflect interest in recreation programs, particularly if individuals return at a later time to engage in other activities.

Qualitative information is also important. As pointed out by Schleien and Ray (1988), "The successful (or unsuccessful) social integration of participants may be determined by observing certain behaviors between participants with and without disabilities. These behaviors may include initiating social interactions, eye contact between peers, physical proximity, appropriate physical contact, sharing" (p. 91).

What is assessed in program evaluation should pertain to the mission, goals, and objectives of the agency. For instance, educators such as Kennedy (1986) and Peterson and Gunn (1984), in addition to well-known practitioners like Janet Pomery from the RCH, Inc., in San Francisco, all suggest that the purpose of recreation programming is to *provide opportunities for fun, enjoyment, satisfaction, and self-expression* within an organized leisure service delivery system. Although community-based recreation programs for persons with disabilities include segregated, transitional, and integrated programs, the goal is to move individuals as far as possible toward independent, leisure functioning within the least restrictive environment.

One useful approach to determine what to evaluate is simply to ask the questions for which you want answers. The following questions reflect this approach.

- Are participants enjoying the activity?
- Are participants gaining social awareness?
- Are participants learning leisure skills?
- Are participants with disabilities interacting appropriately with their peers and/or with nondisabled participants?
- Are attitudes of nondisabled participants changing in a positive direction toward their peers with disabilities?
- How many persons with disabilities participated in recreational programs last year?
- Were the program's goals met?

Types of Evaluation

There are several schemes for classifying the kinds of evaluation used in conducting program evaluations. For example, participant feedback can provide information about how much fun people had during the recreative experience. If learning a social behavior such as sharing was an objective, then a planned observational scheme could be used to measure whether sharing was learned and, if appropriate, was applied in other situations. The following are some typical examples of the types of evaluation that could be used.

- Casual impressions, including comments from participants
- Self-checking or feedback exercises, including simple reaction forms and verbal feedback from participants
- Do-it-yourself evaluations, including follow-up surveys or simple phone surveys
- Impact studies, including carefully designed evaluation studies
- Experimental research, including rigorous studies using standard research designs that control errors

Program Evaluation Steps

As stated earlier, evaluation planning starts when program planning starts, and evaluation is a key step of the program planning process. Each time recreation leaders plan a program, they should (1) decide on the objectives the program is designed to accomplish, (2) establish a plan of action to meet the objectives, (3) identify the program or activities to be conducted, (4) decide which level of evaluation is appropriate for the program, and (5) design an evaluation instrument to accomplish this goal.

There are many approaches to a program evaluation with each having a number of steps. The following is just one example of steps to accomplish a program evaluation:

Before Recreation Program Is Implemented

- Select program to be evaluated and audience from which to gather information
- Identify the audience with whom the evaluation information will be shared
- Decide why this particular program needs to be evaluated
- List and review program objectives
- Decide which level of evaluation is appropriate and feasible
- Decide how the information will be collected
- Develop or obtain the evaluation instrument(s)

After Recreation Program Is Implemented

- Conduct the evaluation (collect data on participants)
- Analyze, summarize, and study results
- Revise future programs accordingly
- Prepare written reports and disseminate results and recommendations

The process of program evaluation is a continuous one. The goal of the evaluation process is to provide better leisure opportunities and to seek ways to improve various aspects of program features.

As mentioned, there are many approaches to the various kinds of evaluation procedures and a multitude of evaluation tools to measure the different phenomena. Records such as attendance sheets can answer questions pertaining to the number of participants and can offer comparisons that reflect any increases or decreases. Schleien and Ray (1988) give examples of skill acquisition forms, social interaction tools, peer acceptance evaluations, and measures of self-concept that can be used with persons with disabilities. Although focusing primarily on the therapeutic process, Peterson and Gunn (1984) give useful information about assessment, documentation, and program evaluation.

The following example highlights the participant feedback approach as a way to evaluate program features.

Importance-Performance Analysis

Obtaining participant input is a primary ingredient in the development and improvement of recreation programs and services. Empirical research has demonstrated that client satisfaction is a function of both *expectations* related to certain important attributes and judgment of attribute *performance* (Meyers & Alpers, 1968; Swan & Coombs, 1976).

Guadagnolo (1985) has applied importance-performance analysis to the recreation and parks field. There has been success in utilizing this approach to market and evaluate programs for adults who were mentally retarded (Guadagnolo, Godbey, Kerstetter, Kennedy, Farrell, & Warnick, 1984), for persons with physical disabilities (Kennedy, 1986), and for the elderly (Gillespie, Kennedy, & Soble, 1989). In all instances, the respective audiences have been willing and able to complete forms and to demonstrate the necessary understanding of the process.

The first step in importance-performance analysis is determining what specific program features are important to measure. The features list should reflect those items over which an agency has some degree of control. The quality of the information collected is dependent on the program features list; therefore, ample time should be devoted to its development.

Various qualitative research techniques such as focus groups and unstructured interviews have been used to identify important program features. In a swim program, for example, the features list could be initiated by the recreation staff. Once the features list is drafted, staff members could talk with two or three potential participants or to parents of children with disabilities, if appropriate. Based on these conversations, a features list can be finalized. A list for a swim program might look like the following:

Safety	Family involvement
Privacy	Length of swim session
Transportation	Temperature of the water
Program location	Ratio of staff to participants
Pool accessibility	Instructor's teaching skill

Once the features list is developed, the next step is the development of the importance-performance (I-P) scale. The I-P scale usually consists of two Likert scales, one measuring importance and the other, performance. The features are rated on a scale ranging from "not important" to "very important." Similarly, performance or satisfaction is rated. In the example provided, a 5-point scale is used. However, shorter scales (3 points) and longer ones (7 points) can be used. Also, faces depicting feelings have been used with young children as well as with adults who are mentally retarded.

Importance Scale

Feature	Not Important		Somewhat Important		Very Important
Safety	1	2	3	4	5
Family involvement	1	2	3	4	5

Labanowich, S. The psychology of wheelchair sports. *Therapeutic Recreation Journal, 12*(1), 11–77, 1978.

LeFevre, D. *New Games for the Whole Family.* New York: Perigee Books, 1988.

Mager, R. F. *Preparing Instructional Objectives.* Palo Alto, CA: Fearon Publishers, 1962.

Mager, R. F., & P. Pipe. *Analyzing Performance Problems* or '*You Really Oughta Wanna.*' Palo Alto, CA: Fearon Publishers, 1970.

McDowell, F., Jr. Toward a healthy leisure mode: Leisure counseling. *Therapeutic Recreation Journal, 8*(3), 96–104, 1974.

McGill, J. Training for integration: Are blindfolds really enough? *Journal of Leisurability, 11*(2), 12–15, 1984.

McKechnie, G. E. Psychological foundations of leisure counseling: An empirical strategy. *Therapeutic Recreation Journal, 8*(1), 4–16, 1974.

Meyers, J. H., & M. I. Alpers. Determining attributes: Meaning and measurement. *Journal of Marketing, 32*(4), 13–20, 1968.

Mirenda, J. *Mirenda Leisure Interest Finder.* Milwaukee, WI: Milwaukee Public Schools, Dept. of Municipal Recreation and Adult Education, 1973.

Overs, R. P. A model for avocational counseling. *Journal of Health, Physical Education and Recreation, 41*(2), 36–38, 1970.

Perrin, B. Community recreation for all: How to include persons with disabilities in regular leisure and recreation. *Journal of Leisurability, 19*(4), 28–36, 1992.

Perrin, B., K. Wiele, S. Wilder, & A. Perrin. *Sharing the Fun: A Guide to Including Persons with Disabilities in Leisure and Recreation.* Toronto: Canadian Rehabilitation Council for the Disabled, 1992.

Peterson, C. A. *State of the art activity analysis. Leisure Activity Participation and Handicapped Populations: Assessment of Research Needs.* Arlington, VA: National Recreation and Park Association and Bureau of Education for the Handicapped, U.S. Office of Education, April 1976.

Peterson, C. A., & S. L. Gunn. *Therapeutic Recreation Program Design: Principles and Procedures* (2nd ed.). Englewood Cliffs, NJ: Prentice-Hall, 1984.

Rynders, J. E., & S. J. Schleien. *Together Successfully.* Arlington, TX: Association for Retarded Citizens of the United States, 1991.

Sable, J. Collaborating to create an integrated camping program: Design and evaluation. *Therapeutic Recreation Journal, 26*(3), 38–48, 1992.

Schleien, S. J. Access and inclusion in community leisure services. *Parks and Recreation, 28*(4), 66–72, 1993.

Schleien, S. J., & M. T. Ray. *Community Recreation and Persons with Disabilities: Strategies for Integration.* Baltimore: Brookes, 1988.

Schleien, S. J., J. E. Rynders, L. A. Heyne, & C. E. S. Tabourne, Eds. *Powerful Partnerships: Parents and Professionals Building Inclusive Recreation Programs Together.* Minneapolis, MN: University of Minnesota, 1995.

Swan, J. G., & L. J. Coombs. Product performance and consumer satisfaction: A new concept. *Journal of Marketing, 40*(2), 25–33, 1976.

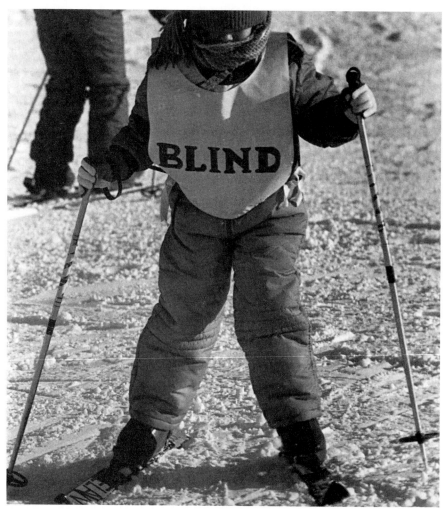

(Courtesy of Courage Center, Golden Valley, MN)

8

Inclusive and Special Recreation Programs—Exemplaries

. . .

This chapter presents seven examples of special recreation programs offering leisure services to individuals who have disabilities. The programs, selected because of their positive features, represent a variety of services and structures. They were chosen from different states across the country, primarily larger cities. It is hoped that by learning what kinds of programs and services exist in different areas of the United States, readers will be better prepared to organize their own programs.

AUSTIN PARKS AND RECREATION DEPARTMENT, ADAPTIVE PROGRAMS

Introduction and Background

The "Special Populations Program" was established in June 1974, as a city-funded operation within the Community Recreation Division of the City of Austin Parks and Recreation Department. The program name was changed to Adaptive Programs in January 1978. From the onset, the focus of the Adaptive Programs has been toward an integrated program of mainstreaming individuals with disabilities into existing programs.

Since 1977, the Adaptive Programs section has had three or more full-time staff members, allowing expanded programming. A neighborhood community program was started in 1979 to complement existing citywide programs. Volunteers have been used extensively in an effort to maintain a lower participant-leader ratio and to offer more variety in programming and quality of supervision.

Information in this section was taken from materials furnished by the Austin Parks and Recreation Department (M. A. Lord, personal communication, 1989).

Goals and Objectives

Adaptive Programs stresses choice, involvement, and self-direction while offering recreational experiences, new challenges, and friendships. The recreation staff attempts to parallel recreation programs so that when skills are learned in Adaptive Programs, they will carry over into existing general recreation programs.

Participants and Programs

Those served by Adaptive Programs include persons 3 years old and older with, but not limited to, the following disabling conditions: physical disabilities including visual and hearing impairment, mental retardation, emotional disturbance, learning disabilities, and those eliciting delinquent behaviors.

Adaptive programs are divided into three phases: integrated, transitional, and adaptive (specialized segregated). The integrated phase provides assistance in getting the person with a disability into existing regular programs and classes. The transitional phase is a "one-shot" experience to introduce the individual to recreational programs and to orient the person to the philosophy of recreation while encouraging participation in regular recreation activities. The third phase is for the person who has little recreational experience and needs encouragement, behavior intervention, or skill development to participate and interact with nondisabled individuals. Within the Austin Parks and Recreation Department, transitional activities have typically included theater productions, hayrides, canoeing and backpacking trips, ice cream socials, and bowling. Special adaptive classes offered have included sewing for individuals with visual impairments, developmental gymnastics, T-ball, cooking, dance, soccer, camping, aquatics, and therapeutic horseback riding.

The Adaptive Programs Section has entered into several cooperative agreements with other agencies in an effort to (1) reduce duplication, (2) enhance the quality of programs, (3) provide additional facilities, and (4) provide more services to more persons with disabilities in the Austin area. For example, cooperative arrangements have been made with Criss Cole Rehabilitation Center for the Blind, the Austin Independent School District, and the Austin-Travis County Mental Health–Mental Retardation Center. The Criss Cole Center shares facilities and programs while the Austin-Travis County MH–MR Center and the Austin Parks and Recreation Department cooperatively operate a day camp for youngsters with emotional disturbances.

The following are some activity highlights that reflect the Adaptive Programs offerings.

Adaptive Programs Summer Highlights

- *At Your Leisure*—A learning-through-leisure program that emphasizes socialization and development of recreational activity skills and attitudes, and promotes independent, self-directed use of leisure. Meets Mondays.
  Fee: Annual registration fee.
- *Cooking Basics*—A basic introduction that will focus on menu planning, food preparation, and table etiquette. Two 6-week classes for teens and adults are held.
  Fee: The participants will prepare a meal for a guest of their choice on the last class night.
- *Creative Movement*—This program emphasizes body awareness, gross motor skills, fitness, and self-expression, and will introduce some basic dance movements designed for youth 6–12 years of age. Two 3-week sessions meet on Tuesdays and Thursdays.
- *Kaleidoscope*—This program is held Monday through Friday and is for youth 6–12 years old. Activities for each 2-week session include crafts, nature study, creative dramatics, group sports and games, "special" days and water play at Bailey Park, and one overnight.
- *Kid Kapers*—A wide variety of activities for youth 6–12 years old. Activities include crafts, creative dramatics, group sports and games, puppetry, storytelling, and others.
- *Leisure Lunchbox*—Bring a sack lunch to eat, and afterward enjoy leisure activities for adults led by an Adaptive Programs staff member. Socialization and fun are the main emphasis of this program. Meets for 6 weeks on Tuesdays.
- *Pottery*—A basic introduction to handbuilding pottery techniques for teens and adults.
- *Swimming*—Specially trained instruction in a small class setting, working on basic skills for the more involved handicapped individual, or those who need some special skill development before moving into the integrated "Learn-to-Swim" program. There are three 3-week sessions for youth (6–16 years).
- *Adult Swimming*—Sessions are 3 weeks in length, 2 nights per week.
- *Teen Trek*—This program is held Monday through Friday for teens 13–19 years old. Activities for each 3-week session include a wide variety of leisure programs, with the main emphasis on leisure education, career exploration, and socialization.
- *Walking for Fitness*—The emphasis of this 6-week program for disabled teens, adults, and family is on fitness, conditioning, and socialization. A warm-up exercise program will be developed for each participant. Meets on Thursdays.
- *Weight Conditioning*—Use of a universal gym for teens and adults, specifically designed to meet the needs of the disabled. Meets Tuesdays and Thursdays.
  Fee: Annual registration fee.

Adaptive Programs Summer Special Events

- *Tubing on the San Marcos River*—This family outing takes place on a Saturday. Transportation, inner tubes, and life jackets are provided. Bring your bathing suit, towel, sun lotion, any snacks you may desire, and enough money for an ice cream cone on the way home.
- *Balloon Day and Water Play*—A lot of fun with activities using balloons and refreshing water play in the afternoon. For youth (6–12 years). Bring a sack lunch and your swimsuit.
  Fee: Free.

CINCINNATI RECREATION COMMISSION, DIVISION OF THERAPEUTIC RECREATION

Introduction and Background

In 1968, the Cincinnati Recreation Commission established the Division of Therapeutic Recreation to offer a variety of community recreation programs to children, teens, and adults with disabilities. The purpose of the division is to provide recreation services for persons living in the Greater Cincinnati Area who are ill or disabled. The budget is made up of city tax dollars and has grown from less than $3,000 in 1968 to more than $200,000. More than 100 unique and varied recreational programs are offered on a yearly basis. Nominal fees are assessed for the Division's programs in addition to a yearly membership fee. The Division of Therapeutic Recreation works with children ages 6 and up and employs a supervisor and four full-time program coordinators who initiate and organize the programs as well as train and supervise staff and volunteers.

Goals and Objectives

The philosophy of the Cincinnati program involves elements of the continuum method, employs principles of normalization, and cooperates with parents and agencies serving people with disabilities. The goals of the program are to aid in individual growth and development, to contribute to the quality of life, and to enhance a leisure lifestyle.

Information in this section was taken from materials furnished by the Cincinnati Recreation Commission, Division of Therapeutic Recreation.

Participants and Programs

Program formats vary according to the seasons, disabilities, and participants' ages and functional levels. The unique and varied program formats currently being implemented by the division include the following:

1. *Activity Programs:* May incorporate music and dance, movement exploration, arts and crafts, nature lore, creative dramatics, game, physical fitness activities, field trips, and swim instruction.

2. *Sports and Athletics:* Seasonal clinics teach tennis, golf, soccer, floor hockey, basketball, flag football, racquetball, and neighborhood games. Fall/winter bowling leagues and spring/summer softball teams are also offered annually.

3. *Adapted Aquatics:* Programs consist of swim instruction, water games, swim and diving meets, and aquatic shows. A weeknight "posttherapy swim" is offered for teens and adults with physical disabilities. In the summer, swim instruction is an integral part of the eight-week day camp program.

4. *Outdoor Adventures:* Consists of high-skill-level nature activities that may include canoeing, camping, backpacking, rappeling, horseback riding, cross-country skiing, and orienteering.

5. *Socials and Special Events:* Include dances, clubs, banquets, parties, holiday events, and experiences in the community such as moviegoing or restaurant dining.

6. *Specialized Skill Programs:* A sample of these leisure life skills offered on a seasonal basis may include ceramics, dance instruction, carpentry, and trimnastics.

Concern for meeting the individual needs of program participants prompted the development of a program skill level continuum (see Table 8.1). The skill levels are used by the staff in developing goals and objectives, planning programs, and assessing individuals.

The first skill level described by the Therapeutic Recreation Program Skill Level Continuum is Level I. Level I activities are geared to persons with developmental disabilities who need a 1:1 or 1:2 staff-participant ratio to learn basic sensory motor and self-help skills. Lists of appropriate skills for each level are used by staff for goal setting and assessment. These listings have been termed *skill sheets* by the staff. Level I skill sheets are used as a guide for planning program objectives and activities and for assessing the skills of children, teens, or adults with severe or profound disabilities as well as young children with physical disabilities. An individual who is severely mentally retarded may need to work on Level I skills his or her entire lifetime, whereas a young child who is mildly mentally retarded or is physically disabled may use skills learned in Level I as a bridge to grow and to develop skills presented in Levels II through IV. Specific skills included in the Level I skill sheets involve body awareness, sensory stimulation and discrimination, and basic visual perception activities. Sequential self-help skills are also presented on the Level I skill sheets in the areas of eating, toileting, personal hygiene, and dressing.

Table 8.1 Cincinnati Recreation Commission Division of Therapeutic Recreation Program Skill Level Continuum

Level I	Level II	Level III	Level IV
Programs for persons exhibiting basic needs who need a 1:1 or 1:2 staff ratio, working on the development of basic socialization, sensory motor, self-help, and motor coordination skills.	Programs for persons possessing sensory motor skills, able to function in group situations and to begin refining basic fine and gross motor and self-help skills for high-level recreation activities.	Programs for persons possessing skills necessary to learn high-level recreation activities.	Integration

Evaluation Requirements	**Evaluation Requirements**	**Evaluation Requirements**	
■ Sensory motor skill assessment ■ Sequential motor development skill assessment ■ Self-help skill assessment ■ Socialization skill assessment ■ Attitudes, values, and emotional development skill assessment ■ Mobility assessment (for physically disabled individuals only) ■ Body awareness and sensory motor (for physically disabled) ■ Self-help (for physically disabled) ■ Sequential Motor Resource Sheet	■ Sequential motor development skill assessment ■ Self-help skill assessment ■ Socialization skill assessment ■ Attitudes, values, and emotional development skill assessment ■ Mobility assessment (for physically disabled individuals only) ■ Cognitive development skill assessment (for individuals with learning disabilities only) ■ Self-help (for physically disabled) ■ Sequential Motor Resource Sheet	■ Sports/leisure activity skill assessment ■ Outdoor Adventure skill assessment ■ Self-help skill assessment ■ Socialization skill assessment ■ Attitudes, values, and emotional development skill assessment ■ Mobility assessment (for physically disabled individuals only) ■ Cognitive development skill assessment (for individuals with learning disabilities only) ■ Self-help (for physically disabled)	

Level II activities are geared to persons who possess sensory motor skills and who are able to begin functioning in a group situation. Individuals at Skill Level II are ready to learn basic fine and gross motor skills that are prerequisite to learning high-level recreation activities. An adult who has severe mental retardation may work on refining the skills presented in Level II indefinitely, whereas a young teen who has mild retardation may use fine and gross motor skills learned in Level II to play a team sport that is classified by the continuum as a Level III activity. Specific skills included on the Level II skill sheets involve individual socialization skill assessment as well as fine and gross motor and basic activity skills.

Level III programs are geared to children, teens, and adults who possess skills necessary to learn high-level recreation activities. Activities included on the Level III skill sheets involve team sports, specific leisure skills, and outdoor adventure skills. A teenager who has mental retardation may participate in a softball league sponsored by the Division of Therapeutic Recreation to refine skills and learn the rules necessary to eventually compete on a public team in the community. For some individuals involved in Level III programs, being integrated into a community softball league (Level IV on the continuum) is a challenge and a true possibility. For other individuals, integration would not be the most appropriate least restrictive environment. Their individual needs would best be met by continuing in Level III activities sponsored by the Division.

Integration is the fourth and final skill level on the Division of Therapeutic Recreation's program level continuum. Integration is attained by individuals with disabilities when they leave a program sponsored by the Division of Therapeutic Recreation to become a participant in a community recreation program. Such a program has specially trained staff or volunteers who program for, or work with, individuals with special needs. During the various stages of integration, the involvement of the division staff becomes that of facilitator, trainer, consultant, and advocate. It is the philosophy of the division that once an individual is successfully integrated into a community center program, he or she is no longer at a disadvantage (handicapped) in relation to the specific skill he or she is performing.

The continuum is unique because many individuals who are learning skills presented in Levels II and III of the continuum may, at the same time, be working on basic self-help skills presented in Level I. For example, an individual who is in an Outdoor Adventure (Skill Level III) program may also be working on his or her personal hygiene and toileting skills, which are classified as Level I. General recreation programs group individuals into the most appropriate skill levels to meet individual needs. A day camp program, therefore, may divide into specific skill level groups to work on the competencies listed on the assessment sheets. However, the entire group will get together to eat lunch and participate in scheduled group socialization activities.

As different programs use the continuum as a guideline for planning program objectives and activities, the flexibility of the continuum becomes apparent. In some general activity programs, for example, children benefit from skills listed in more than one level.

For those in the process of moving from Level I to Level II, the most appropriate activities for them might be a mixture of skills listed in both levels. An individual could be learning the gross motor skills presented in Level II and at the same time benefit from the tactile stimulation activities presented in Level I. A teen with a severe physical disability who, because of his or her physical involvement, is in Skill Level I may become involved in a Level III program because it best fulfills his or her cognitive, social, and emotional needs. For example, a teenager with a degenerative disease and severe physical involvement may no longer benefit from Skill Level I and II activities. Therefore, he or she may become part of the Level III Outdoor Adventure Program for teens with physical disabilities because it gives the opportunity to learn more about the community and to socialize with peers.

CITY OF MIAMI DEPARTMENT OF RECREATION, PROGRAMS FOR PERSONS WITH DISABILITIES

Introduction and Background

With the thought that it is the responsibility of municipal government to provide services to citizens who are disabled, the City of Miami has developed a comprehensive system to serve persons with disabilities. Programs for Persons with Disabilities was formed in 1973.

The City of Miami has been a national leader in obtaining funding from outside sources to support special recreation services. Monies were obtained, for example, from the U.S. Department of Education Office of Special Education and Rehabilitation Services for Project STAR (Staff Training for Adapted Recreation). The purpose of Project STAR was to develop an in-service training model to be used by public park and recreation departments to prepare their staff to include citizens with disabilities as participants in their programs. City of Miami recreation staff members, of course, were able to benefit from training provided through Project STAR.

Another example of a project funded by an outside source was Project CARE (Continuum of Adapted Recreation Education). Project CARE was designed to address leisure education needs of citizens with disabilities who live in the greater Miami area. This project, too, was funded by a grant from the U.S. Department of Education Office of Special Education and Rehabilitation Services.

Information in this section was taken from materials furnished by the City of Miami, Department of Recreation, Programs for Persons with Disabilities.

Project CARE was based on a full-spectrum participation philosophy. According to this philosophical position, no member of society, including the estimated 60,000 citizens with disabilities residing in Miami, should be denied the right to participate in and benefit from a full range of leisure education experiences.

Goals and Objectives

The following goals exemplify the interests of this program.

1. Monitor and ensure the city's compliance with the Rehabilitation Act of 1973, as amended by the Americans with Disabilities Act (ADA), and other state, federal, and local legislation that impacts the city's services.
2. Give impetus to the City of Miami ADA Board.
3. Coordinate city services that relate to the community's people with special needs.
4. Monitor compliance with city building and housing codes and the sensitivity of these to the needs of people with disabilities.
5. Serve as a communication link between the City of Miami government and citizens who have disabilities.
6. Secure state, federal, foundation, and private funding for the provision of existing and additional services.

Participants and Programs

The following are five types of services provided by the Programs for Persons with Disabilities:

1. *Barrier-Free Design*—Assist with the development of plans for the removal of architectural barriers from the community's park and governmental facilities. Acquire funds to complete this work.
2. *Leisure Services*—Provision of leisure-time services and special events to citizens with disabilities who are not able to become involved in programs with the general population.
3. *Work-Oriented Activity Center*—Activities in self-help skills, prevocational aptitude, academics, and supported employment to improve the independence of previously institutionalized citizens as well as those living at home or in sheltered living arrangements.
4. *Community Relations*—Information source for community members in areas related to various groups with special needs.
5. *Training for Adapted Recreation*—The in-service training of general recreation staff to recognize the attitudinal and architectural barriers that prohibit the delivery of equal services to persons with disabilities in a recreational setting.

The City of Miami developed a continuum flow pattern for appropriate placement in leisure and education programs. The level of advancement begins with the Leisure on Wheels program in the homes of individuals who are homebound. Leisure on Wheels focuses on participants who are not in an organized program because of behavioral problems or functional level. This homebound program serves the individual for two hours per day, two days per week. A parent or guardian of the homebound individual is encouraged to become involved with the program on a regular basis.

The next phase of the flow pattern is the Transitional Training Program. This segment is designed to transfer the homebound participant into a more involved community skills program designed to expand the participant's successful inclusion into the general community. The final phase in the flow pattern, prior to total integration into the mainstream of the community, is the general recreation program offered by Programs for Persons with Disabilities. Components of this program include, but are not limited to, activities such as creative arts, sports and fitness, outdoor education, aquatics, and special events.

As can be readily surmised, the City of Miami Programs for Persons with Disabilities has many thrusts. The primary focus, however, remains that of providing citizens with special needs in the Miami area with equal access to recreation services.

DISTRICT OF COLUMBIA DEPARTMENT OF RECREATION, SPECIAL PROGRAMS DIVISION

Introduction and Background

The Program for the Mentally Retarded & Physically Handicapped (MRPH), later changed to Special Programs Division, was initiated in 1954 by the District of Columbia Department of Recreation. A three-week summer day camp was established for 30 elementary-age children with orthopedic impairments on a budget of $2,161 donated by United Cerebral Palsy. The development of services evolved in four major phases: the initial years, 1954–1961, which depicted the growing pains of the program; the developmental years, 1962–1965, in which potential and actual growth in services occurred; the expansion years, 1966–1969, which saw major financial aid to the program; and the reorganization years, 1970–1974, which provided cohesive management and administration of the program. Today the program provides comprehensive therapeutic recreation services involving a continuum of care to an enrollment of more than 3,000 with a year-round staff of 40 (both certified therapeutic recreation specialists and assistants) and an

---

Information in this section was taken from materials furnished by the D.C. Department of Recreation, Special Programs Division.

additional summer staff of 70 (mostly high school and college students). Service components offered by the program include programming, counseling, job placement, referrals, transportation, outreach, training and technical assistance, media/material services, and consultation. The program operates six centers and four day camps that are school, park, and recreation-based settings located throughout the city in wards I, II, III, IV, and VI of the District of Columbia's 630 square miles (Mitchell, 1975).

The Special Programs Division Managers/Directors meet yearly in April with organizations, agencies, and various other groups to advise, to exchange information with colleagues, to pool community resources, and to initiate plans to encompass recreation services to people with disabilities. The centers also maintain communication in working with parent clubs, allied disciplines, and community advisers; they confront them personally on areas of specific concerns, they present program data results of individual and group achievements in conferences, and together they discuss and suggest methods needed to achieve program effectiveness.

Various sheltered programs are available for persons with severe to profound involvement. The program provides a wide range of activities and programs centered on the following areas of development: basic independent functioning, perceptual motor skills, socialization and communication (which are exclusively in therapeutic recreation settings with programmed interaction with other levels of services), and participation in prescribed, closely supervised activities.

Transitional programs are designed specifically to assist the clients who are ready to move toward more independent recreation and leisure pursuits. The Community Awareness Program (CAP) and Mainstream Project are the major vehicles for client transition. Intramural sport teams, D.C. Special Olympics, high-risk activities, wheelchair sports, and Boy Scout and Girl Scout clubs are also highly utilized.

A significant step toward meeting the recreation and leisure interests of persons with disabilities in the District of Columbia has been the opening of the D.C. Center for Therapeutic Recreation. This publicly funded municipal recreation center, opened in 1977, was specifically planned and designed for use by individuals with disabilities, with the ultimate goal of fostering the mainstreaming of participants into regular programs.

From the center's beginning, the major disability groups enrolled in the program have been persons who have mental retardation or orthopedic and health related disabilities. Over the last few years, the participants at the center have also included persons with hearing impairments and visual, emotional, and health problems.

Architectural barriers were taken into account in the design of the D.C. Center for Therapeutic Recreation. There are no steps except to mechanical areas. Even in shower areas and outside doors, all sills are flush. Parking spaces for persons with physical disabilities are close to building entrances. All outdoor sport areas were designed for wheelchair users—including a unique miniature golf course with access slots along the curbs allowing wheelchairs free mobility on and off the course. All sinks and drinking fountains are designed and located for use by persons with disabilities. In areas where counters are required, at least a portion of these have been placed at wheelchair height. These include kitchen counters, washroom areas, arts and crafts counters, and shop counters. The specially designed swimming pool includes many features that make it accessible:

- A ramp was provided on the deck into the pool for easy direct access by wheelchairs.
- The floor of the pool was designed with a minimum slope from 2 ft 6 in. to 3 ft so that the wheelchair users with additional muscular disabilities in hands and arms would not, by gravity, roll into water over their heads.
- A deep-water alcove was provided for special training. This was protected from shallow areas by underwater railings. It is protected from ridges on the deck by a continuous bench that also serves as a wheelchair transfer point into deeper water.
- Removable guide rails were provided at one end of the pool to assist in therapy and swimming instruction.
- The pool deck was sloped back toward the pool (contrary to usual practices) to reduce water collection and slipping on the deck.

Goals and Objectives

The Special Programs Division offers a continuum of programs and services aimed at maintaining and developing basic independent functioning, perceptual motor skills, socialization, and communication skills. The division's transitional programs are directed toward moving individuals with disabilities to more independent leisure functioning.

In concert with the D.C. Public Schools' special education criteria, namely behavioral levels and functional abilities, the Special Programs Division provides the following levels of services to children, youth, and adults:

Level I. Assessment of leisure function; recreation/leisure services in community recreation centers; leisure counseling/guidance (facilitation); recreation/leisure in nonpublic sector; limited use of special recreator or therapeutic recreation services when needed, e.g., travel, special events. Fifty percent of their recreation services in regular recreation programs.

Level II. Twenty-five percent of their recreation services in regular recreation programs.

Level III. Participants in closely supervised activities such as special events, sports, etc.

Level IV. Close supervision in settings; attention to fundamental motor/movement skills development.

Participants and Programs

A variety of programs are conducted by the Special Programs Division. Included in the program offerings are programs developed through federally funded projects (e.g., PREP and "I CAN").

PREP and "I CAN." A children's project, referred to as the Preschool Recreation Enrichment Program (PREP)[1] and the "I CAN"[2] system, has been employed by the staff within the Special Programs Division. The purposes of PREP are to foster the development and use of the child's fine and gross motor, social, self-help, cognitive, and language skills. The program is structured so the child can both learn and practice new skills through everyday life experiences, particularly play activities. "I CAN" is an individualized instructional management system with resource materials for teaching physical recreation and associated skills to those preschool children through youth with special needs. As a system, "I CAN" is built around a set of objectives correlated to diagnostic assessment instruments, prescription instruction through diagnosis, evaluation, and planning individualized instruction. The child is guided through a continuum of skills that are needed for health and fitness.

An example of a program schedule of activities follows.

Example of a Program Schedule, D.C. Center for Therapeutic Recreation

Monday thru Friday

8:30 A.M.–2:30 P.M.	Preschool	2 1/2 to 5 years
8:30 A.M.–6:00 P.M.	Day Care	3 to 5 years
9:00 A.M.–10:00 A.M.	Infant Stimulation	6 mos to 2 years
10:00 A.M.–11:00 A.M.	Activity/Swimming (St. Elizabeth's)	ADULTS
2:00 P.M.–4:00 P.M.	Life Skills (St. Elizabeth's)	20 years & above
6:00 P.M.–8:00 P.M.	Community (Gym)	20 years & above

---

1. Designed and developed by Karen Littman of the Maryland National Capital Park and Planning Commission through a grant from the Bureau of Education for the Handicapped. Office of Education, U.S. Department of Health, Education, and Welfare.

2. The "I CAN" system was developed by Dr. Janet Wessel of Michigan State University through a grant from the Bureau of Education for the Handicapped. Office of Education, U.S. Department of Health, Education, and Welfare.

Monday thru Wednesday

9:30 A.M.–11:30 A.M.	Activity/Swimming (St. Elizabeth's)	20 years & above
1:30 P.M.–3:30 P.M.	Workshop/Auto	20 years & above
6:00 P.M.–8:00 P.M.	Mechanics (Disabled & Able-bodied)	
(Feb–Apr)		

Monday and Thursday

11:00 A.M.–12 noon	Preschool	2 1/2 to 5 years
9:30 A.M.–12:15 P.M.	Swimming Program (MR)	20 years & above
5:00 P.M.–6:00 P.M.	Basketball Practice (CYO)	9 to 16 years

Tuesday

8:30 A.M.–2:30 P.M.	Infant Stimulation	6 mos to 3 years

Tuesday and Thursday

9:30 A.M.–12:15 P.M.	Adult Activity	20 years & above
11:30 A.M.–12:30 P.M.	Activity/Swim Community	ADULTS
12 noon–1:00 P.M.	Activity/Swim Hope Village	ADULTS
1:00 P.M.–2:00 P.M.	Infant Swim	6 mos to 2 years
1:30 P.M.–3:30 P.M.	Activity/Swim Community	ADULTS
5:00 P.M.–6:00 P.M.	Activity/Swim Area B Community Mental Health	ADULTS
6:00 P.M.–8:00 P.M.	Activity/Swim	ADULTS
	Open Swim	ALL AGES
	Walk-in Swim	
	(Handicapped Hospital for Sick Children)	

Tues., Wed., & Thursday

6:00 P.M.–8:30 P.M.	Basketball Practice (wheelchair)	20 years & above

Thursday

9:30 A.M.–3:30 P.M.	Community/Activity	20 years & above

Tuesday & Thursday

3:30 P.M.–4:45 P.M.	Community/Non-handicapped)	9 to 16 years

Wednesday

1:30 P.M.–3:30 P.M.	Activity/Swim (St. Elizabeth's)	ADULTS
5:00 P.M.–6:00 P.M.	Activity/Swim (Mamie D. Lee)	ADULTS
6:00 P.M.–8:00 P.M.	Walk-in Swim	ADULTS

MAINE-NILES ASSOCIATION OF SPECIAL RECREATION (ILLINOIS)

Introduction and Background

Several special recreation associations have been established in Illinois since the early 1970s. The Maine-Niles Association of Special Recreation (M-NASR) is one of several such associations established because member park districts recognized that the leisure needs of individuals with disabilities were not being met. Committed to the idea that individuals have the *need* and *right* to make productive and enjoyable use of their leisure time within their own communities, in 1972, seven park districts and one municipal agency (withdrew in 1981) became supportive members of Maine-Niles Association of Special Recreation. M-NASR was formed under special legislation in the state of Illinois that permits two or more park districts or municipalities to join together to form a special recreation association to serve persons with disabilities.

M-NASR is dedicated to providing comprehensive leisure services for children and adults having diverse disabling conditions. Persons with various levels of mental retardation, physical disability, emotional disturbance, hearing impairments, visual impairments, and multiple disabilities are provided opportunities for quality leisure activities specifically oriented toward individual ability levels and limitations.

It must be realized that not every individual who has a disability is in need of specialized recreation services. M-NASR has taken the position of selecting and evaluating the programs of the member park districts on their appropriateness for individuals with disabilities. As the Americans with Disabilities Act became federal law, M-NASR became proactive in integration programming by forming a task force to study integration with member park districts. The Youth Baseball Team and Latchkey program were developed to provide for better integration. Other integrated programs have been designed for those individuals able to participate in some of the ongoing park district programs. In those cases, consultation and professional input from the M-NASR staff is provided. By offering recreation programs in the mainstream of the community and by providing opportunities for involvement in new situations and environments, individuals with limiting conditions can learn and become comfortable with leisure opportunities that they will later be able to pursue independently.

Information in this section was taken from materials furnished by the Maine-Niles Association of Special Recreation.

Goals and Objectives

The mission of the Maine-Niles Association of Special Recreation is to facilitate growth and self-direction, achieved by active participation in enjoyable leisure opportunities for those individuals with special needs. M-NASR programs emphasize the development of appropriate social skills, foster creative expression, and promote physical fitness, resulting in an appreciation of one's own value. All individuals are encouraged to seek the fullest possible independent community involvement. Recreational involvement may take place through parallel programming (where M-NASR provides the program within the community for individuals of similar abilities and age) or through integrative programming (where M-NASR provides support services to integrate appropriate individuals with disabilities into member district programs).

The staff at the Maine-Niles Association has developed these basic program philosophies:

1. *Programs may be leisure-oriented.* This will allow opportunities for relaxing, self-motivated leisure experiences that can eventually be pursued independently.
2. *Programs may be individualized and goal-oriented.* These programs can be structured to meet individual therapeutic or remedial needs.
3. *Programs may be an extension of the educational program in which the participant is involved.* Information can be obtained from classroom teachers and professional school staff members. A leisure program can then be structured to reinforce educational objectives.

Participants and Programs

Funding for M-NASR is primarily through special legislation that allows park districts to tax up to 4 cents per $100 of assessed valuation to fund programs for individuals with disabilities. M-NASR operates on a budget of contributions from local member park districts and other sources. Sources such as foundation and corporate gifts, grants, fees, and charges make up approximately one quarter of the operating budget. M-NASR has received grants from the American Camping Association, the Illinois Department of Mental Health, and the Illinois Arts Council; such grants have kept program fees to a minimum.

Many of the children's programs stress *cooperation, skill development,* and *positive self-image.* Even with the tremendous amount of variety in programming, individual participants get plenty of attention. A much-needed volunteer core of community residents provides more than 3,000 hours a year of free service, making possible a ratio of one staff member to every four participants. Nevertheless, M-NASR policy dictates that a trained recreation specialist supervise every program.

M-NASR programs have been designed to meet the individual needs of every participant with age-appropriate activities. Recreation and leisure services are offered to all ages and disability groups year-round. In addition to more than 250 programs and some 75 special events offered annually, M-NASR sponsors leisure education programs, several day camps, overnight camping trips, and SOAR (Special Outdoor Adventure Recreation).

More than 200 children and some 100 adults enroll in camp programs each summer. A leisure education program takes place during the academic school day and includes nature activities, bowling, music, sports, and many other activities. Whenever possible, children are mainstreamed into affiliate park district programs. For example, seven children from one of M-NASR's ice skating classes were placed into the regular Park Ridge Recreation and Park District ice skating program for eight weeks. At the end of the session, three of these children performed in the Annual Ice Show.

The Maine-Niles Association of Special Recreation provides cooperative programs with many agencies, including Lutheran General Hospital and Forest Day School. A recent development is a statewide burn camp being planned with the Illinois Fire Safety Alliance. In addition, Special Recreation Associations (SRA) work very closely with the special education districts, fostering a total interdisciplinary approach to integrating children with disabilities into the community as active participants. This total concept incorporates the philosophy of community outreach as an integral part of SRA services.

The Maine-Niles Association of Special Recreation has received recognition from numerous sources as an outstanding program. The Association received awards from the Illinois Therapeutic Recreation Society (1978) and was named 1981 winner of the National Gold Medal Award for "Outstanding Community Achievement for Disabled Citizens" by the Medalist Industries.

MONTGOMERY COUNTY RECREATION DEPARTMENT, THERAPEUTIC RECREATION SECTION

Introduction and Background

Montgomery County Department of Recreation is located in Silver Spring, Maryland. The Therapeutic Recreation Section of the Montgomery County Department of Recreation conducted a needs-assessment survey in 1984 to collect data that were used to determine program needs and direction. A lack of mainstreaming opportunities was identified as a major gap in service and became a focal point.

The Mainstreaming Initiative has been strongly endorsed by the Montgomery County Executive and County Council as well as the County's Commission on Handicapped Individuals. Billie Wilson points out that "This initiative goes beyond a single program or activity and includes a process which uses 'special' programs which are segregated in nature as stepping-stones to more normalized and integrated experiences" (B. Wilson, personal communication, 1990).

Information in this section was taken from materials furnished by the Montgomery County Recreation Department.

The Mainstreaming Initiative of Montgomery County, Maryland, was developed to provide non-segregated and age-appropriate recreation services for all citizens with disabilities. (Courtesy of Montgomery County Department of Recreation, Silver Spring, MD)

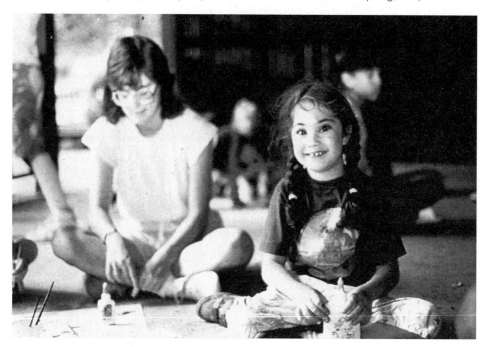

Goals and Objectives

Program goals were developed and include the following:

1. Provide the range of options necessary to meet individual needs of all recipients in the areas of recreation activities and leisure opportunities.
2. Provide access to nonsegregated recreation services for all citizens with disabilities appropriate to their chronological age.
3. Promote access to recreation services that encourages interaction with nondisabled peers, using, whenever possible, the principle of natural proportion (i.e., citizens with disabilities shall, whenever possible, be integrated into community-based services, activities, and programs in the same proportion as disabling conditions appear in the wider community). The ratio of disabled persons to nondisabled persons is 1:10.
4. Develop strategies for the meaningful participation of citizens with disabilities in recreation and leisure activities.
5. Provide a coordinating staff committed to high-quality services, activities, and programs, and the enhancement of cooperation at all levels of the service system that would monitor the provided services.
6. Promote meaningful participation of all consumers, especially in the determination of programs and services and their development and evaluation.

Figure 8.1. Challenge levels of Montgomery County (MD) Therapeutics Recreation Section.

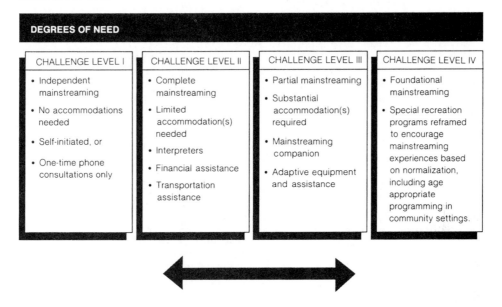

DEGREES OF NEED

CHALLENGE LEVEL I	CHALLENGE LEVEL II	CHALLENGE LEVEL III	CHALLENGE LEVEL IV
• Independent mainstreaming • No accommodations needed • Self-initiated, or • One-time phone consultations only	• Complete mainstreaming • Limited accommodation(s) needed • Interpreters • Financial assistance • Transportation assistance	• Partial mainstreaming • Substantial accommodation(s) required • Mainstreaming companion • Adaptive equipment and assistance	• Foundational mainstreaming • Special recreation programs reframed to encourage mainstreaming experiences based on normalization, including age appropriate programming in community settings.

Participants and Programs

To operationalize the mainstreaming process, challenge levels were used as a means to identify an individual's abilities and determine accommodations needed for participation in specific programs or activities. Accommodations can include transportation assistance, mainstreaming companions, and financial assistance.

Since people are at different ability and functioning levels, each time an individual with a disability is mainstreamed into a general recreation program or activity, the process is unique to that situation. Even the same individual may choose a more independent mode for one recreation program and opt for less independence for another activity.

The Therapeutic Recreation Section has developed the concept of challenge levels to depict the mainstreaming process (see Figure 8.1 and Table 8.2). When participating in a particular activity, an individual's degree of need determines the amount of support required to make a mainstreaming experience successful. The challenge levels do not reflect a continuum but are treated as separate entities wherein activity choice is the primary concern.

Staff members of the Therapeutic Recreation Section believe that leisure education must be an integral part of the mainstreaming process because educating individuals about various leisure resources and available accommodations enhances their integration

Table 8.2 Foundational Mainstreaming Opportunities (Challenge Level IV)

(Challenge Level IV): Special Recreation Programs

Adult Activities

Adult clubs include dances, parties, community trips, and social opportunities.
Adult Social Club—Adults who are mentally retarded.
Adult Swim—Adapted aquatics for adults with disabilities.
Confidence Bound—Club for young adults (ages 18–25) who are mentally retarded.
Inwood House—Leisure education and ongoing workshops for adults with disabilities.
MCARC Square Dance—Monthly dances for adults who are mentally retarded.
Open Door—Club for adults who are emotionally recovering.
Socializers—Club for adults with learning disabilities, physical disabilities, and vision and hearing impairments.
Stroke Club—Adults with disabilities resulting from strokes.

Teen Activities

Teen clubs offer weekly activities including outdoor activities, dances, parties, and community trips.
Ballet—Weekly class for youth and young adults who are mentally retarded.
Discovery Teen Club—Teens with physical disabilities.
Teen Scene—Club for teens who are mentally retarded.
TIME Teen Club—Teens with learning disabilities.
(Civiteens is a twin club cosponsored with the City of Rockville, Department of Recreation. Rockville residents are given first priority.)

Children's Activities

Children's programs are structured to include creative activities involving the arts, physical fun, and social interaction.
After-School Programs—For children and teens with disabilities (at various locations).
Expressive Arts and Sports Program (EASP)—Children (ages 6–12) with disabilities.

Summer Programs

Day camps for children and teens include swimming, nature lore, outdoor activities, arts and crafts, cooking fun, and community trips.
Beep Ball—Softball league for children and adults with vision impairments.
Camp Blackfoot—Children (ages 6–12) with learning or emotional disabilities.
Camp Chickadee—Preschool children (ages 2–6) with language delays.
Camp Apollo—Children (ages 7–12) who are mentally retarded.
Camp Chesapeake—Teens (ages 13–21) who are mentally retarded.
Camp Sligo Woods—Preschool children (ages 3–6) with developmental disabilities.
Crafts Workshops—A selection of craft specialties offered to adults with disabilities.
Creative Afternoons—UCP Camp for children with severe and profound mental and physical disabilities.
Project Discovery—Individual camps for children and teens with physical disabilities.

into community recreation programs. A comprehensive eight-week leisure education curriculum has been developed and used in a variety of settings (e.g., group homes, day treatment programs) to have greater impact in the area of leisure awareness. Staff members believe that what makes this education endeavor so profitable is the intended "ripple" effect that has been built into the planning.

The mainstreaming initiative undertaken in Montgomery County has demonstrated that it is possible to integrate persons with disabilities into community-based recreation programs. The staff members have done a nice job advertising their programs via flyers and other promotional materials with the invitation, "Recreation is for everyone . . . and that means you!"

The following comment from a parent says it all: "Ben has had very successful experiences at summer camp because of the Mainstreaming Program. He has a lot of fun, is excited about the activities, and, most of all, enjoys the opportunity to be 'just one of the kids.'"

RCH, INC. (FORMERLY RECREATION CENTER FOR THE HANDICAPPED, INC.), SAN FRANCISCO, CALIFORNIA

Introduction and Background

RCH, Inc., established in 1952 by Janet Pomeroy, is recognized nationally and internationally as a pioneer program and a model in developing community recreation for persons with disabilities. The center was founded with private funds in one room of an old pool building owned by the San Francisco Recreation and Park Department, with six teenagers with physical disabilities enrolled and with only volunteer help. When the center moved into a newly constructed facility in 1973, enrollment had increased to 650 children, teens, and adults with a wide range of disabilities, served by a paid professional staff of 80 and a corps of 120 volunteers. Today the center is a major provider of services to persons with disabilities in the City and County of San Francisco, with an enrollment of more than 1,800 and a professional staff of more than 150 workers.

A large proportion of the operating budget is raised annually by the board of directors through personal solicitation of individuals, service clubs, and groups; by letter solicitation of individuals; and by working with groups who conduct benefits for the center. Fund-raising events such as horse shows, luncheons, and bazaars are conducted annually by these groups. It should be noted that parents of participants as well as some persons with disabilities themselves assist the board in all fund-raising events. For example, one major contribution made by parents is a yearly donation of a bus as a result of fund-raising activities.

Information in this section was taken from materials furnished by RCH, Inc.

Goals and Objectives

From the beginning, the center has changed and evolved to keep pace with changing conditions and community needs. The center is a community-based facility that serves individuals of all ages and disabilities. The mission of RCH, Inc., embodies the following objectives:

- to provide programs in recreation and leisure, vocational rehabilitation and supported employment, adult development, children's services, and respite care services for individuals of all ages who have all types of disabilities
- to promote the development of the recreation and social skills appropriate and necessary for successful participation in community life
- to promote the development of vocational training skills needed for successful community-based employment
- to create and provide programs designed to give people with disabilities the opportunity to live and work safely in the least restrictive environment
- to educate the community by serving as advocates for the rights of persons with disabilities, and by training professionals in methods to meet the community's changing needs

Participants and Programs

In 1970, the center initiated an Outreach Program to serve the needs of children, teens, and adults who could not participate in programs at the center. Social recreation programs are now being offered to persons in their own homes, in board and care homes for individuals with mental retardation, and in residential care homes. These include "travel groups" designed to integrate groups into the community and "Project 1:1," which provides volunteers on a 1:1 basis for those who are homebound. The center's "Playtime" program offers services to children with chronic and terminal illnesses in home and hospital settings.

Many groups with special needs are represented among those who participate at the center or through the Outreach Program. The majority of participants have mental retardation or physical disabilities. A growing population at the center are people with acquired head injuries who participate in the "Brainstorm" program. In addition, the center has seen an influx of children with emotional disorders, as well as adults who are dually diagnosed with mental retardation and developmental disability. The center also has special programs designed to meet the needs of people with spinal cord injuries, arthritis, and multiple sclerosis.

The center is located on 5 1/2 wooded acres adjacent to a lake, near the ocean and the San Francisco Zoo. Accessible facilities include a large main hall and stage that is home to "Theatre Unlimited," the center's famous mainstreamed theater company. Related facilities include a full-service kitchen, arts-and-crafts-room, and four multipurpose rooms. The center also has an indoor therapeutic swimming pool heated to 95° and measuring 25 ft × 75 ft, as well as a full-size gymnasium and wooded day camp area. The center utilizes a variety of community facilities, including a YMCA Camp in the Santa Cruz Mountains, which plays host to the center's Residential Camp Program for children and adults. Their Outdoor Environmental Education Program also uses such natural resources as national parks and forests for senior retreats and adventure trips.

Primary day, evening, and weekend programs are offered through five departments providing direct service to center participants. Those departments include Adult Development, Children and Teens, Community Leisure Training, Leisure/Outreach, and Adult Behavior. Support services are provided by Aquatics/PE, Social Services, and Transportation. The center owns and operates 26 vehicles, including lift vans providing services to more than 300 participants on a regular basis. Department programs include such therapeutic recreation activities as nutrition education, music, and sports and games adapted for participants of all ages and abilities.

Their new Children's Annex, dedicated in April, 1989, provides preschool, infant, and respite-care programs. The pre-school program serves children ages 3 to 5 in a mainstreamed setting, with infant care for those with special needs. The respite-care program offers 24-hour services in four beautifully designed respite-care rooms. The annex was built through the charitable contributions of several foundations and individuals who were interested in helping the Center achieve its goal of "meeting the needs of the community."

RCH, Inc., has many unique programs that have not been discussed. One such program, Theatre Unlimited, is discussed in considerable detail in Chapter 10. Also, it is important to point out that the center has been dynamic and progressive throughout the years. As Janet Pomeroy indicated in their 40th anniversary report,

> Access to Success—the theme of this Anniversary Report—reflects our basic goal of helping people push beyond any limits imposed by disabilities to live full, rewarding lives. At RCH, Inc., success is measured individually. For some participants, it means standing upright without assistance. For others, it might mean learning to dress and groom themselves. And for still others, success can be measured by developing skills, getting a job, doing it well and becoming self-sufficient. Our greatest joy has also been our greatest accomplishment: an estimated 16,000 Center participants have successfully integrated into community life since 1952. (*Anniversary Report*, 1992)

SUMMARY

By briefly reviewing different special recreation programs, including two that have "centers" (Washington, D.C., and San Francisco), it should be apparent that similarities and differences exist in all programs. For example, philosophically all programs tend to aim toward integrating individuals with disabilities into the mainstream. Yet, some programs offer fewer segregated activities than others. The Cincinnati Recreation Program purports to offer a fairly structured program skill level continuum and the Montgomery County Recreation Department has developed the concept of challenge levels to depict the mainstreaming process. The Austin and Miami Programs also tend to provide noteworthy continua, ranging from adaptive recreation services to integrated programming. Others offer a range of programs even though they may not be organized along a formal continuum. Although programs tend to focus on individual growth and development, family programs are included in programming efforts.

The emphasis on therapeutic effects also tends to vary from program to program. While some programs focus almost exclusively on the recreative experience, others give more emphasis to therapeutic benefits.

A full range of activities is being offered. Programs range from infant stimulation and preschool recreation (PREP) to senior citizen aquatics. Reflective of the varied nature of recreation programming designed to meet the needs, interests, and abilities of the specific population, programs address self-help skills, athletics and fitness, health education, home economics, arts, music, and drama among other areas.

Interagency cooperation was specifically illustrated in most program descriptions. Such cooperation is important to the success of special recreation services in the community.

In 1985, Schleien and Werder put forth recommendations for future special recreation programming. These included better networking with other community agencies, expanding activity offerings, more integrating of individuals with disabilities into recreation programs with nondisabled participants, increasing the number of specially trained personnel, and improving the accessibility and availability of special recreation programs and services.

Programs like the ones discussed in this chapter have set the tone for new and improving programs and services for the 1990s and beyond.

For individuals who desire further information, the agency addresses for the programs referenced in this chapter are as follows:

- Adaptive Programs
  Austin Parks and Recreation Department
  Municipal Building, Eighth at Colorado
  P.O. Box 1088
  Austin, TX 78767

- Division of Therapeutic Recreation
  Cincinnati Recreation Commission
  222 East Central Parkway
  Cincinnati, OH 45202

- Programs for People with Disabilities
  Department of Leisure Services
  City of Miami
  P.O. Box 330708
  Miami, FL 33133

- Therapeutic Recreation Services
  D.C. Department of Recreation
  3149 Sixteenth Street, N.W.
  Washington, DC 20010

- Maine-Niles Association of Special Recreation
  7640 Main Street
  Niles, IL 60648

- Therapeutic Recreation Section
  Montgomery County Recreation Department
  12210 Bushey Drive
  Silver Spring, MD 20902–1099

- RCH, Inc.
  207 Skyline Boulevard
  San Francisco, CA 94132

SUGGESTED LEARNING ACTIVITIES

1. Obtain information about community-based recreation programs for individuals with disabilities in your own community, and present your findings orally or in writing.
2. Given specific demographic factors in your community, indicate how you would implement a special recreation program for persons with disabilities.
3. Invite local recreation personnel into class to discuss their program philosophy, goals, and activities. Then compare their offerings and themes to those outlined in this chapter.

REFERENCES

Anniversary Report (40 years). San Francisco: RCH, Inc. 1992.

Mitchell, Helen Jo. *The History of Recreation Services for the Mentally Retarded and Physically Handicapped in the District of Columbia Department of Recreation: 1954–1974.* Unpublished master's thesis, University of Maryland, 1975.

Schleien, S. J., & J. K. Werder. Perceived responsibilities of special recreation services in Minnesota. *Therapeutic Recreation Journal, 19*(3), 51–62, 1985.

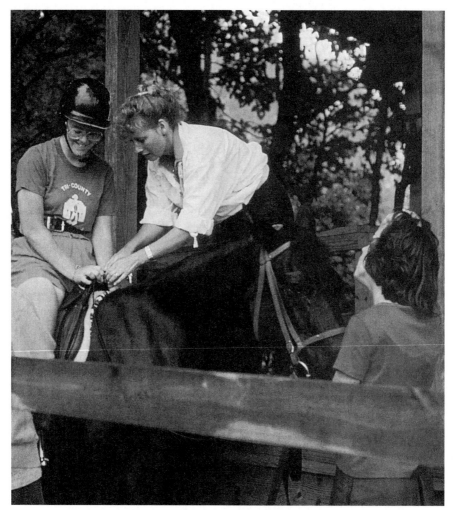

(Photo courtesy of Bradford Woods, Indiana University)

PART THREE

INCLUSIVE AND SPECIAL RECREATION PROGRAM AREAS

The following section highlights activities and successful programs that enable people with disabilities to pursue their recreational interests. Chapter 9, Camping and Wilderness-Adventure Experiences, describes actual and potential contributions that organized camping and wilderness experiences offer to people who have disabilities. The importance of qualified and enthusiastic leadership is stressed, and a detailed presentation on wilderness-adventure programs is included. Chapter 10, The Arts—for Everyone, outlines the benefits of arts participation for everyone. A special section features information on Very Special Arts. The chapter concludes with two examples that emphasize the deep, personal meaning that comes from participation in the arts. Selected sports programs for people with disabilities are covered in Chapter 11, Competitive Sports. The pros and cons of competitive sports programs are discussed, and detailed information on wheelchair sports, the Special Olympics, and the Barrie Integrated Baseball Association is provided.

The emphasis of Part III is on the benefits to people with disabilities of well-organized and professionally directed recreation activities. Most of the activities presented are easily incorporated into inclusive programs. Some of these activities, however, such as wheelchair sports and Special Olympics, restrict participation to people with disabilities. Including such examples in no way implies that we advocate segregated programming for most people who have disabilities. To the contrary, we feel that each person with a disability should participate in the least restrictive recreational environment. We have highlighted some segregated recreation programs solely because they allow us to identify more clearly the benefits of a given recreational activity for all people with disabilities.

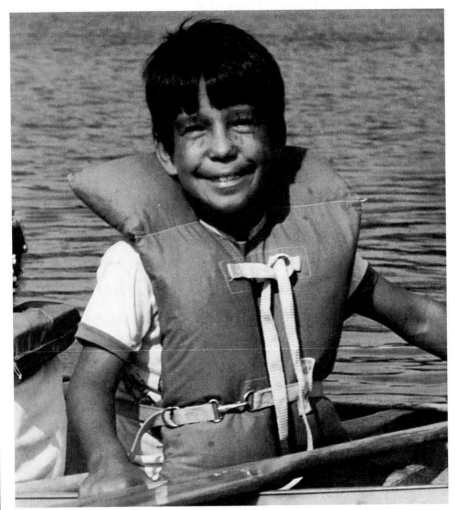

(Courtesy of The League: Serving People with Physical Disabilities, Inc., Baltimore, MD)

9

Camping and Wilderness-Adventure Experiences

If you ask a group of people to define *camping,* you might get as many definitions as there are people in the group. To one person, camping might mean backpacking through California's High Sierras. To another, it may bring back memories of childhood scouting trips to lakeside woods. Yet another person may picture himself or herself sitting in an elaborate recreational vehicle parked in a neatly arranged campground. In truth, the word *camping* has come to refer to a wide variety of outdoor experiences. The equipment may range from simple to sophisticated; the surroundings, primitive to developed; and the activities, nature based to indoor oriented. Camping means many things to many people. This chapter, however, is concerned with *organized* camping programs and their potential for benefiting individuals with disabilities.

As the term implies, *organized camping* refers to outdoor living experiences that are carefully structured and supervised. The American Camping Association (ACA), a nationwide organization dedicated to organized camping, provides the following definition:

> [Camping is] a sustained experience which provides a creative, recreational and educational opportunity in group living in the out-of-doors. It utilizes trained leadership and the resources of natural surroundings to contribute to each camper's mental, physical, social, and spiritual growth. (American Camping Association, 1980, p. 8)

Clearly, then, camping as referred to in this textbook does not pertain to "escaping" urban living in recreation vehicles with all the comforts of home, nor does it apply to the solo backpacker who sets out on an extended hiking expedition. Each of these activities may meet the needs of its participants, but neither contains all of the essential components of an organized camping experience. Betty Lyle (1947) wrote that five components are common to any definition of organized camping, including (1) out-of-doors, (2) recreation, (3) group living, (4) education, and (5) social adjustment. Despite the fact that her observation was made more than 45 years ago, the similarity between her remarks and the current ACA definition is striking. Adding one critical component to Lyle's list, trained leadership, provides an understanding of how organized camping differs from casual outdoor experiences. It is a *directed* experience that combines the unique properties of nature with the developmental potential of human group interaction. As an editorial in *Camping Magazine* (American Camping Association, 1985) stated:

> [Organized camping] is living in a community of people. It is face-to-face contact with the ebb and flow of human life—it is the civilizing, socializing, humanizing process of people working and playing and living together, closely, intimately. It is experimenting with hopes and aspirations, joys and sorrows, laughter and tears, successes and failures, moods and temperaments, and all humanity. It is *group* living—strong, virile, robust living together in the realm of people. Minus this human element, it is not organized camping. (p. 22)

Camping is fun, but equally important, it offers unlimited opportunities for human interaction and personal growth. Each year, thousands of campers go to summer camps expecting to become more comfortable with nature; most return more comfortable with themselves.

CAMPING AND PEOPLE WITH DISABILITIES

Until recently, most camping opportunities for persons with disabilities have been confined to segregated experiences. Camps were designed and built to accommodate the unique needs of children and adults with disabilities; moreover, programs were developed to facilitate each camper's personal growth within the "protected" social environment of peers with similar disabilities. Recent legislation, however, especially the Individuals with Disabilities Education Act (IDEA) and the Americans with Disabilities Act (ADA) (see Chapter 3), has helped to expand inclusive camping opportunities for people with disabilities.

Segregated Camping Programs

Camping for people with special needs is traced to the 1880s, but it was not until the 1930s that a concerted effort was made to provide segregated camping opportunities for large numbers of people with disabilities. At first, these programs focused on therapy and treatment for children, but the camp environment's potential to aid personal growth of the *total* individual was eventually recognized by camp leaders. Since the 1960s, most camps for people with disabilities have closely paralleled camps for the general population. Their goals, objectives, activities, and organizational structures are similar. Although the camper-staff ratio may vary (segregated camps for individuals with disabilities usually have fewer campers per counselor), the emphasis is the same: development of the total person through enjoyment of the out-of-doors.

The similarity between most camps for people with disabilities and so-called regular camps can be detected in the following general concepts listed by a National Easter Seal Society task force:

1. Persons with special needs should be afforded the same rewarding experiences that are available to [campers without disabilities].
2. Special programs can play a major role in the rehabilitation or habilitation of persons with special needs.
3. The sociorecreational values to be derived from association with nature through camping are inherently therapeutic without regard to any concomitant medical or paramedical benefits that may accrue.
4. Group living and working or playing situations provide social and psychological opportunities not available in the clinical or educational setting. (Hardt, 1968, p. 2)

Clearly, the unique value of a segregated camping experience is enhanced because the camp's leadership accepts a holistic view of the individual (Robinson & Skinner, 1985). All aspects of the person's life, from eating habits to activity selection, contribute to his or her personal fulfillment. Therefore, camps should provide quality opportunities in as many aspects of life as possible if the potential of a camping experience is to be fully realized. The girl who receives extensive physical therapy at camp undoubtedly benefits from the therapy. Does she, however, receive maximum benefit from all that camping has to offer? One long-time leader in the field of camping for persons with disabilities, Jeanne Feeley from Pennsylvania, emphasized the importance of camping—not therapy—in her personal philosophy statement. Her words summarize the underlying theme of this chapter.

> I believe every person, handicapped [*sic*] or not, should have at least one camp experience. . . . I believe in the intrinsic value of camping. We need to preserve these values for our children and our children's children. Let all people whether mildly, moderately, or severely handicapped know what good camping is. (Feeley, 1972, pp. 44–45)

Feeley did add one warning that should be kept in mind, however: Not everyone will enjoy camping. Some individuals will discover that outdoor activities and group living are perfectly suited to them; others will learn that the out-of-doors is not for them. The important thing is that everyone, whether having a disability or not, has the *opportunity* to experience camping. Only through personal experience can one discover the potential benefits of a camp experience. As one teenaged camper remarked recently, "I can't believe it! I didn't even want to go on this (camping) trip; now I wish I could *live* in the woods!" Opportunity enables discovery. Unfortunately, the percentage of children and adults with disabilities who have experienced camping appears to be very small; and those who have had camping opportunities were generally provided those experiences at segregated camps designed specifically for individuals with disabilities. Historically, the importance and value of segregated camps is undeniable; moreover, they continue to provide valuable opportunities for children and adults who are, for whatever reason, not prepared for inclusion into regular camping programs. Nevertheless, we agree with Havens's (1992) statement that integrated experiences "should be the priority in most cases and segregated experiences considered an alternative, or 'stepping stone'" (p. 16).

Inclusive Camping Programs

Few camps currently promote inclusion of persons with disabilities into their regular camping programs (Sable, 1992); moreover, integrated camping opportunities for persons with severe disabilities are extremely rare (Rynders, Schleien, & Mustonen, 1990). As noted earlier, however, recent legislation (i.e., IDEA, ADA) has and will continue to increase inclusion of persons with disabilities within the mainstream of society. These legislative mandates will also help to expand integrated camping opportunities for persons with disabilities. As noted by Sable, "Although in its infancy, it is encouraging to see private camp directors, youth service agencies, and parents creating inclusionary environments for children. Such environments prevent parents from being faced with the dilemma of returning to a segregated summer program for their child after intensely advocating for the integration of their child within the school program" (p. 39).

One progressive effort to integrate children with disabilities into a regular camping program was described by Sable (1992). This program, which was a cooperative venture of the University of New Hampshire's Leisure Management and Tourism Department, the Easter Seal Society of New Hampshire, and a local Boy Scout council, successfully integrated about 20 youngsters with disabilities into two camping programs at a Boy Scout facility. Except for sleeping arrangements, campers with disabilities were fully integrated in all aspects of the camping programs, including bonfires, meals, archery, swimming, sailing, and, of course, traditional "snipe" hunts. Whenever necessary, modifications and adaptations were made by counselors to facilitate participation by campers with disabilities. According to Sable, "Counselors learn early in the summer never to be very far from a supply of duct tape" (p. 41). Overall, this inclusive camping program was seen by parents of campers as a model for others to emulate, and its success is reflected in the following statement:

> Although no metric tool to measure friendships was developed, we have collected anecdotal information which supports our belief that inclusion breaks down barriers and creates a fertile environment for emerging relationships. . . . In discussing their week at camp, Scouts relate to their parents that the best thing about camp that year was getting to know some of the [campers with disabilities]. . . . Campers exchange addresses and correspond with each other after camp. . . . Scout Troops have included more boys with disabilities into their troops. (p. 42)

As camp directors fulfill their legal mandate to provide programs that are accessible to persons with disabilities, inclusive camp environments will undoubtedly expand. With this expansion will come increased awareness of the benefits that inclusion offers to *all* campers.

Camp Objectives

Each camp, whether segregated or inclusive, should establish its own general objectives. These objectives are used to guide staff decision making in all aspects of the camp, including activity selection, food preparation, discipline techniques, personnel policies, and administrative procedures. The philosophy of the camp's governing body is usually reflected in the list of general objectives. It is important, therefore, that all objectives be clearly stated in writing. Wilkinson (1981) provided a list of six general objectives that reflect a holistic view of a camp's purpose. These general objectives, developed by the American Camping Association, are appropriate for most camps, no matter how many of their campers have special needs:

1. To provide each camper with the opportunity for wholesome fun and adventure in a safe and supervised outdoor program.
2. To help develop a concept of safe and healthful living by stressing wholesome daily health habits; by stressing safety in camp skills; by offering a change for increasing strength, vitality, and endurance; and by fostering freedom from mental tensions.
3. To contribute to the development of "at-home-ness" in the natural world by imparting an understanding of and appreciation for the world of nature, by fostering an understanding of human dependency on nature and a sense of responsibility for conservation of natural resources, and by increasing the ability to use basic camping skills.
4. To increase a camper's concept of spiritual meaning and values through encouraging the development of a kinship with the security in an orderly universe, and through gaining an understanding of and appreciation for persons of other religions, cultures, nationalities, and races.
5. To encourage the development of skills and knowledge that can contribute to wholesome recreation during later years.
6. To contribute to the development of the individual through adjustment to group living in a democratic setting by instilling in him a sense of worth of each individual, by helping him to function effectively in a democratic society, and by helping him to develop a sense of social understanding and responsibility. (pp. 10–12)

Robinson and Skinner (1985) also provide some general objectives that give direction for camps that integrate campers with disabilities into traditional camp programs. These include developing positive relationships, promoting camper independence, encouraging social integration, teaching leisure skills, and having fun.

One goal of most organized camping programs is to provide group living experiences that enhance social understanding and responsibility. Camp is an ideal setting for cooperative activities that promote "togetherness" among disabled and nondisabled campers. (Courtesy of The League: Serving People with Physical Disabilities, Inc., Baltimore, MD)

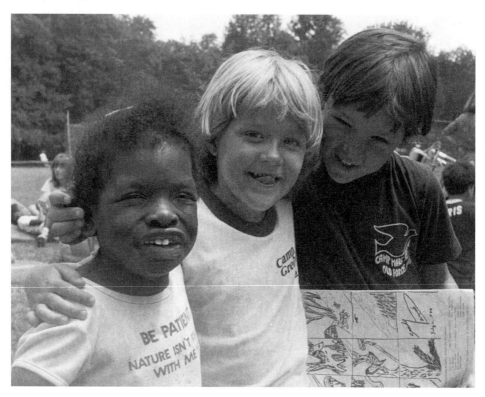

Naturally, the preceding list of general objectives may not be ideal for all camps. Also, each camp should develop specific objectives that are more limited in scope and easier to measure than general objectives. Many camps are organized by sponsoring organizations to use the outdoor setting as a way of promoting specific special interests or outcomes. Religious camps, weight-control camps, and computer camps are just a few examples of special-interest camps. General and specific objectives also may vary according to the type of camp. Day camps, resident camps, wilderness-adventure camps, trip camps, and family camps are examples of different camp types. Each type has its own advantages, and these should be emphasized within the written objectives.

Properly written and publicized camp objectives are exceedingly important because they serve two purposes. First, as stated earlier, they provide direction to all camp staff members. Thus, consistency and quality of services are more easily maintained. Second, written objectives provide essential information to parents and campers. If maximum enjoyment is to occur, the programs and operations of the camp must be well suited to the camper's individual interests. Written objectives help provide a basis for selecting the most appropriate camp. Vinton, Hawkins, Pantzer, and Farley (1978) provide five basic principles for camps serving children. The principles should help any camp create an appropriate atmosphere for achieving its objectives. They are

- Emphasize what the [child with a disability] can do rather than what he or she cannot do. Provide programs that are within range of abilities of the child.
- Stress both the fun and the educational potential of each experience equally.
- Provide a flexible program that is geared to the needs of each individual child.
- Provide a situation that is as normal as possible, deviating or adapting only when necessary.
- Stress participation in the democratic processes. Environmental education and camping should be a doing process, involving the child in all levels of planning and implementing the program. (p. 8)

Camp Leadership

Objectives provide direction in any camp program, but the camp's staff has responsibility for achieving these objectives. Anyone who has attended or worked in an organized camp can testify to the importance of a competent and enthusiastic staff. This is especially true in a camp that has campers with disabilities. It is easy for a counselor to become frustrated if the pace of camp is slowed by campers with physical disabilities, or if maintaining discipline becomes difficult because of behavioral disorders among campers. How counselors deal with these frustrations helps determine their job effectiveness, and effective counselors are critical to a camp's success.

Rodney and Ford (1971) emphasized the unique role of a camp counselor who supervises children:

The child-adult relationship at camp is a very unusual one, for in this particular setting the adult in the role of camp counselor is considered neither teacher, regulator, disciplinarian, minister, nor parent. Yet, he is a combination of all, and at the same time he is a companion and a pal. (p. 14)

Whether working with children or adults, the qualities, or personality traits, of an ideal camp counselor are almost endless. Some, however, are more important than others. Kimball (1980) emphasized "flexibility, a high degree of perseverence and tolerance for frustration, an ability to empathize, and a sense of humor" (p. 31). Creativity is certainly another vital characteristic, as is good judgment. Of course, knowledge of how to manage the special needs of campers is essential when a camp includes campers with moderate to severe disabilities. However, the single most important characteristic for any camp counselor is a genuine interest in and love for the campers. When counselors are "into" their campers, the camp's atmosphere is alive and exciting for everyone, and possibilities for personal fulfillment abound.

Effective camp counselors enable a camp to achieve its objectives. Counselors who are dedicated to the well-being of their campers provide experiences that foster personal growth and self-discovery. (Courtesy of The League: Serving People with Physical Disabilities, Inc., Baltimore, MD)

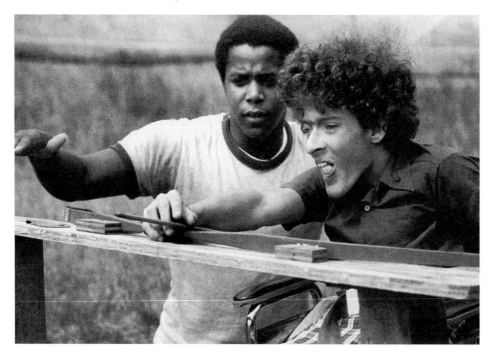

One experienced director of a camp for children with disabilities confided that he and his administrative staff once sat around a campfire discussing the attributes of previous counselors. "We selected an 'all-star' staff made up of the best counselors we had seen during the preceding 10 years," he said. "Afterwards, we tried to identify what qualities made them so exceptional. Their ages and personalities varied, but one characteristic was common to all—they *loved* being with the campers." These counselors showed their love in a variety of ways; they put the campers' needs above their own desires, they asked for the campers' ideas and tried to implement them, they were alert to risks but never over-protected the campers, and, above all, they established an atmosphere of sharing between themselves and the campers. "They all stayed a few summers and then moved on," the director said, "but their campers will never forget them." After a brief pause, he added, "And I know they will never forget their campers!"

Good counselors enable a camp to fulfill its potential. They serve as role models for the campers and promote personal growth within their group. Successful camps select their counselors wisely, and they provide them with the best possible training. As most camp directors acknowledge, a camp is only as good as its counselors.

Staff Training

One outcome of Project REACH, a federally funded program to upgrade training techniques in camping and environmental education for individuals with disabilities, was a *Camp Staff Training Series*. These publications were designed to "assist camp personnel to gain a better understanding of the nature of their jobs and to acquire those skills and competencies needed to perform their duties in an effective and professional manner" (Pearce, Vinton & Farley, 1979, p. 1).

The portion of the *Camp Staff Training Series* devoted to preparing camp counselors was particularly exciting. It included six separate instructional "modules" that were prepared by a variety of experts in the field of camping. Each module, or unit, was field tested at six different sites. The resulting publication, *Camp Counselor Training Series* (in six volumes), was packed with useful written materials and learning exercises. The six volumes included (1) "An Orientation to Camping and the Camp," (2) "Knowing the Campers," (3) "Camp Program Planning and Leadership," (4) "Camp Health and Safety Practices," (5) "Dealing with Camper Behavior," and (6) "Evaluating the Camp Experience." There is little doubt that completion of this or a similar comprehensive training program would help any counselor improve his or her skills as a camp counselor in a camp serving individuals with disabilities.

Formal staff training should also include leadership opportunities for persons with disabilities. For example, at the University of Indiana's Bradford Woods Outdoor Education, Recreation, and Camping Center, formal camp-related leadership training is provided to people with disabilities. Robb and Shepley (1988) note that leadership development programs for people with disabilities have lagged behind similar training in traditional residential and other camp settings. They emphasize: "Leadership begins with recognizing the intrinsic value of each person, and with that recognition comes the equality and integration of all people" (p. 21). They urge continued development of formal leadership training programs "so that in return we may benefit from the leadership skills and potential of everyone" (p. 21).

Whether or not a standardized training program is used, staff training is of vital importance. Each training program should do the following: include some "hands-on" experience, provide practical tips and information, specify policies and procedures, stress safety and health, and clarify program philosophy. In short, camp training must prepare staff members for all aspects of their jobs. Of primary importance, however, is preparation for being with the campers.

Knapp (1984) emphasized the need for staff training to develop interpersonal skills with campers. Reporting the results of a survey of midwestern camp personnel, Knapp listed knowledge of group dynamics, leadership skills, and techniques for building camper self-esteem as the three most important staff training topics. He added:

> Camp leaders recognize that their staff need both people skills and activity skills to perform their roles effectively. Because of time limitations, they are forced to decide what topics are most important to include in pre-camp educational workshops. The results of this study reveal that the respondents viewed the development of people skills as more important than activity skills. (p. 24)

Byrd (1972) outlined three aspects of preparation for being with campers that are unique to camps serving people with disabilities. First, information about disabilities and special needs should be simple and basic. "If a counselor is going to have a camper with muscular dystrophy," wrote Byrd, "he does not need to know the detailed population incidence of [muscular dystrophy], its etiology and medical research summaries to date. He does need to know what help the [camper with muscular dystrophy] will need and how best to give it. . . . If he is fed quantities of technical medical and psychological jargon in professional terms in pre-camp, he is apt to think of the impending (carefully chosen word) camper less and less as a person, and more and more as a medical case—thus defeating one of our main purposes in camp" (pp. 140–141).

Byrd's second point was that all areas of difference between campers with disabilities and those without disabilities need to be specified. The nature of the campers' disabilities or special needs would, no doubt, determine what information should be included in this aspect of camp training. Byrd urged that physical, psychological, social, and emotional differences be specified, but he included a warning that "the danger exists of exaggerating differences and potential individual problems to the point of painting the camper as a potential monster!" (p. 141). We strongly support Byrd's caution and feel that emphasizing differences between campers with and without disabilities is generally inadvisable.

The third unique aspect offered by Byrd is the need for "empathy" training. Empathy means that you not only recognize another's situation, but you identify with that person to the point of actually experiencing his or her thoughts or feelings. It means that you *really* understand what someone else is experiencing. Byrd suggested that discussions and role playing (simulations) are two ways to achieve empathy. Some films and videotapes may be effective, too. Whatever techniques are used, however, empathy is one of the most important qualities a counselor can possess. Every camp training program should include activities designed to foster empathy, thus enabling the formation of positive attitudes toward campers who have disabilities. As noted by Stearn (1984), staff attitude is the first aspect to be analyzed when ensuring that a camp is accessible to people with disabilities.

Proper training refines the skills and attitudes of all camp staff members and enables them to offer the best possible experience to all campers, including those with disabilities. If campers are to receive the maximum benefit from their stay at camp, a well-trained staff is essential.

Benefits of Organized Camping

Camping offers many potential benefits to individuals with disabilities. Both parents and health professionals agree that the camp environment offers a unique setting for personal growth. Many individuals with disabilities have limited life experiences because of the barriers they face. Camp, however, gives a chance for exploration of oneself and the environment. It allows the flexibility to express creativity, yet provides sufficient structure for feelings of security. Above all, it offers a chance for independence of thought and action to individuals who are, regretfully, too often forced to assume a dependency role.

Table 9.1 Benefits of Camping for Persons with Disabilities: A Codified Statement

Primary Benefits	Functional Benefits
Attitudes	**Educational**
independence/self-confidence	learning opportunities
motivation	learn new skills and activities
self-awareness	opportunity for success
heightened morale	improved verbalization
improved behavior	higher academic achievement
improved discipline	creativity
improved cooperation	
respect for others	**Physical**
	activities of daily living
Social	increased opportunity for participation
socialization/informal group participation	improved coordination and physical
group identity	fitness
relationships with adults of a	
nonprofessional nature	**Vocational**
get along with others	organizing own activities
opportunity for sharing	camping as possible future employment
	initiating own activities
Environmental	
expanded environment	**Recreational**
heightened community	activities
interest/awareness	fun
opportunity for normal experiences	education for leisure
adapt to community	
adapt to family	

Advocates attribute numerous benefits to an organized camping experience. Hansen (1972) analyzed 50 references and listed the most frequently mentioned benefits. He also divided the statements included in his resources into two categories, primary benefits and functional benefits. Table 9.1 shows these categories, as well as the benefits included in each. McCormick, White, and McGuire (1992) used a statistical procedure (factor analysis) to assess the benefits that parents perceived camping offered to their children with mental retardation. Their results revealed "six dimensions of benefits of an ideal summer camp program" (p. 32). These dimensions are social skill development, social competence, respite care, cognitive development, expressive development, and physical competence. They added, "Overall, the most important benefit of summer camp, as perceived by parents of campers with mental retardation, appears to be social growth" (p. 34).

It is hoped that camp's many benefits interact to help campers with disabilities increase their own feelings of self-worth. Thus, their self-concepts are strengthened. Lundegren (1976) observed that an individual's self-concept is influenced both by interaction with others (especially significant others) and by interaction with the environment. She added, "Camping has the unique opportunity to contribute in all aspects here" (p. 263). A number of self-concept studies have supported Lundegren's statement (Hourcade, 1977; Robb, 1971; Sessoms, 1979; Shasby, Heuchert, & Gansneder, 1984), but the evidence is far from conclusive. Nevertheless, the skills and activities available in camping activities are ideally suited to self-concept improvement. Camps offer new skills to novice campers and almost unlimited opportunities for skill improvement among experienced campers. As noted by Iso-Ahola, LaVerde, and Graefe (1988), skill development and continued skill enhancement appear to be fundamental to improvements in self-concept.

Unfortunately, most of the benefits that are claimed by camping enthusiasts have only limited research support. Weaknesses in research methodology and use of questionable measures have limited the results of many camping studies. Also, some authorities doubt that short camp sessions, with young and often inexperienced counselors, could produce significant changes in campers. Still others caution that returning from camp to an institution may have negative consequences, particularly for those with psychological disorders (Polenz & Rubitz, 1977; Ryan & Johnson, 1972).

There is still much research that needs to be done, but almost everyone who has worked in camps with individuals who have disabilities can cite examples of personal growth among campers. They are convinced, as we are, that organized camping programs offer many benefits to campers, irrespective of disabilities or special needs. As Sessoms (1979) concluded, "What is known is that a purely recreationally oriented program does have value and consequences [for campers with disabilities]. It stands on its own merit; need we say more" (p. 42).

WILDERNESS-ADVENTURE PROGRAMS

One of the most exciting developments in camping and outdoor-related activities for people with disabilities has been the recent emphasis on wilderness-adventure programs. These programs provide a challenging experience for any action-oriented individual, irrespective of disabling condition (Dattilo & Murphy, 1987). They also offer participants many opportunities for physical expression and personal achievement that are *not* based on complex language skills or abstract thinking processes. Wilderness-adventure programs include challenges that can be understood in concrete terms, and they take place in an outdoor environment that maximizes feelings of personal freedom. It is precisely these qualities that make wilderness-adventure programs the ideal leisure experience for many people with disabilities.

While wilderness-adventure programs vary in format and techniques, most have been adapted from the model established by the Outward Bound program (Hollenhorst & Ewert, 1985). In the early 1960s, Outward Bound opened this program to people with special needs by incorporating "delinquent" youth into the program. By the 1980s, Outward Bound was offering challenging outdoor experiences to many individuals with disabilities. People with cerebral palsy, paraplegia, multiple sclerosis, amputations, muscular dystrophy, and many other disabilities were being given the chance to participate in Outward Bound groups composed of four nondisabled people and four individuals with disabilities (Goodwin, 1978). Other programs were also emerging, many willing to accept people who were considered too disabled by some Outward Bound programs. Wilderness Inquiry in Minnesota, C. W. Hog in Idaho, and Paraplegics on Independent Nature Trips (POINT) are a few examples of such programs. Through activities such as rock climbing, white-water rafting, canoeing, spelunking (caving), backpacking, and so on, these programs and others like them provide personal challenge at the same time that they foster interpersonal interaction and small group cooperation.

Wilderness-Adventure Experience Components

Philosophy, format, and techniques vary from program to program, but there are some components common to most, if not all, wilderness-adventure programs open to people with disabilities. The following components, although listed separately, are interrelated and combine to form an experience that, it is hoped, has lifelong meaning to participants.

1. *The experience takes place in the out-of-doors.* Most people in technological societies experience a variety of artificially constructed constraints in their daily lives. Windowless rooms in modern buildings shut out "distractions"; city lights and signs tell people when to cross the street, where to park their cars, what products to buy, and so on; schools restrict movement by insisting that each student sit at a desk until a bell rings its approval to move (usually to another desk). Examples of these constraints are limitless. People with disabilities experience all of these constraints as well as many barriers that do not limit people who do not have disabilities. Wilderness settings, however, offer a chance to overcome barriers that have not been imposed by other human beings. Adaptive behavior is required by mother nature, not by architects or school officials. For people who have disabilities that do not limit mobility, such as learning disabilities, the wilderness also offers an important chance for freedom of movement and expression while, at the same time, providing a natural, yet orderly, environment.

2. *Small group cooperation and trust in others is emphasized.* Some individuals with disabilities by necessity devote much of their daily lives to individual challenges. Not only must they overcome obstacles that do not confront their peers without disabilities, but they also may find their contributions to a group or family effort ignored or devalued. It is little wonder, therefore, that some people with disabilities have limited experience in cooperative efforts. Wilderness-adventure programs, however, provide for group experiences that require cooperation and trust. Each participant has the opportunity to

Wilderness-adventure activities offer participants personal challenges that demand discipline, concentration, and trust in others. Rapelling, for example, requires both individual skill and dependence upon fellow participants. (Courtesy of Wilderness Inquiry and Erin Broadbent/Photo by Greg Lais)

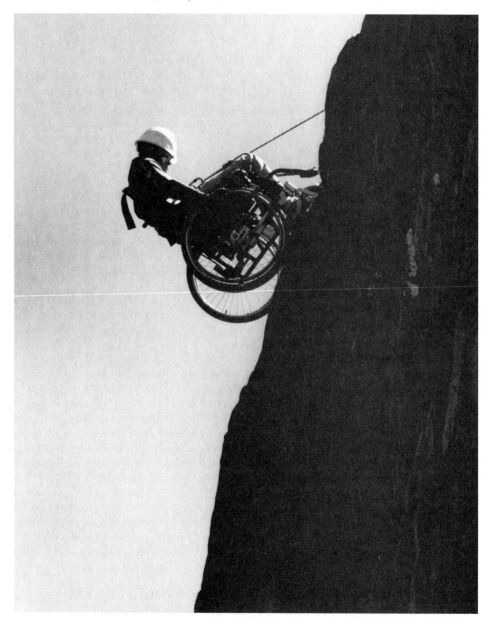

contribute to a clearly defined group goal, and because the group is small, that contribution is evident to everyone. The freshly caught fish frying over an open fire will be shared among those who caught the fish *and* those who gathered the firewood. Everyone learns that his or her efforts were of value; there could not have been a meal without *each* person's contribution. In time, a series of such activities results in a cohesive group characterized by members who not only cooperate with each other, but also trust that everyone will do his or her part. As noted by Hollenhorst and Ewert (1985), "Activities that emphasize the importance of the individual's contribution and responsibility to the group and that involve camaraderie, friendship, group decision making and problem solving should be an integral part of the [wilderness-adventure] program" (p. 33).

3. *Stressful objectives are systematically presented and successfully achieved.* In Robert Frost's poem *The Death of the Hired Man,* a farm worker who is elderly is referred to as being in a hopeless situation. He has nothing in his past to be proud of, and his future holds no hope for improvement. Unfortunately, some people feel like they are in the same situation. Their lack of success in the past, whether in school or in other aspects of their lives, has resulted in a feeling of futility toward the future. As one youth expressed emphatically, "Why should I try, man? I'd just [mess] up again!" Wilderness-adventure programs offer the participant much more than a hodge-podge of outdoor experiences. They are composed of activities that are carefully selected and systematically introduced. Whether these challenges are contrived, as with some Outward Bound activities, or occur naturally in the process of an expedition, each requires the accomplishment of a specific objective. Each objective is challenging enough to induce feelings of stress, but not so difficult that it should result in failure. To cross a stream by use of a fallen tree, the young woman with a disability must overcome her fear of falling. As important, however, is the fact that she may also be making progress toward overcoming her fear of *failing.*

4. *The group's leader is critical to program effectiveness.* Leading wilderness-adventure activities requires a great deal of experience and skill, especially when the activities involve stressful situations in unfamiliar surroundings. The leader of a wilderness-adventure group must guide the group so that objectives are achieved *by the group members themselves.* As Dattilo and Murphy (1987) point out, "The leader should systematically reduce the amount of assistance while encouraging the participants to accept more and more responsibility for making decisions that allow them to meet the challenges encountered in adventure recreation" (p. 19). At the same time, the leader needs to remain alert to the optimum level of stress for the group. Too little stress prevents a feeling of accomplishment, but too much stress can result in feelings of failure. As noted by Kimball (1980), "There is only a small difference between tension that is creative and growth oriented and tension that is defeating" (p. 12). The leader must be able to anticipate events and likely reactions of group members. He or she must not only know the techniques for accomplishing group goals, but *when* to use them. McAvoy (1987) emphasized the importance of leadership, noting that "without well-qualified leaders, [wilderness-adventure] activities and programs become dangerous to the participant, a threat to the existence of the sponsoring agency, and pose a real danger to the integrity of the natural environment where the activity takes place" (p. 460).

Project Adventure, one of the leading organizations focusing on adventure-based programming and counseling, includes two important concepts in all of its challenge activities. They are *Full Value Contract* and *Challenge by Choice*. The Full Value Contract is not a written contract; rather, it is "the process in which a group agrees to find positive value in the efforts of its members. This positive value is expressed in encouragement, goal setting, group discussion, a spirit of forgiveness, and confrontation" (Schoel, Prouty, & Radcliffe, 1988, p. 33). The Full Value Contract means that group members agree, in advance, to work together toward group goals, adhere to safety and appropriate group behavioral guidelines, and both give and receive constructive feedback (positive and negative). Challenge by Choice is a separate, but interrelated, concept. Challenge by Choice provides the student with:

- A chance to try a potentially difficult and/or frightening challenge in an atmosphere of support and caring.

- The opportunity to "back off" when performance pressures or self-doubt becomes too strong, knowing that an opportunity for a future attempt will always be available.

- A chance to try difficult tasks, recognizing that the attempt is more significant than performance results.

- Respect for individual ideas and choices. (Schoel et al., p. 131)

Project Adventures activities also include a debriefing, which is essential for complete understanding among participants of the meaning and outcomes of an activity. The debriefing answers three simple questions: *What?* (discussing the facts of what occurred); *So What?* (discussing what is the meaning of what happened, thus giving participants the chance to abstract and generalize what was learned); and *Now What?* (discussion used to introduce the next activity and/or focus on how what was learned may be applied in participants' daily lives).

Leading a wilderness-adventure program provides immense personal reward because behavior changes and personal growth among participants become clearly visible as the experience progresses (Crase, 1988; McAvoy, Schatz, Stutz, Schleien, & Lais, 1989; Witman, 1987). The wilderness-adventure program leader is the catalyst who enables these positive results to occur. Fortunately, many wilderness-adventure programs provide an opportunity for experienced participants who have disabilities to assume leadership of groups. Wilderness Inquiry, for example, presently has several previous participants with disabilities leading their challenging expeditions. C. W. Hog and POINT, on the other hand, were formed by persons who have disabilities *and* extensive experience in the out-of-doors.

Wilderness-Adventure Activities and Outcomes

Hollenhorst and Ewert (1985) found that the most important activities to Outward Bound participants without disabilities included expeditions and group-oriented challenges. Since people with disabilities generally participate in wilderness-adventure programs for

Overcoming nature's challenges requires cooperation and interdependence among participants. In addition, such experiences provide unparalleled feelings of personal control and accomplishment. (Courtesy of **POINT;** Photo by Gary Hagar)

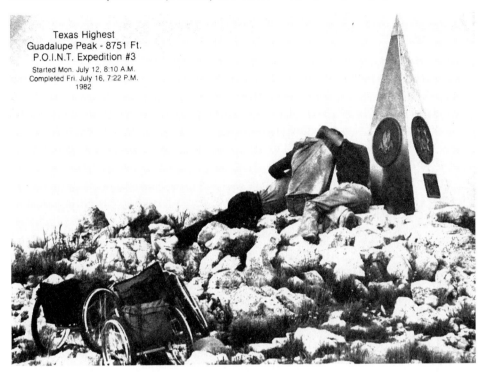

Texas Highest
Guadalupe Peak - 8751 Ft.
P.O.I.N.T. Expedition #3
Started Mon. July 12, 8:10 A.M.
Completed Fri. July 16, 7:22 P.M.
1982

the same reasons as individuals without disabilities (Lais & Schurke, 1982; Richardson, 1986; Robb & Ewert, 1987), these same activities predominate among programs with participants who have disabilities. Examples include a 19-day trip to the Yukon (Lais, 1985), dogsled rides into the Idaho wilderness (Wittaker, 1984), a 16-day raft trip through the Grand Canyon (Szychowski, 1993) and the dramatic climb of rugged Guadalupe Peak (8,751 feet in elevation) by a group of POINT members with spinal cord injuries. In 1989, one individual with a disability captured the nation with his climbing prowess. Mark Wellman, a rock climber with paraplegia, scaled the face of 3,200-foot El Capitan in Yosemite National Park. The ascent required Wellman to execute 7,000 pull-ups as he advanced only 6 inches at a time. In 1993, Wellman and Jeff Pagels, who also has a spinal cord injury, completed a 50-mile cross-country ski trip through the snow-covered Sierra Nevada mountains. *Sports 'n Spokes* described their trip as follows:

> Hauling their own food, water, and supplies on sleds behind sit skis, they encountered 50-mph winds, 50° temperature extremes, avalanches, extreme sunburn, and deep snow. In addition to

the hardships, the two U.S. Disabled Ski Team members experienced stupendous scenery, a better understanding of the technology that can allow wheelchair users the freedom to access the wilderness, a heightened awareness of self-reliance, and a natural high that is the reward for pushing to the limits and succeeding. ("Avalanche of Adventure," 1993, p. 41)

Inclusive Wilderness-Adventure Activities. Havens (1992) wrote, "It is time for Adventure leaders to consider the inclusion of persons with disabilities in community-based Adventure programs—not just via a physical presence but with social interaction and acceptance" (p. 2).

Both the Yukon and Idaho trips mentioned earlier were inclusive experiences in which individuals without disabilities participated along with people who had disabilities. Such expeditions need to be organized with careful attention to group structure in order to ensure social interaction and acceptance. Describing Wilderness Inquiry canoe trips into the boundary waters along the U.S.-Canada border, Lais and Schurke (1982) noted that:

> A usual group would include two people who use wheelchairs, two who are sensory impaired, three "able-bodied" persons, one who uses crutches and two group leaders. Consideration is given so that groups are intergenerational, balanced in the number of men and women, and include persons from a wide variety of occupations and lifestyles. (pp. 25–26)

Schleien, McAvoy, Lais, and Rynders (1993) state that the "underlying goal of integrated high adventure programs is to provide positive experiences for everyone in the group in settings that empower them to expand perceived limitations" (p. 10). They also indicate that adventure programs provide participants with opportunities:

- To experience social integration in settings far removed from the everyday environment
- To increase self-esteem and self-confidence
- To promote independent living skills for persons with disabilities
- For persons without disabilities to look beyond disabilities and to discard negative stereotypes
- To recognize similarities between people with and without disabilities (p. 10)

Inclusive wilderness-adventure programs enable each group member to use his or her unique skills and abilities. People with disabilities are generally accepted for their abilities (Lais, 1985), and participants without disabilities accept the responsibility for performing tasks that are difficult or impossible for people who have disabilities. It is a learning experience for everyone, and each person is expected to respond to the challenge at hand. As one participant with cerebral palsy explained, "You are encouraged to do things you never thought possible but, with a little effort and ingenuity, you find out that you can do them" (Lais & Schurke, 1982, p. 27). Moreover, such integrated experiences have been demonstrated to have positive outcomes for *all* participants, irrespective of the presence of a disabling condition. Samples of individuals with and without disabilities who participated in Wilderness Inquiry trips were found to have reduced trait anxiety after the trip. Both groups also reported posttrip improvements in a number of important areas, including interpersonal relationships, attitudes toward persons with disabilities, confidence levels, willingness to take risks, feelings about self, and tolerance of stress (McAvoy et al., 1989).

Segregated Wilderness-Adventure Activities. Some expeditions, such as the POINT climb of Guadalupe Peak and Wellman and Pagels's cross-country ski trip, are composed exclusively of participants with disabilities. One goal of such trips may be the feeling that participants receive from successfully "going it alone," or not depending on nondisabled companions to assist with difficult tasks. Successfully overcoming wilderness challenges can increase a person's self-confidence (McAvoy et al., 1989; Wright, 1983) and overcoming them without the aid of participants without disabilities can provide unparalleled feelings of personal control and achievement. Despite the fact that only three of the six POINT members who began the ascent of Guadalupe Peak actually reached the summit, all participants shared in the joy of accomplishment.

Outcomes of Wilderness-Adventure Activities. The outcomes of any successful wilderness-adventure program are similar, whether or not they include people with disabilities. Participants enjoy the beauty and wonder of nature, share experiences with other human beings, develop skills, and overcome challenges that enable feelings of self-worth and personal control. The presence of people with disabilities in such programs may intensify these outcomes for everyone. As Corty (1979) wrote, on returning from one expedition, "Looking around the table at those faces I have come to know so intimately, I realize that we have been voyageurs not only through the boundary waters, but through the hearts of ourselves and each other. . . . It has been a voyage that will continue long after the paddles are put away" (pp. 10–12). We hope the outcomes of a wilderness-adventure experience will help all participants, including those with disabilities, enjoy smoother and more satisfying voyages through life.

SUMMARY

Organized camping and wilderness-adventure experiences offer everyone, including people with disabilities, unique opportunities for enjoyment and personal growth. Experts have attributed many beneficial outcomes to participation in these experiences, including improved interpersonal skills, increased strength and endurance, greater independence, and enhanced feelings of self-worth. Despite these benefits, however, only a small percentage of people with disabilities in the United States and Canada have had the opportunity to participate in organized camping and wilderness-adventure programs. As these programs expand to accommodate more people with disabilities, it is essential that they (1) have clearly stated objectives, based on a sound philosophy, (2) provide effective staff training that emphasizes empathy for participants, and (3) offer well-organized and safe activities that are consistent with the skills and interests of *all* participants.

SUGGESTED LEARNING ACTIVITIES

1. Identify eight topics that you feel should be included in any orientation program for a camp with persons who have disabilities. Develop a learning activity for one of these topics.

2. Interview the director of a residential camp or wilderness-adventure program. What does he or she feel are the *unique* benefits that can be derived from participating in the program?

3. Vinton and coworkers (1978) list five basic principles for camps to follow to create an appropriate atmosphere for achieving its objectives. Discuss how each principle facilitates the personal growth of campers with disabilities.

4. List 10 qualities that are important for a camp counselor to exhibit. Discuss the importance of each.

5. Name the four experience components that are common to most wilderness-adventure programs. Discuss the benefits to participants provided by each component.

REFERENCES

American Camping Association. *Standards for Accrediting Camps.* Martinsville, IN: Author, 1980.

American Camping Association. What is the role of camping? *Camping Magazine, 57*(4), 22–24, 1985.

Avalanche of adventure. *Sports'n Spokes, 19*(2), 41–45, 1993.

Byrd, J. D. Selecting and training staff in a camp for handicapped children. In J. A. Nesbitt et al., *Training Needs and Strategies in Camping for the Handicapped.* Eugene: University of Oregon Press, 1972, pp. 136–143.

Corty, J. Disabled blaze new trails in the wild. *The New York Times,* October 21, 1979, pp. 10–12.

Crase, N. Wilderness on ice. *Sports'n Spokes, 14*(1), 7–12, 1988.

Dattilo, J., & W. D. Murphy. Facilitating the challenge in adventure recreation for persons with disabilities. *Therapeutic Recreation Journal, 21*(3), 14–21, 1987.

Feeley, J. E. Should every handicapped person have a camping experience? In J. A. Nesbitt et al., *Training Needs and Strategies in Camping for the Handicapped.* Eugene: University of Oregon Press, 1972, pp. 44–45.

Goodwin, G. Outward Bound. *Sports 'n Spokes, 4*(1), 1978, 5–7.

Hansen, C. C. Content analysis of current literature on camping for handicapped children. In J. A. Nesbitt et al., *Training Needs and Strategies for the Handicapped.* Eugene: University of Oregon Press, 1972, pp. 32–37.

Hardt, L. J. *Easter Seal Guide to Special Camping Programs.* Chicago: The National Easter Seal Society for Crippled Children and Adults, 1968.

Havens, M. D. *Bridges to Accessibility: A Primer for Including Persons with Disabilities in Adventure Curricula.* Hamilton, MA: Project Adventure, 1992.

Hollenhorst, S., & A. Ewert. Dissecting the adventure camp experience: Determining successful program components. *Camping Magazine, 57*(4), 32–33, 1985.

Hourcade, J. Effect of a summer camp program on self-concept of mentally retarded young adults. *Therapeutic Recreation Journal, 11*(4), 178–183, 1977.

Iso-Ahola, S. E., D. LaVerde, & A. Graefe. Perceived competence as a mediator of the relationship between high risk sports participation and self-esteem. *Journal of Leisure Research, 21,* 32–39, 1988.

Kimball, R. O. *Wilderness/Adventure Programs for Juvenile Offenders.* Chicago: University of Chicago, School of Social Service Administration, 1980.

Knapp, C. E. Staff education: Balancing people and activity skills. *Camping Magazine, 56*(6), 22–24, 1984.

Lais, G. Paddling the Yukon. *Sports 'n Spokes, 10*(6), 9–12, 1985.

Lais, G., & P. Schurke. Wilderness Inquiry II. *Sports 'n Spokes, 8*(2), 25–27, 1982.

Lundegren, H. Self-concepts of special populations. In B. van der Smissen, compiler, *Research Camping and Environmental Education.* State College: The Pennsylvania State University, 1976, pp. 253–273.

Lyle, B. *Camping—What Is It?* Martinsville, IN: American Camping Association, 1947.

McAvoy, L. H. Education for outdoor leadership. In J. F. Meyer, T. W. Morash, & G. E. Welton, *High Adventure Outdoor Pursuits.* Columbus, OH: Publishing Horizons, 1987, pp. 459–467.

McAvoy, L. H., E. C. Schatz, M. E. Stutz, S. J. Schleien, & G. Lais. Integrated wilderness adventure: Effects on personal and lifestyle traits of persons with and without disabilities. *Therapeutic Recreation Journal, 23*(3), 50–64, 1989.

McCormick, B., C. White, & F. A. McGuire. Parents' perceptions of benefits of summer camp for campers with mental retardation. *Therapeutic Recreation Journal, 26*(3), 27–37, 1992.

Pearce, B. O., D. A. Vinton, & E. A. Farley. *Directory of Agencies Concerned with Camping and the Handicapped.* Lexington: University of Kentucky (Project REACH), 1979.

Polenz, D., & F. Rubitz. Staff perceptions of the effects of therapeutic camping upon psychiatric patients' affect. *Therapeutic Recreation Journal, 11*(2), 70–73, 1977.

Richardson, D. Outdoor adventure programs for physically disabled individuals. *Parks and Recreation, 21*(11), 43–45, 1986.

Robb, G. M. A correlation between socialization and self-concept in a summer camp program. *Therapeutic Recreation Journal, 5*(1), 25–29, 1971.

Robb, G. M., & A. Ewert. Risk recreation and persons with disabilities. *Therapeutic Recreation Journal, 21*(1), 58–68, 1987.

Robb, G. M., & S. G. Shepley. Forging partnerships: The real challenge. *Camping Magazine, 61*(2), 18–21, 1988.

Robinson, F. M., & S. S. Skinner. *A Holistic Perspective on the Disabled Child: Applications in Camping, Recreation, and Community Life.* Springfield, IL: Charles C Thomas, 1985.

Rodney, L. S., & P. M. Ford. *Camp Administration.* New York: John Wiley & Sons, 1971.

Ryan, J. L., & D. T. Johnson. Therapeutic camping: A comparative study. *Therapeutic Recreation Journal, 6*(4), 178–180, 1972.

Rynders, J., S. Schleien, & T. Mustonen. Integrating children with severe disabilities for intensified outdoor education: Focus on feasibility. *Mental Retardation, 28*(1), 7–14, 1990.

Sable, J. Collaborating to create an integrated camping program: Design and evaluation. *Therapeutic Recreation Journal, 26*(3), 38–48, 1992.

Schleien, S. J., L. H. McAvoy, G. J. Lais, & J. E. Rynders. *Integrated Outdoor Education and Adventure Programs.* Champaign, IL: Sagamore, 1993.

Schoel, J., D. Prouty, & P. Radcliffe. *Islands of Healing.* Hamilton, MA: Project Adventure, 1988.

Sessoms, H. D. Organized camping and its effects on the self-concept of physically handicapped children. *Therapeutic Recreation Journal, 13*(1), 39–43, 1979.

Shasby, G., C. Heuchert, & B. Gansneder. The effects of a structured camp experience on locus of control and self-concept of special populations. *Therapeutic Recreation Journal, 18*(2), 32–40, 1984.

Stearn, S. Accessible programs. *Camping Magazine, 56*(7), 12–15, 1984.

Szychowski, E. River of dreams. *Sports 'n Spokes, 18*(1), 19–22, 1993.

Vinton, D. A., D. E. Hawkins, B. D. Pantzer, & E. M. Farley. *Camping and Environmental Education for Handicapped Children and Youth.* Washington, DC: Hawkins & Associates, 1978.

Wilkinson, R. E. *Camps: Their Planning and Management.* St. Louis, MO: C. V. Mosby, 1981.

Witman, J. P. The efficacy of adventure programming in the development of cooperation and trust with adolescents in treatment. *Therapeutic Recreation Journal, 21*(3), 22–29, 1987.

Wittaker, T. C. W. Hog: A journey into the unknown. *Sports 'n Spokes, 9*(5), 8–11, 1984.

Wright, A. N. Therapeutic potential of the Outward Bound process: An evaluation of a treatment program for juvenile delinquents. *Therapeutic Recreation Journal, 17*(2), 33–42, 1983.

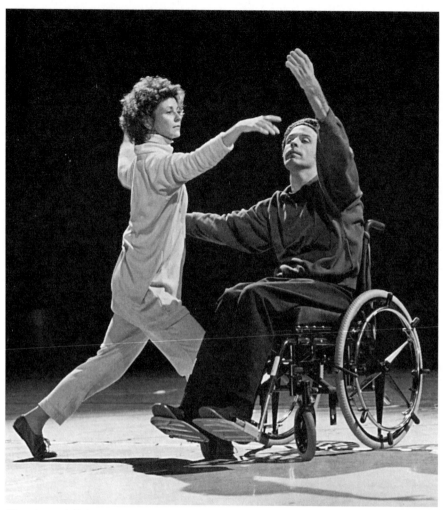

(Courtesy of *Palaestra,* 1989, Vol. 6, No. 1, Dr. Boni Boswell and Mike Hamer/Photo by Tony Rumple)

10

The Arts—for Everyone

■   ■   ■

The more a person travels around the world, the more he or she becomes aware of the cultural differences among human beings. Behaviors that are acceptable, or even rewarded, in one country are taboo in another. Ideas that are received with acclaim by members of one culture are rejected as absurd by people with different heritages. Yet, despite many differences, people throughout the world demonstrate similar desires for aesthetic experiences. Appreciation of beauty, in its many forms, appears to be universal. Enjoyment of beauty created by human beings is so fundamental to human existence that the right "to enjoy the arts" is included in the United Nations' Universal Declaration of Human Rights. Through the arts, people are offered an opportunity for interaction on an aesthetic level. Such interaction, which is based on positive feelings for beauty, is a very important part of human society. In fact, much of our knowledge about the customs, values, and beliefs of ancient societies is based on archeological analysis of their artwork. The arts, it seems, help to form and also to reflect the national character (ethos) of a society.

Because the arts are so essential to a society, they make an important contribution to individual development. Hayman (1969) underscored this importance in the following statement:

> Art can and should be an experience shared by all [people] every day of their lives; this does not mean that all [people] must be painters, architects, authors, composers, nor does it mean that they must spend all of their days in museums, their evenings in theatres and concert halls. Rather, it means that [people's] innate sensitivities to the arts must be allowed to develop and, by early encouragement and education, must be given opportunity for growth so that the whole [individual] can emerge. (p. 11)

The arts are essential to each citizen's life. From the small child drawing with crayons to the senior citizen reflecting on a lifetime of experiences through poetry, the arts provide a basis for discovery, self-expression, and human growth. Access to and participation in the arts is important for *all* persons in our society. Moreover, the Americans with Disabilities Act mandates that U.S. society realize its obligation to ensure that arts-related programs and services are accessible to everyone.

WHAT CONSTITUTES "THE ARTS"?

The term *the arts* is used frequently in everyday conversation, yet defining this term is exceedingly difficult. As Roehner (1981) pointed out, "On the one hand, the arts are those human endeavors that are known as art, dance, drama, filmmaking and photography, music and writing. On the other hand, the arts is also a whole battery of working methods of styles and constantly developing skills. . . . The arts embody a way of working and learning" (p. 6). "The arts," therefore, has more than one definition. The term refers to a set of creative activities, but it also implies a concept that encompasses many methods and processes.

Regardless of art form, the arts is founded upon one essential element—creativity. Participation in the arts, on any level, provides the individual with an opportunity to organize, interpret, and express his or her *own* perceptions of the world. In other words, the arts offer a uniquely personal experience to everyone. Creativity, as noted by Diamondstein (1974), "involves the capacity to be open to experience, to welcome novelty, to be intrigued by discovery, and to exercise new dimensions of imaginative thought" (p. 15).

The National Institute on Disability and Rehabilitation Research (1991) cites research by Teresa Amabile of Brandeis University that examines the basic ingredients of creativity in the arts. These ingredients include "(1) *expertise*—information, talent, and technical ability in relevant fields; (2) *creativity-specific skills*—a work style characterized by concentration and persistence plus a thinking style conducive to generating new possibilities; and (3) *intrinsic task motivation*—the most important component—delight in doing something for its own sake" (p. 1). Dr. Amabile's research indicates that creativity, unlike many human behaviors, cannot be operantly conditioned because extrinsic rewards appear to reduce creativity.

Creativity in the arts is not necessarily limited to the act of developing an artistic creation. Someone else's effort, such as a musical score, offers the chance for creativity, too. For example, a pianist may play his or her own interpretation of another's creation. Carrying this idea a little further, some authorities even insist that merely perceiving a work of art is, in itself, a creative act. Paraphrasing one of his friends, Shaw (1980) stated that "once you have really experienced Shakespeare's *King Lear,* you cannot even fry the breakfast bacon in quite the same way again" (p. 73). Perhaps Shaw was exaggerating, but his point is an important one. Participation in the arts offers a person the chance to have an aesthetic experience on one (or more) of three levels—as the *creator,* the *performer,* or the *perceiver* of a work of art.

The *creator* of an artwork, no matter what medium is used, is providing an expression of his or her own being. The creator gives form to symbols or objects in such a way that beauty results, and this beauty is shared with, and affects, others. The *performer* takes a creator's efforts and, through his or her own artistic feelings and skill, transmits the work of art to others. As noted above, the *perceiver* views the performance or work of art and experiences it in a creative way. The perceiver "feels" the artistic effort, but unlike the creator

Participation in the arts enables a person with a disability to "create" an expression of his or her own being. (Courtesy of Hospital for Sick Children, Washington, DC/Photo by Rhoda Baer)

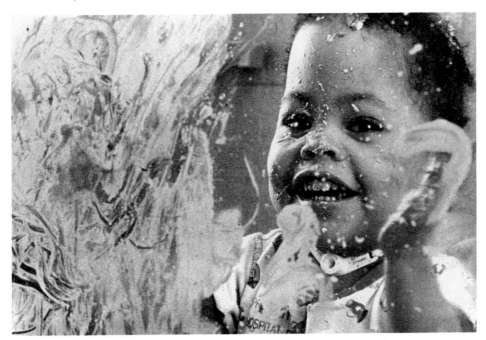

and performer does not share with others what is felt. Of course, it is not necessary (or possible in some cases) for all three levels of participation to be offered by a given work of art. The painter does not need a performer to transmit his or her work of art to an audience. Also, the same person may be involved on different levels, as when a poet recites his or her own poems. Nonetheless, the arts cannot be fully understood without recognizing the presence of these three levels of participation.

It is especially important for people associated with special recreation services to recognize that three levels of participation are offered through the arts. Rehabilitation professionals, advocacy groups, and people with disabilities themselves complain that people who have disabilities are too often spectators while others perform. This is a valid complaint. Every effort should be made to ensure that individuals with disabilities are provided opportunities through the arts to experience creativity as both creators and performers. But it should be recognized, also, that "spectators" of the arts are *active* perceivers of a creative work of art. Moreover, observing a performance or work of art may inspire the perceiver to later become a creator or performer (Tomlinson, 1982).

All three levels of participation are important and offer unique opportunities for everyone, including individuals with disabilities. The woman with mental retardation who paints a sunset provides a lasting testimony to both her talent and her personal view of the world. She is a creator. The youth with a visual impairment who faithfully practices his guitar lessons may use his musical talents to entertain others. In so doing, he brings the composer's work to life and provides enjoyment to the listeners. He is a performer. The man with cerebral palsy who attends a ballet performance can appreciate the agility and grace of another's movement. He has an emotional reaction to the ballet's beauty that is uplifting and deeply moving. He is a perceiver. All three of these participants are engaged in "the arts," and all three are receiving the many benefits that arts participation provides.

BENEFITS OF ARTS PARTICIPATION

The benefits received from participation in the arts are not necessarily different for individuals with and without disabilities. However, barriers may limit opportunities for persons with disabilities to participate in community arts activities. Thus, people who have disabilities may not receive as many personal growth experiences as their nondisabled peers. If arts programs are made available to *everyone,* however, the three levels of arts participation offer limitless opportunities for enjoyment and satisfaction, as well as personal growth. Baer (1985), who uses a motorized wheelchair because of quadriplegia, used her personal experiences to conclude that art experience "represents a valuable coping tool for human beings, particularly those living with debilitating and irreversible physical conditions" (p. 213). An examination of the following six benefits of participation reveals why the arts are so important to everyone in the community.

Self-Discovery

Creativity, which is the cornerstone of arts participation, requires that an individual get in touch with his or her own feelings and perceptions. Participation in the arts, therefore, may enable a person to become more aware of his or her own individuality. Diamondstein (1974) emphasized the importance of self-discovery through involvement in the arts by noting that it can "open new windows on the world and enable [the participant] to perceive his world more richly" (p. 3). Dance, for example, may provide the opportunity for a young man with a psychological disorder to focus on the sensations of muscle relaxation and tension. Once focused on these sensations, the connection between his own emotional feelings and muscular responses may become clearer to him. Such discoveries may not only aid in self-awareness, but may also make future happiness a more realistic goal (Williams, 1977). The importance of song, for example, was expressed by U.S. Navy veteran Angela Walker in a promotional letter from the National Veterans' Creative Arts Festival. She said, "In every person's life there is joy, pain and hope. When I sing, it takes away the pain, and it fills me with hope."

Creativity forms the foundation for arts participation. The girl with a disability who writes a poem is offering an expression of her own being; the beauty that results from her creativity may be shared with others. (Courtesy of The League: Saving People with Physical Disabilities, Inc., Baltimore, MD)

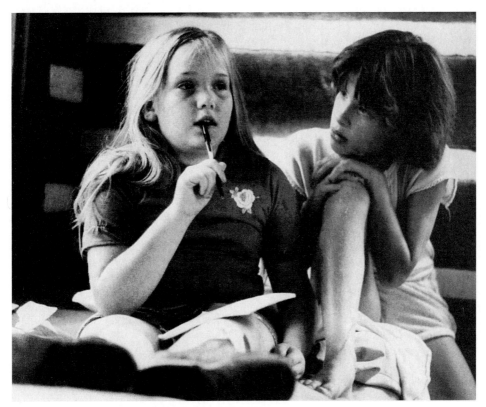

Viewing the arts as an essential means of self-discovery for people with disabilities is summarized in the following statement by Jean Kennedy Smith (1987):

> What are the educational needs of individuals who face severe physical and mental challenges? Their needs are simple and profound: opportunities to develop self-confidence; a chance to take "safe risks" and learn from the results; and the challenge of physical and recreational activities that let them improve their condition and explore their sense of play. They, like all of us, need outlets for imagination, expression, and joy. How do the arts meet those needs? Because they emphasize process over product, divergence rather than convergence, creative choice more than conformity, they provide uniquely appropriate strategies for developing the social, educational and occupational potential of students with special needs.

Communication with Others

Both the creator and performer levels of arts participation provide unique opportunities for an individual, particularly one with a disability, to communicate with others. For example, people who cannot speak distinctly may use novels, poems, and so on, to share ideas, thoughts, and feelings with others. The late Christy Brown (1932–1981), an Irish author and poet with severe cerebral palsy, was an excellent example of such communication. Able to type only by using the little toe on his left foot, Christy Brown published a renowned novel entitled *Down All the Days*. This book, a fictionalized version of his auto-biography, *My Left Foot,* was a powerful personal statement by a talented and perceptive man. In it he was able to express the challenges and frustrations he faced while living with a severe physical disability. Similarly, Tomlinson (1982) noted that the theater "allows for enlightenment and education; it is a tool whereby the reality of disability and the realities of people who have disabilities can be introduced, demonstrated and discussed" (p. 13). As Dr. Earnest Boyer (1987), president of the Carnegie Foundation for the Advancement of Learning and Chairman of the Board of Directors of Very Special Arts has said, "It is my deep conviction . . . that the arts are one of mankind's most essential forms of language. And I believe that if we do not educate all children in the symbol system called the arts, we will lose not only our culture and civility, but our humanity as well."

Kennedy (1985) provided an example that brings Boyer's statement to life. Describing the reaction of a blind Canadian woman who was asked to draw a picture, Kennedy wrote:

> she protested: "How can I make a picture? I've never seen anything, let alone a picture, in my life!" But she soon discovered for the first time that she had an ability and a talent she had never used and never suspected she had. She found she could communicate with and learn from pictures—and she did not have to be taught to do so. (p. 165)

Improved Self-Concept

The way an individual feels about himself or herself is a critical factor in adjustment to life's many stresses. Therefore, activities that provide for successful participation and offer a chance to exert personal control of a given situation are especially important. Arts activities are ideally suited for both success and personal control. Most, for example, do not have a right or wrong way of doing things. Whether painting on canvas or dancing to music, the participant should be developing his or her own personal style. Arts activities encourage individuality and are noncompetitive in nature. There is no winner or loser. Participation itself can be the measure of "success." Perhaps more important than success, however, is a perception of being in control of the situation. The arts offers a unique opportunity for an individual with a disability to be in control. A participant in an arts activity is constantly presented with decision-making opportunities, and the individual himself or herself controls the outcome of each decision. Personal control is reflected in the photographer's adjustment of a camera's lens, the musician's decision to hold a particular note, and the painter's selection of colors. In the following testimony to a U.S. Congressional committee, Laureen Summers (1988), a talented weaver who has cerebral palsy, emphasized both the feelings of control and the self-confidence offered by arts participation:

> Weaving afforded me many new opportunities to explore and develop a sense of myself. Although my disability affects my coordination, I was able to figure out how to manage yarns and strings and create pleasing textures and designs. The encouragement I had to experiment with materials and ideas on my own helped me feel confident about exploring and defining other areas of my life. I gained confidence because I had proven that I could succeed in an area that was admired and respected by others. I learned to take risks, make choices, and trust myself to know what was right for me. In time I fulfilled my dreams of having my own family, my own career, my own life.

Skill Development

The many activities included within the arts offer opportunities to develop and improve on daily living skills. To cite a few examples, painting and sculpture emphasize fine motor tasks; dance promotes increased coordination, endurance, and flexibility; and literature and drama teach one to communicate through written words and verbal expression. Cognitive, psychomotor, and affective skills may all be enhanced through arts participation. Although the following statement by Smith (1981) refers to children with learning disabilities, it is obvious that it is valid for any child who has a disability.

> Through all the arts forms, a child can be helped to sort out one color, one shape, one form, one sound from another; discriminating through the hands, the body, the eyes, the ears, and all the senses is part of artistic experience. Learning to look, learning to listen, remembering what is seen, remembering what is heard—problem areas for the learning disabled—are emphasized in the arts. These skills help organize experience. They help make sense of the world, make sense of the messages coming in through the senses. That's what perception is all about—making sense of the environment, organizing it to have meaning. (p. 84)

The process of organizing nonverbal experiences is essential, and provides the foundation for subsequent skill development through the arts. Appell (1978) examined research that focused on the arts and concluded that the effects of arts programs include "improved social response, gains in school achievement, self-confidence gained by personal achievement, and a better and more integrated existence" (p. 14). The Office of Disabled Student Services at California State University, Northridge, also documented marked improvements in social growth and artistic skill development among participants in its Artistic, Cultural, and Entertainment Program (National Institute on Disability and Rehabilitation Research, 1991).

The Arts in Education Project, conceived by Very Special Arts, formerly the National Committee, Arts for the Handicapped (NCAH), developed a conceptual model that illustrates the use of an arts program for skill development (National Committee, Arts for the

Handicapped 1981). This model, which has been modified to include literary activities, appears in Figure 10.1. The primary purpose of the model is to show that basic learning abilities and aesthetic development are interrelated, and both are enhanced through participation in the arts.

Societal Recognition and Awareness

The arts have proven especially well suited for people with disabilities to share their exceptional talent with others. Christy Brown (literature—cerebral palsy), Stevie Wonder (music—blindness), Joni Eareckson (art—quadriplegia), Sylvia Plath (literature—psychological disorder), Itzhak Perlman (music—polio), and Marlee Matlin (drama—deafness) are just a few of the people with disabilities who have received national and international acclaim through the arts. Their successes also have helped make the general public aware that individuals with disabilities have a great deal to offer society. Tomlinson (1982) observed that during theater performances by actors with disabilities, "the very act of controlling the particular medium for a certain period of time in front of a largely passive, captive crowd, actually does allow for the possibility of clearing away much of the mythology that has been created about disability" (pp. 11–12). Such public education is of benefit to all people with disabilities, regardless of their artistic talents.

It should be noted also that the arts has proven to be an excellent vehicle for public education when the subject (irrespective of the creator and performer) refers to disability. The Kids on the Block, for example, is a puppet troupe that provides outstanding entertainment while at the same time focuses on issues of disability. It is a joy to observe the audience react positively to these puppets, most of which portray youngsters with disabilities.

Following most performances, youngsters in the audience wave their hands in anticipation, hoping to ask questions about the puppets' disabilities during a question-and-answer session. Janus (1981) emphasized the value of the Kids on the Block program. Advocating the use of a specially prepared kit to aid teachers, she wrote:

> When one considers the implications of Bill 82 in Ontario [Canada] schools, which provides for education for every child in his/her least restricted environment, the problem of immediate integration of disabled people into society becomes apparent. The Kids on the Block Teachers' Kit, used as a medium for the creation of positive attitudes toward disabled peers and their integration into the visible majority, is a move toward the solution. The message is clear. It hits *home.* (p. 35)

The message of social awareness provided by arts participation also "hit home" with high school students without disabilities in Ontario, Canada. Performing in a Theatre Ashbury production about persons with hearing impairments, these students found the need to know more about deafness and individuals with hearing impairments. They "asked for six hours a week of instruction [in sign language]—an immersion in deaf culture" (Mangiacasale, 1993, p. 55). In an earlier production of *One Flew Over the*

Figure 10.1. Arts for learning conceptual model. (Modified from: *Very Special Arts, Arts Resource and Training Guide.* Washington, DC: NCAH, p. 59.)

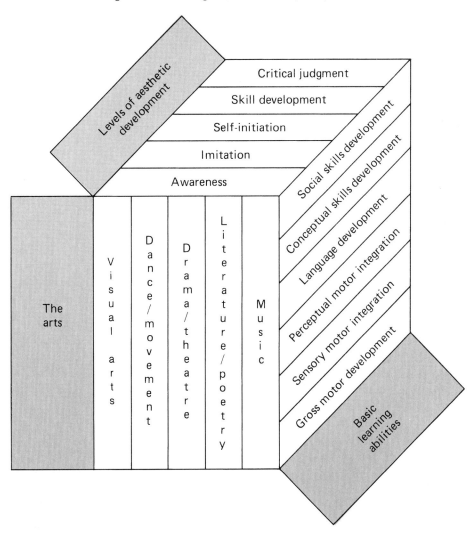

Cuckoo's Nest, Theatre Ashbury's student actors and actresses also immersed themselves in study about psychological disorders. As Molloy (1978) pointed out, "The arts reflect and inspire the hopes and struggles of society. Struggling for their place in society, [people with disabilities] can infuse the arts with a completely new range of human experiences, and through the arts inspire the public to accept them for their gifts rather than their needs" (p. 39).

Social Interaction

The arts offers tremendous potential as a medium for socially integrating people with disabilities into the mainstream of society. Most arts activities offer cooperative tasks that lend themselves to small group efforts using each participant's unique skills and abilities. These activity characteristics are ideal for successful integration (Hutchison & Lord, 1979; Johnson & Johnson, 1980; Schleien & Ray, 1988). Schleien, Rynders, and Mustonen (1988) have provided support for the use of arts-related activities to promote social integration for individuals with disabilities. They reported on a three-year project (separate investigations) that utilized a variety of strategies to integrate children with moderate to severe cognitive disabilities into community-based museum activities. These studies found (1) significant improvements in attitude among nondisabled children toward their peers with disabilities; (2) significant increases in positive social interactions by children without disabilities toward peers with disabilities; (3) significant increases in appropriate behavior among younger children with disabilities; and (4) slight increases in cooperative behaviors among participants with and without disabilities. Although more studies of this nature are needed, it is apparent that the arts can help to achieve social integration.

The six benefits of arts participation are not all-encompassing, of course. Nor, as noted by Ross (1980), should they be interpreted to mean that everyone benefits equally from artistic pursuits. Just as some people display more artistic talent than others, some benefit more than others from arts involvement. It was stated previously that the benefits of arts participation are similar for both people with and without disabilities. The *degree* of benefit may differ, however. Spencer (1978) described the importance of art lessons in a German concentration camp during World War II, and proposed that the need for art increases during times of crisis. For many people with disabilities, the challenges of daily life approach crisis proportions, so their need for arts involvement may be much greater than that of their peers without disabilities. Regardless of whether their need is greater or the same as everyone else's, however, two important principles should be recognized: (1) Everyone, including people with disabilities, can enjoy and benefit from participation in the arts; and (2) each art form can benefit from the unique perspective offered by participants who have disabilities.

VERY SPECIAL ARTS

Because of the many benefits offered by the arts, the Joseph P. Kennedy, Jr., Foundation provided funding in 1974 to support a national conference on arts for persons with mental retardation. The interest created by this conference eventually resulted in the formation of Very Special Arts by Jean Kennedy Smith, who remains a guiding force in the organization today. Very Special Arts, previously known as the National Committee, Arts with the Handicapped, is an educational affiliate of the John F. Kennedy Center for the Performing Arts and receives support from the U.S. Department of Education as well as from a wide variety of private sector sources. Its main function is the coordination of nationwide efforts to provide arts programs for individuals with disabilities. This function is reflected in the following mission statement:

> The mission of Very Special Arts is to ensure that individuals with disabilities have equal opportunity to participate in programs which demonstrate the value of the arts in the lives of all individuals and provide opportunities for the integration of people with disabilities into society.

Very Special Arts has five goals that demonstrate the organization's dedication not only to program development and implementation in the arts, but also to research, training, technical assistance, public awareness, and interagency coordination. Very Special Arts' goals are as follows:

> *Goal 1.* To support the initiation and expansion of arts-related programs that enhance learning and enrich the lives of persons with disabilities.
>
> *Goal 2.* To initiate and support research, development, and evaluation activities relating to programming in the arts for persons with disabilities.
>
> *Goal 3.* To provide arts-related training and technical assistance to those agencies and individuals who provide services to persons with disabilities.
>
> *Goal 4.* To develop and implement systems that demonstrate effective interagency cooperation and community involvement in providing services in the arts for individuals with disabilities.
>
> *Goal 5.* To expand international awareness and to provide a system for sharing information about existing programs in the arts for persons with disabilities.

Among the many exciting programs supported by Very Special Arts is the Very Special Arts Festival program. This program offers opportunities for youngsters with and without disabilities to develop their talents in the visual and performing arts. Thus, in preparing to demonstrate their artistic skill before an audience, the children are placed in an ideal situation for promoting integration. All participants are encouraged to express their own individuality in a noncompetitive way. In addition, working toward the annual festival requires a year-round cooperative effort from everyone involved. This unique blending of individual expression with collective cooperation toward a group goal provides the perfect environment for lasting integration of persons with and without disabilities.

Very Special Arts Festival program's impact extend well beyond the young participants, too. Parents, artists, teachers, and spectators all benefit from a variety of arts experiences. Demonstrations, workshops, exhibits, and a multitude of performances are all part of the annual festival that concludes a year of preparation. In-service training is a special emphasis of the Festival program, so everyone connected with the festival's educational efforts is well prepared for his or her role. Spectators leave the festival with a new appreciation for the abilities that artists who have disabilities possess, and through such experiences the general public becomes more aware of the valuable contribution made by the arts to the lives of all persons. The Very Special Arts Festival is, indeed, a very special program.

In 1984, Very Special Arts expanded its programs internationally. International Very Special Arts Festivals are now held in more than 50 countries around the world, including Brazil, India, Italy, and Kenya. Additionally, Very Special Arts sponsors many special projects that research, develop, and document new initiatives that may be included among Very Special Arts' programs. The following are just a few examples of these special projects:

Theater. The *Young Playwrights Program* provides opportunities for students aged 12–18 to develop their interest and skills in writing for the stage. Students participate in workshops to learn about theater arts and are encouraged to write plays addressing an aspect of a disability.

Dance. The *New Visions Dance Project* is designed to teach dance and movement skills to people who are blind or visually impaired. First piloted in cooperation with the Alvin Ailey American Dance Center, the project is now implemented by dance companies and schools throughout the country.

Music. The *Itzhak Perlman Award* is given annually to an outstanding musician under the age of 21 who has a physical or mental disability. Career assistance through a scholarship award is provided to encourage the artist's further studies in the performing arts.

Literature. The *Creative Writing Project* provides hospital patients and institution residents with opportunities to explore and express their feelings and experiences through poetry and prose. The *Creative Writing Project* encourages self-expression and increases communication and writing skills.

Visual Arts. Call to Rise is Very Special Arts' national museum exhibition of works by American artists who have physical disabilities. Sponsored in part by The Humana Foundation, the exhibition travels to a variety of conferences, including the International Very Special Arts Festival.

Integrated Arts. The *Early Childhood Project* stimulates the development of social and learning skills of infants and preschool children with special needs through the introduction of the arts in early education. Participatory activities such as puppetry, storytelling, theater games, painting, dance, and music are offered, and training and instruction relevant to the child's daily surroundings and later life is provided to parents, siblings, and caregivers. Another special project is *Transition Through the Arts* for high school students with developmental disabilities leaving the educational system. Very Special Arts state organizations work closely with community leaders to develop arts workshops to strengthen vocational, motor, communication, and independent living skills.

LEADERSHIP IN THE ARTS

More arts programs that include individuals with disabilities can be achieved only through knowledgeable, energetic, and effective leadership. Personnel working with persons who have disabilities need adequate training, both in the arts and in how to lead arts activities effectively. It is not possible, within the scope of this chapter, to provide a comprehensive guide for leaders of arts activities that would encompass all art forms and all types of disabling conditions. We may, however, offer a few essential principles for successful leadership of an arts program that includes participants with disabilities. These principles are essentially the same as leadership principles for any inclusive recreational activity and include the following:

1. *Determine Program Goals.* What you are trying to accomplish through your arts program should be expressed as written goals. These program goals, to a large extent, will guide decision making in such matters as the amount of integration desired, leadership style employed, whether cooperative group projects are more desirable than individual efforts, and so on. One area of special concern in the arts is the relative importance of the final product in comparison with the *process* used to achieve the final product. Although there will be some situations that require a strong emphasis on the finished product, we agree with the following statement by Roehner (1981):

   > a [child with blindness] working with finger paint may express a feeling of being loved by making magnificent circles in finger paint. The product may not be aesthetically pleasing but the kinesthetic treatment of the soft paint with circular motions indicates that the student perceives something of emotion, love, and is responding to it and to the medium. It is the art of expressing that is important, not the product. (p. 6)

   Putting the final sentence of Roehner's commentary into a written goal statement would help ensure that program leaders approach all arts activities in a consistent way.

2. *Encourage Creativity.* Moran (1979) contended that the creative talents of individuals are "often thwarted, ignored, or tossed aside by [others] on the grounds that they work against long established human traditions" (p. 48). The arts, however, should provide activities that encourage, rather than discourage, creative expression. Prefabricated or highly structured arts activities should be minimized or eliminated, and program leaders should emphasize flexibility in each activity. The leader's importance in fostering creativity cannot be overemphasized. The leader can serve as a role model by expressing his or her own individuality while, at the same time, communicating to each participant that there is no such thing as failure in the arts (Kunkle-Miller, 1981). Successful integration is much easier to attain when creativity is emphasized. Children with mental retardation, for example, may be able to achieve high status in an integrated arts group because they do not differ significantly from their nonretarded peers on nonverbal measures of creativity (Sherrill & Cox, 1979). Ross (1980) also stressed the importance of creativity and stated that arts leaders should create conditions of creativity by:

   1. establishing the sanctity of mutual truthfulness.
   2. developing trust (trustworthiness and mutual trustfulness).
   3. being free enough to free students to act playfully, to explore and invent an atmosphere that is nonjudgmental, where error is essential to trial.
   4. providing conditions of psychic safety—being compassionate.
   5. being devoted to the child's learning and growth. (p. 110)

   Unless creativity is allowed to flourish, many of the benefits of arts participation will be lost.

3. *Individualize Activities.* Each arts activity should be geared, as much as possible, to the skill level and personal needs of each participant. The demands of a given activity should be compared with the participant's capabilities, and modifications made when appropriate (Copeland, 1984). The following are a few considerations for offering arts activities to participants with disabilities:

   1. Time, space, and materials may need to be limited to meet specific needs.
   2. Emphasis should be placed on the senses by using appropriate materials—i.e., sand, finger paints, soft cloth or yarn, aromatic fragrances, audible devices, etc.
   3. Small group size is often preferable to larger groups, and forming a circle increases feelings of unity in some activities, such as dance.
   4. A logical progression of skill development should occur, starting with tasks that have been mastered and proceeding to more difficult ones.
   5. Reinforce accomplishments with appropriate praise. This rewards participation and gives the individual a feeling of success.

   Harlan (1992) also notes that open-ended projects should be used because they "allow the participant to determine the outcome of the art experience to as great an extent as possible" (p. 2). Ananda Coomaraswamy, an Indian writer, is credited with stating that "the artist is not a special kind of man, but every man is a special kind of artist" (Shaw, 1980, p. 73). Individualizing arts activities brings out the "specialness" in each participant, irrespective of disability.

4. *Plan for Access.* In *Arts and the Handicapped: An Issue of Access,* the Educational Facilities Laboratories (EFL) and the National Endowment for the Arts (NEA) (1975) stated, "the vast majority of [people with disabilities] still perceive the arts as an inconvenient obstacle course strewn with rules, regulations, revolving doors, and inaccessible opportunities" (p. 6). Public laws have helped improve this situation (see Chapter 3), but it often is necessary to make special preparations to ensure that arts programs are accessible to and usable by people with disabilities. Architectural barriers often limit participation by those who have disabilities, but public attitudes are important, also, when planning for access. The EFL and NEA (1975) noted that the use of "tactile" art galleries, which allow artifacts to be handled by individuals who are blind, is criticized by some museum officials because "they fear that artifacts will be at worst destroyed and at best soiled by repeated handling" (p. 20). Sadly, such attitudes serve to prevent people with disabilities from becoming patrons of the arts. Access depends on both removal of physical obstacles *and* change of attitudinal barriers.

5. *Attend In-Service Training Programs.* As the arts participant increases in skill, his or her changing needs may require a change in teaching methods and materials. Similarly, the leader of an arts program should continue to grow by seeking relevant and informative in-service training opportunities. Unfortunately, many such programs focus solely on awareness or sensitivity training in one specific arts area. Selecting *quality* in-service programs, however, can result in benefits. The NCAH (1981), now Very Special Arts, cautioned potential in-service participants, "the frequency and length of individual training sessions has much less to do with effectiveness, than the quality of the instructor, format and resources" (p. 169). Careful selection is required, but in-service training for arts leaders can result in better arts programs for everyone.

Modifications may be required to allow successful arts participation. For example, attaching a brush to a helmet can enable a participant (who has upper extremity limitations to experience) the joy of painting his *own* crafts project. (Courtesy of The League: Serving People with Physical Disabilities, Inc., Baltimore, MD)

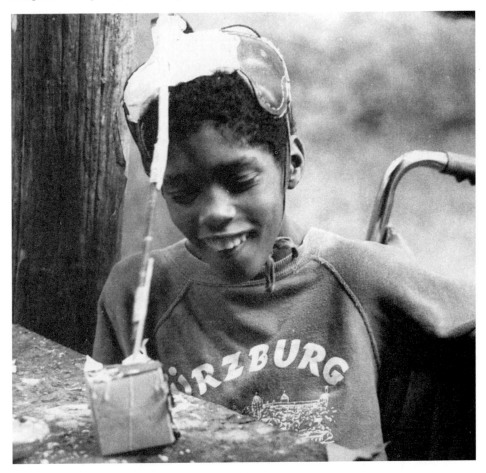

ARTS PARTICIPATION—EXAMPLES

This chapter has provided information about the arts and people with disabilities, but to really understand the *personal* nature of arts involvement we need to examine actual examples of arts participation. We have selected two in-depth examples that reveal the meaning of arts participation to persons with disabilities. One of these focuses on an individual participant, Claudia Fowler, and the deep personal fulfillment she received from writing poetry. The other, Theatre Unlimited, presents group participation in the arts (theater), and highlights creative expression, attitude change, and integration through the arts. These two examples are followed by brief descriptions of other noteworthy arts programs that include persons with disabilities.

Claudia Fowler

Claudia Fowler died on December 11, 1981. In most ways, Claudia's life was not exceptional, but she had cerebral palsy and scoliosis which, for all of her 32 years, resulted in almost complete dependency on others. She could not walk; neither could she dress, bathe, eat, or use the toilet unassisted. Claudia could speak, but only people who spent a great deal of time with her could understand her. Many whose lives touched Claudia's thought she had severe mental retardation—they did not take the time to find out if she could comprehend what they were saying. "Claudia couldn't understand why people who knew her, even some relatives, would speak to her as if she were a child," commented her mother, Catherine L. Fowler. "That's something I will never understand, either," she added, slowly shaking her head.

Feelings

People are not just specimens of the physical anatomy,
*   they consist of mysterious and unpredictable things which*
*   are known as feelings.*
Feelings aren't something that we can control
*   although sometimes we'd give anything if we could;*
*   they're a part of life which is involuntary.*
Occasionally, we become timid about expressing our feelings,
*   and they grow into a whirlpool of frustrations within us.*
To share our feelings with someone,
*   is like releasing a herd of wild mustangs;*
*   it places our innermost soul in a state of tranquility*
*   and freedom.*

(Claudia, 1978)

Claudia attended "special" elementary and junior high schools in the Baltimore, Maryland, area. It was many years before PL 94-142 (Education for All Handicapped Children Act), however, so the regular high schools were not accessible to individuals using

---

Claudia's poems are reprinted courtesy of Catherine L. Fowler.

wheelchairs. Denied the right to attend high school, Claudia was taught by home tutors until she received her high school diploma in 1968. Home instruction did enable Claudia to develop her cognitive abilities, but it deprived her of one very important aspect of the teen years—social interaction with peers.

Remedy for Loneliness

Today, pearl-gray clouds fill the sky,
*   making the solitude seem more intense,*
Loneliness is the most agonizing sickness,
*   with no chemical pain reliever known;*
*   it is the slowest form of suicide*
Being lonely and withdrawn from people,
*   is just as poisonous as any*
*   type of malignancy.*
This senseless illness has the simplest remedy in the world,
*   a friend.*
One other thing is also needed,
*   a willingness to trust your fellow man.*

(Claudia, 1977)

Community programs developed exclusively for individuals with physical disabilities became Claudia's primary source for social interaction. Many of these programs, however, required that she conform to the leader's plans, rather than allowing her the freedom to pursue her own interests. "Claudia became very frustrated with some of the programs she attended," her mother recalled. "A woman at one program *insisted* that she participate in a cooking class. After the class Claudia said to me, 'Mother, I'll never be able to cook! Why can't I be allowed to do what I want?'" Few of these programs could offer her the freedom she desired—the freedom to express her individuality in her own way. This need for self-expression was met when Claudia began to write poetry.

"My first attempts at writing poetry began in 1974," wrote Claudia. "It is a bit difficult to describe just how I come up with a poem. It builds up inside of me, but not in my mind, until I start to type. The words just keep coming 'til I type the last word in a poem. It is sort of like giving birth." Most of the thoughts included in Claudia's poems evolved while she lay in bed at night reflecting on her favorite themes of animals, nature, and human emotions. In the morning, her poems were "born" at an electric typewriter. Claudia could not use her arms and hands to type, of course, but she did have some control of her head movements. She painstakingly pecked at the typewriter keys using a metal pointer attached to a head band. As with many people who have cerebral palsy, the amount of muscular control Claudia possessed varied from moment to moment. The more relaxed she was, the better she was able to type. She wrote, "To type a poem takes me anywhere from half an hour to a week depending on the length of the poem and how nervous I feel. Of course, some days are better than others." Claudia could relax best when she was able to spend time outdoors. Whether she was sitting behind her rural home overlooking acres of fields and woods, or on a hike at the resident camp she loved, Camp Greentop, Claudia was fascinated by the wonders of nature.

Perfect Day

If a mystical person suddenly materialized to grant me one perfect day,
I know exactly the things I would order.
it would be a bright, warm, late Spring day,
with the birds singing their songs in the meadow-green shade
of the rich, new foliage of the trees;
as the honeybees and butterflies dart and dash from flower
to flower as though they were on a city-wide shopping spree.
The first thing I'd wish to do would be to soar through the clouds,
and let the golden eagle act as my guide.
To have the creatures of the forest as my teachers,
so I may learn their many secrets;
and I promise not to tell a single soul.
Let me follow the wild mustangs
as they race with the wind of the plains.
May I be given the privilege of accompanying the white-tail deer,
while they quench their thirst at a clear, spring-fed stream.
I would observe as many activities of nature as time would allow,
and request that you share it all with me.

(Claudia, 1979)

It was at Camp Greentop, located in western Maryland, that Claudia met Peter Setlow and his wife, Barbara. Pete, the camp's program director, appreciated Claudia's intellect and took a sincere interest in her. The friendship between Claudia and the Setlow family, particularly Pete, continued year-round until Claudia's death. The importance of friendship in anyone's life cannot be overestimated, but to someone with a severe disability the joy of having a genuine friend may transcend all other emotions. Pete, Barbara, and later their children, Barry and Jenny, added much happiness to Claudia's life. But, as the Setlows are quick to point out, knowing Claudia also enriched their lives immensely.

Never a Stranger, Again

When I first saw you,
you were just a stranger to me.
But you, along with time have,
in some mysterious way;
claimed a segment of my life.
Unlike most of life's gifts which fade with time
the treasure of you in my life will last forever.

(Claudia, 1976)

What You Mean to Me

To peer into your autumn leaf-brown eyes and perceive how much
you care without a single word being spoken,
is something mystical which only you possess.
When your arms tenderly encompass me,
it is as though an invisible fortress materializes to obstruct
life's annoyances and disappointments.
You have taught me many important things,
but among the most invaluable is that someone does care about
me as a person.
Uncertain of whether you are aware of what you mean to me,
I yearn for the day when everything is as tranquil as a
mid-winter's morning;
and there will be time for you to listen to my memorized
inventory of all the wonderful ways that you
supplement my life.

(Claudia, 1978)

Two Important Arrivals
(dedicated to Barry and Jenny Setlow)

The sky is the color of the robin's broken egg shell,
given to me by someone very special.
This fragile gift rests in a small, gray-blue box on
my reference book shelf,
where it becomes a welcome sight from typewriter
keys, papers and books.
Looking into my dresser mirror,
two, important, little people gaze down at me from
a photograph held tightly by the mirror's frame.

It is possible to see you both grow up again and
again.
simply by glancing at the row of photographs
spread
along the middle shelf of my bookcase.
From a Halloween dog and a little hobo,
to two, bright elementary school students.
While looking through some old photographs the
other
night,
I came across a couple of baby pictures.
It is difficult to realize that so many years have
come and gone since the two of you first entered
this world,
but I didn't know what I was missing until
your arrival.

(Claudia, 1980)

The last few months of Claudia's life were spent in the hospital. She was not physically strong, but her faith and friendships sustained her. Finally, however, in late 1981, respiratory failure claimed Claudia's life.

Life

Life is a strange thing,
which can't be explained in just a few words.
It is the happiness found in a new healthy baby,
or the sadness of a senseless death.
The gleam in the eyes of a child as he tried to
blow out the candle on his first birthday cake
or the empty look in the eyes of a lonely old
man as he gazes out the window on his ninety-first
birthday.
That hard struggle of a young intelligent girl lifting
herself from the apathy of the slums,
or the wealthy sophisticated debutante;
who has her desires and goals handed to her
without having to strive for them.
It is seeing and appreciating the beautiful wonders of nature,
and not taking them for granted.
Life is made of these things and so much more,
but above all else, it is the most precious thing
that we will ever have and
it should be cherished.

(Claudia, 1976)

Final Comment

Claudia Fowler was not included in this chapter because she possessed exceptional literary talent. Until now, none of her poems has been published, although a friend did have some of them bound into a volume entitled *A Bridge to My Thoughts*. Claudia was unique because every individual, whether having a disability or not, is unique. The arts simply provided Claudia with a meaningful way of expressing her individuality. A British woman, who had a disability that distorted her facial features and prevented speech, once wrote, "It's my body you see, not my mind." Through her poems, we get a glimpse of Claudia Fowler's bright and sensitive mind.

Theatre Unlimited

Theatre Unlimited[1] is a dramatic ensemble that shatters popular myths about mental retardation. Composed half of actors with developmental disabilities and half of actors without disabilities, the company is dedicated to a creative process that provides a vision; the vision is that of a community of spirit, where love sparks the transformation process allowing the performer to risk and the viewer to perceive in new ways. Through visual and corporeal images, a spectrum of pain and exhilaration is revealed. Theatre Unlimited is changing the context and aesthetics of theatre. Performances throughout the nation provide a model for artists, educators, recreators, and therapists, and present new attitudes and approaches to the general public.

Process. Theatre Unlimited's work is based on transformation and revelation. The ensemble addresses many of its members' needs—physical, emotional, and intellectual—while offering society a model for the future. In addressing these needs, the actors approach a nurturing quality of spirit that, when viewed by an audience, has applications in many realms.

The persona of the actor is central to this process. The actor transforms images of sound and movement and quantities of time and space for the single purpose of exposing a soul in public. As one audience member discovered, "There is someone up there, who is beyond labels, beyond pity and fear—someone who is more like myself than I ever realized."

The roots of Theatre Unlimited lie in developmental theatre. A relatively new approach, this form seeks to prepare the actor physically and vocally, with an extra emphasis on emotional development and group process or ensemble work. Theatre Unlimited defines an ensemble as "a group of supporting players who work together to create a single effect." This ensemble process is reflected in all aspects of the company's work and

1. Theatre Unlimited is a program of RCH, Inc., in San Francisco, CA. The Company's publication, *Theatre Unlimited,* was funded by a grant from the Evelyn J. and Walter Hass, Jr., Foundation, and the Sandy Foundation. The booklet was written by David Morgan, Herb Felsenfeld, and Richard Heus, and appears in modified form with permission of the authors and RCH, Inc.

play. Concentration and focused interactions are nurtured and find expression through sound, movement, and physical contact. Like improvisational theatre (another approach used by Theatre Unlimited), ensemble process demands the development of trust, support, and cooperation. Through this approach emerges a level of honesty and caring that has allowed the company to clearly mature from year to year.

While it is true that an actor without a disability can express a movement or a dramatic gesture with more fluidity than a performer with cerebral palsy, it is equally true that sincerity of ensemble effort achieves artistic excellence. Theatre Unlimited has forged its own identity, and there is much that can be done only by the artists in Theatre Unlimited. The work is built on discipline and imagination, the principal ingredients of theatre art.

Rehearsal. Initially, Theatre Unlimited decided that each three-hour rehearsal would consist of a full hour of physical warm-ups, followed by a half hour of partnered exchanges such as mirror exercises and give-and-take games, an hour for the introduction of ensemble activities, and a half hour at the end for group discussion and sharing: It turned out, however, that too much structure too soon inhibited both growth and the possibility of new discoveries.

While building and maintaining a ritual of starting with group warm-ups, and closing with a circle for discussion and sharing, the company loosened the time in between to allow for spontaneous occurrences and to accommodate specific rehearsal needs.

The warm-up routine incorporated traditional theatre exercises along with the company's collective knowledge of techniques from yoga, T'ai Chi, mime, and dance. Particularly important was the time taken to study and learn the essential skill of relaxation. From a calm basis, sessions continually maintained a flow of energy that rarely demanded a break. From the beginning, energy was high and the intensive level of training produced slow yet steady progress. The ratio (actors with and without disabilities) of the company allowed the participants to become close working partners. At first, some members were confused by the abstract nature of the work. To them, drama meant putting on a play. Common questions were: "What's this mirror for?" or "Why am I relaxing?" Then and today, it is necessary to continually struggle for a common vocabulary, one accessible to all company members. The group concentrated on the basic building blocks of actor training, sound and movement, and began to put more and more imagery to its physical work. By connecting concrete images to movement, understanding began to increase and entire movement combinations were assimilated.

Much early work focused on building the trust necessary to function well as an ensemble. Games and exercises were introduced that demanded this response. Actors leaned on each other with full body weight. They formed a tight circle and took turns falling into waiting arms. One partner led the other, blind-folded, through strange environments. Because these games placed few cognitive demands, success was easily noted.

Learning is frequently divided into three categories: cognitive, affective, and physical. While research shows that those with normal intelligence score significantly higher in verbal measures of creativity—or the cognitive domain—there are no significant differences between people with and without retardation on nonverbal measures of creativity.

Persons with developmental disabilities often show strengths in imaginative behavior and willingness to trust, take risks, and be spontaneous. From its inception, Theatre Unlimited's process has been built on this research and on the belief that a creative theater form that relies on nonverbal activity can evolve.

The mirror game is the best example of this kind of nonverbal activity. With its many variations, it has been an essential part of ensemble training. A partnered exercise of follow-the-leader, the mirror exercise demands great concentration. Often performed to slow, flowing music, it involves both precise imitation as well as creative initiation. As roles are reversed and partners changed, actors begin to know each other as individual expressive people.

At the end of each three-hour session the ensemble sits in a circle and talks. When pressed for reactions to the evening's rehearsal, members with disabilities often find it difficult to articulate specific feelings. It has been particularly gratifying for the company to become close enough for all to share reactions and feelings. Sharing, especially in nonverbal ways, began to balance in importance with the pace of Theatre Unlimited's skill building. One participant stated:

> Here I've learned about timing—after ten years of working with disabled people. I've finally allowed myself the time to wait. It's different timing than I would use. But when someone else uses it, it's unique. Here, I find that disabled people 'can do'. For years we've been told that they can't. The progression is amazing—people are expressing themselves, they are saying things to each other, to the audience. I can take that knowledge of slow steady growth back to my job and use that with my hope that people will change. It may take 2 or 3 weeks, maybe 2 or 3 years.

Performance. Theatre Unlimited views its approach to performance as a direct and logical outgrowth of rehearsals and workshops. Performance is looked at as a way station along a developmental continuum, and the audience is invited to participate in the viewing of this process.

The company's first performed score (an outline of events that occur in sequence around a theme) was called "The Initiation." Its theme involved two groups of strangers learning each other's rituals and eventually coming together. The score was also an accurate reflection of the company's stage of development. Tensions, anxieties, and mistrust existed. Instead of being looked at as problems, these fears were incorporated into the creative process, and solutions, developed through rehearsal, were shared in public. Technical aspects of the piece remained simple—as much out of choice as out of financial necessity. Performing barefoot in leotard tops and drawstring pants against a dark backdrop, the group used masks and live percussion accompaniment.

The outcome of the first year's exploration involved work that was primarily in sound and movement. Work was at a level of physical interaction akin to dance theater. Because of its grounding in improvisation, the company was able to transform mistakes, missed cues, and delayed entrances into appropriate happenings. A style was beginning to evolve. The audience saw that support could be a demanding and exciting physical discipline.

Another level of development happened during the second year. The score grew in complexity. New elements included performing parts of the sequence in American Sign

Theatre Unlimited's performances are a direct and logical outgrowth of rehearsals and workshops. (Courtesy of Theatre Unlimited/RCH, Inc., San Francisco, CA)

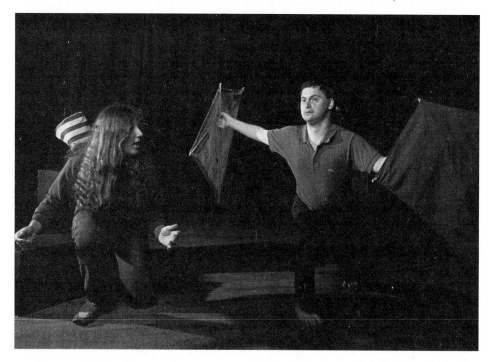

Language; creating a particular place, a playground, through the actors' imaginative skills; refining the company's sound and movement skills to extend into the area of physical and spatial transformation; and integrating song and poetry into the sequence. Audience response—especially during moments when the planned "next move" did not occur—gave the company reassurance. People were once again genuinely intrigued by what they saw. The awkward, the amateurish, were transformed into the deeply human, the deeply affecting. The audience participated in the event. The act of faith *played*.

For Theatre Unlimited, performance is a laboratory where the group can explore and reveal greater understanding of the developmental process. The performance laboratory is a place where ideas, not personalities, dominate.

Workshops. Workshops are the way Theatre Unlimited reaches out and opens its process to the audience. Here the momentum of performance winds down, the fourth wall between viewer and actor opens, and the empty space fills with the activities of revelation.

People—from school-age children on up—are involved in an intensely physical experience. What begins as two groups, actors and viewers, soon coalesces into one group that functions on different levels. The line starts to blur. What of the disability? Does it make any difference?

Here the viewer is put into a unique situation: Working, for example, with a man who has Down's syndrome, is almost nonverbal, and is engaged in bending over to touch the top of his head to his toe. Not knee. Toe. Perception shifts, and the mind moves on to the next level of wonder. A woman with mental retardation shows a university professor how to master an isolation exercise. Ground is broken, and the meaning of the word disability changes.

The most uninhibited reactions, and in many ways the most challenging and gratifying, are those involving schoolchildren. Students in the second and third grades have not learned to label and stereotype. They can hardly wait to share energy and games. As they look to all company members as equals, their learning is accelerated and they are soon involved in a joyful experience. The workshop atmosphere is exciting, with a sense of wonder that is barrier-free, as the following quote attests:

> What I want from the general public is honesty. I see how our process has changed people in our company, because now people are together with those they can trust, we can confide in each other, talk and really feel like we're getting honest feedback. There was not communication, before, between some of these people. You could sit down and listen to people talk, and one person would be talking and the other person would respond on a totally different subject. There was no real communication, there was no feeling. Now I sit and listen to our company talk and it's amazing. It's almost too much. It's "you know, I really like you." All this out front stuff.

Theatre Unlimited functions as a reflection of our particular time and culture, in addition to acting as a model of events about to happen. As long as the model remains healthy, it will point toward a time of unobstructed access to creative tools for all people.

Other Arts-Related Programs

Museum One (Washington, DC). This innovative program was established to encourage adults who are elderly to experience the arts, particularly the visual arts. Museum One, founded in 1982, offers courses and workshops for adults who reside in nursing homes and are unable to travel to art museum locations. Slide programs, videotapes, detailed educational guides, and books bridge the gap between the art museum and the nursing home. Museum One also provides in-facility seminars, as well as practical advice to nursing homes interested in starting arts education programs for residents. As noted by Joan Hart (1991), executive director of Museum One, "A facility-based art appreciation program can create a 'Museum Without Walls,' a gallery of great works which older adults can enjoy and study despite disabilities . . . [it] offers more than a learning experience. It enhances the environment of the nursing facility." Museum One also has a multiarts appreciation workshop series, Creating For Life, which includes visual arts, music, and dance.

Carmel Community (Chandler, AZ). This nonprofit organization provides programs emphasizing a wide variety of arts activities (e.g., dance, movement, music, drama) for persons with disabilities of all ages. Primarily therapeutic in nature, these programs stress cognitive, social, and skill development through arts participation.

Many of Carmel Community's programs, including storytelling, drama, and puppetry, have been offered to schoolchildren with disabilities in Arizona. According to Carmel Community's staff, "We have discovered that through the arts, children with special needs open up and express themselves in ways that they are otherwise unable to do. They become creative and their self-esteem increases."

Young Adults Educational Theatre's Reality Theatre (New York, NY). Sponsored by the Young Adult Institute, this drama group performs plays focused on AIDS enlightenment for persons with developmental disabilities, particularly those with mild to moderate mental retardation. One unique aspect about Reality Theatre is that the performers also have developmental disabilities. By using drama for peer education, Reality Theatre has increased knowledge of HIV and AIDS, homophobia, sexual abuse, and notifying family members of HIV infection (Jacobs, 1992). Each performance is followed by a comprehensive question and answer period. Writing in *The Village Voice,* Finkle (1993) described one of Reality Theatre's plays as "not a show to which traditional critical standards would automatically be applied; the surprise is that they could be. As often as not, the jokes in the improvised script land solidly; the premises . . . are imaginative; the players have developed admirable stage presence; the points are made . . . and gotten" (p. 94).

Famous People Players (Toronto, Canada). Founded in 1974, this touring theatre company features performers with and without mental retardation. "Making wonderful use of blacklight technology, black-garbed, and thus invisible actors and actresses manipulate all sorts of fluorescent puppets and props under ultra-violet lights. . . . The effects they create are amusing and without exception visually arresting, and one leaves the superbly designed theatre feeling happy and uplifted" (Speck, 1986). Famous People Players use puppets of such well-known people as Elvis Presley, Michael Jackson, Barbra Streisand, and Kenny Rogers, as well as a number of fictional characters such as Darth Vader. "It's amazing how [people with disabilities] develop and mature as they gain confidence in the fact that others have confidence in them," stated Diane Dupuy, the founder and artistic director of Famous People Players.

Theatre Access Project (TAP) (New York, NY). Since 1979, this organization has responded to the needs of persons with hearing impairments by providing sign language interpreters for theatre productions. Because of the group's success and the passage of the Americans with Disabilities Act, demand for TAP's services has been increasing dramatically. One significant challenge for interpreters is to allow theatergoers to understand not only what is being said but who is doing the talking. Schaefer (1992) quoted one staff member who said, "You're not acting, but you need to match a character, to give the audience an idea of who's talking now. . . . You're dealing with a ping-pong effect—the audience still needs to be able to watch the play" (p. 12C). TAP is sponsored by New York's Theatre Development Fund and its off-Broadway sister group, Hands-on.

SUMMARY

The arts help to form and also to reflect the national character of society. As a result, it is essential that *all* members of society be provided the opportunity to participate in the arts. Such participation may be through the creation of an original work of art, but it also may be through performing the work of another artist, or even perceiving the artistic efforts of another in a creative way. These three levels of art participation offer limitless opportunities for enjoyment and satisfaction, as well as personal growth. This is especially true for people who have disabilities because their opportunities for personal growth experiences may be more limited than those of individuals without disabilities.

SUGGESTED LEARNING ACTIVITIES

1. Name the three levels of participation in the arts, and give (from your own experiences) specific examples of each.
2. Interview a community recreation arts specialist, and determine the ways in which individuals are encouraged to participate in all three levels of arts participation.
3. Write a poem that expresses your feelings concerning the arts for everyone.
4. Examine the activities offered by a local recreation center. Specify five arts activities that could be incorporated into the program, and discuss the benefits of each activity.
5. Discuss why it is important for individuals without disabilities to experience the artistic efforts of people with disabilities.
6. Discuss ways that community recreators can use the arts as a tool to allow individuals with disabilities to express their own feelings or needs.

REFERENCES

Appell, M. J. An overview: Arts in education for the handicapped. In *The Arts and Handicapped People: Defining the National Direction.* Washington, DC: National Committee, Arts for the Handicapped, 1978, pp. 13–17.

Baer, B. The rehabilitative influences of creative experience. *The Journal of Creative Behavior, 19*(3), 202–214, 1985.

Boyer, E. Unpublished speech given at the Very Special Arts Princeton Symposium on Early Childhood, Princeton, NJ, June 1987.

Copeland, B. Mainstreaming art for the handicapped child: Resources for teacher preparation. *Art Education, 37*(6), 22–29, 1984.

Diamondstein, G. *Exploring the Arts with Children.* New York: Macmillan, 1974.

Educational Facilities Laboratory and the National Endowment for the Arts. *Arts and the Handicapped: An Issue of Access.* New York: Educational Facilities Laboratory, 1975.

Finkle, D. Act-Hunger: MR/DDs are no longer overlooked. *The Village Voice,* pp. 94, 96, April 20, 1993.

Harlan, J. E. *A Guide to Setting Up a Creative Art Experiences Program for Older Adults with Developmental Disabilities.* Bloomington, IN: Institute for the Study of Developmental Disabilities, 1992.

Hart, J. Art appreciation courses can become "Museums Without Walls." *Provider,* p. 39, May 1991.

Hayman, d'A. Introduction. In United Nations Educational, Scientific and Cultural Organization, *The Arts and Man: A World View of the Role and Functions of the Arts in Society.* Englewood Cliffs, NJ: Prentice-Hall, 1969, pp. 11–26.

Hutchinson, P., & J. Lord. *Recreation Integration.* Ontario, Canada: Leisurability Publications, 1979.

Jacobs, R. YAI APEP develops peer education drama group: Reality Theatre. *HIV/AIDS and Mental Hygiene, 2*(2), 4–5, 1992.

Janus, C. The Kids on the Block: An effective medium for positive attitude change. *Journal of Leisurability, 8*(4), 32–35, 1981.

Johnson, D. W., & R. T. Johnson. Integrating handicapped students into the mainstream. *Exceptional Children, 47*(2), 90–98, 1980.

Kennedy, J. Insight into blindness. In E. Bernstein, Ed. *1985 Medical and Health Annual.* Chicago: Encyclopedia Britannica, 1985, pp. 154–165.

Kunkle-Miller, C. Handicapping conditions and their effect on the child's ability to create. In L. H. Kearns, M. T. Ditson, and B. G. Roehner, Eds. *Readings: Developing Art Programs for Handicapped Students.* Harrisburg, PA: Arts in Special Education Project of Pennsylvania, 1981, pp. 8–20.

Mangiacasale, A. The sounds of silence. *Disability Today, 2*(2), 54–55, 1993.

Molloy, L. Public facilities and handicapped patrons. In *The Arts and Handicapped People: Defining the National Direction.* Washington, DC: National Committee, Arts for the Handicapped, 1978, pp. 37–39.

Moran, J. Mainstreaming severely and profoundly handicapped children. In C. Sherrill, Ed. *Creative Arts for the Severely Handicapped.* Springfield, IL: Charles C Thomas, 1979, pp. 47–56.

National Committee, Arts for the Handicapped. *Art Resource and Training Guide.* Washington, DC: Author, 1981.

National Institute on Disability and Rehabilitation Research. Disability and the arts. *Rehab Brief: Bringing Research into Effective Focus, 8*(6), 1991.

Roehner, B. G. What is an arts program? In L. H. Kearns, M. T. Ditson, & B. G. Roehner, Eds. *Readings: Developing Arts Programs for Handicapped Students.* Harrisburg, PA: Arts in Special Education Project of Pennsylvania, 1981, pp. 5–7.

Ross, M., Ed. *The Arts and Personal Growth.* New York: Pergamon Press, 1980.

Schaefer, S. Theatre interpreters give signs of progress for the deaf. *USA Today*, p. 12C, December 10, 1992.

Schleien, S. J., & M. T. Ray. *Community Recreation and Persons with Disabilities: Strategies for Integration*. Baltimore: Paul H. Brookes, 1988.

Schleien, S. J., J. E. Rynders, & T. Mustonen. Arts and integration: What can we create? *Therapeutic Recreation Journal, 22*(4), 18–29, 1988.

Shaw, R. Education and the arts. In M. Ross, Ed. *The Arts and Personal Growth*. New York: Pergamon Press, 1980, pp. 69–78.

Sherrill, C., & R. Cox. Personnel preparation in creative arts for the handicapped: Implications for improving the quality of life. In C. Sherrill, Ed. *Creative Arts for the Severely Handicapped*, Springfield, IL: Charles C Thomas, 1979, pp. 3–11.

Smith, J. K. Testimony for reauthorization of Very Special Arts before Senate Subcommittee on Education, Arts and Humanities, July 16, 1987.

Smith, S. The arts in the education of learning disabled children. In *A Collection of Interest*. Washington, DC: National Committee, Arts for the Handicapped, 1981, pp. 80–90.

Speck, G. Handicapped make delightful "Magic" at Lyceum. *New York City Tribune*, p. B-6, October 29, 1986.

Spencer, M. J. A case for the arts. In The Rockefeller Foundation, *The Healing Role of the Arts*, New York: The Rockefeller Foundation, 1978, pp. 1–9.

Summers, L. Testimony before Congressional subcommittee on Americans with Disabilities Act, September 23, 1988.

Tomlinson, R. *Disability, Theatre, and Education*. Bloomington, IN: Indiana University Press, 1982.

Williams, R. M. Why children should draw. *Saturday Review*, pp. 101–106, September 3, 1977.

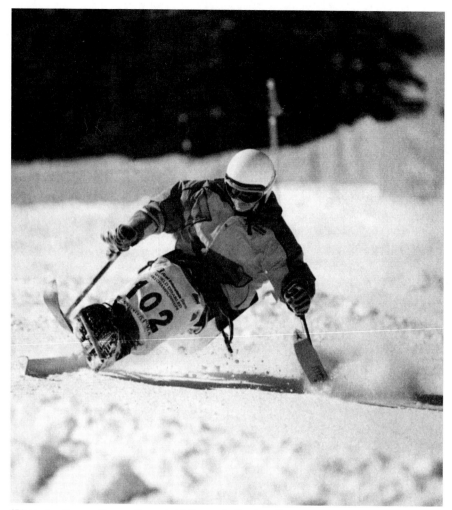

(Photo by Nancy Crase. Copyright Sports'n Spokes/Paralyzed Veterans of America)

11

Competitive Sports

■   ■   ■

You only have to pick up a newspaper or turn on a television to be reminded of the importance of competitive athletics in North America. Game results for local sports teams are often noted on the front page of major metropolitan newspapers, and it is not unusual for local television news programs to devote 20 percent or more of their air time to sports topics. But the influence of organized sports on our culture goes much deeper than merely the reporting of athletic events by the mass media. Indeed, there are few areas of modern society that are not influenced in some way by the presence of sport.

SPORTS FOR PERSONS WITH DISABILITIES

Despite the widespread influence of sport in our society and the recognition of its contribution to individual growth and development, the role of sport in the lives of persons with disabilities has received relatively little attention. In his interesting and widely read book, *Sports in America,* James Michener (1976) covers many fascinating aspects of sport. In-depth chapters are included on the role of sport in the lives of children, minorities, and women. Yet, although Michener's book is more than 500 pages long, the subject of sports for people who have disabilities is virtually ignored. Occasional articles on sports for athletes who are disabled may appear in newspapers or other publications, but they rarely appear in the sports sections and are usually treated as "human interest" stories rather than genuine examples of competitive sporting events. Even the major network television sports shows, which seem anxious to televise almost anything remotely resembling sport, have generally failed to provide coverage of organized and highly competitive sports competition among athletes who have disabilities.

On June 27, 1989, Natalie Bacon, the first female wheelchair athlete to compete in the New York Marathon, lost her battle with cancer. This chapter is dedicated to Natalie's memory and to her incredible competitive spirit.

Why, with sport's influence so important in our culture, has society's acceptance of competitive sports programs for athletes with disabilities been so slow to develop? Perhaps one reason is the comparative newness of organized sports for people with disabilities. Although sports historian Earle Zeigler (1979) dated the first recorded sports competitions as occurring during the Early Dynastic period of the Sumerian civilization (3000–1500 B.C.), organized sports for people with disabilities is largely a 20th-century phenomenon. In fact, most sports programs for individuals who are disabled are less than forty years old.

Newness alone does not account for the lack of public attention, however. Probably a more fundamental reason for the absence of public awareness and interest in sports for people with disabilities is the widespread belief that such programs are solely "therapeutic." The needs and motivations of athletes who have disabilities are often viewed as different from their nondisabled counterparts, and the primary emphasis of such competition is seen as rehabilitation. While the rehabilitative potential of sports involvement is undeniable, emphasizing this aspect to the exclusion of the other benefits to the individual participant is unfortunate. Such emphasis merely strengthens the public's view of individuals with disabilities as "different" or "abnormal." Rather than stressing differences, the desire for sports participation among many people who have disabilities is, in fact, a classic example of the *similarity* of *all* people.

Professor Timothy Nugent (1969), longtime director of the University of Illinois Rehabilitation-Education Center until his retirement in 1985, emphasized this point in the following statement:

> Let us recognize that, individually and collectively, [people with disabilities] have the same aspirations, interests, talents and, in most instances, the same skills as all people. They have the same basic social-psychological needs and would like to travel the same avenues that you and I have been privileged to travel in fulfillment of these needs. It is the fault of our society as a whole, and more particularly, of the apathy, lack of awareness and sensitivity of our professional leaders that these individuals have not been privileged to travel these avenues. It is not the fault of the disability or the individual with the disability. (pp. 20–21)

As noted earlier, sports is an important part of our society and, as such, it is one of the major "avenues" for needs fulfillment mentioned by Nugent. Providing sports opportunities for athletes who are disabled is not necessarily rehabilitation, but it is certainly a contribution that enables the participant to receive the same physical, social, and psychological benefits that organized, competitive sports programs offer to *all* participants.

Fortunately, there is evidence that athletes with disabilities are beginning to receive the recognition they deserve. In the late 1980s, a U.S. postage stamp was issued paying tribute to athletes who compete in the Winter Special Olympics. Sharon Hedrick, recipient of the prestigious Southland Olympia Award, was seen on worldwide television winning her second consecutive Olympic gold medal (exhibition 800-m wheelchair dash). And Craig Blanchette, a talented wheelchair athlete, was the subject of both a five-page article in *Sports Illustrated* and a "Just Do It" television commercial for Nike athletic shoes. Additionally, prize money supplied by corporate sponsors now attracts wheelchair athletes from around the world to compete in some major sports events. The appearance of published compendiums on sports for people with disabilities, such as *Sports and Recreation for the Disabled: A Resource Handbook* (Paciorek & Jones, 1994) and *Go for It* (Kelly & Freiden, 1989) also demonstrates increased public acceptance of and interest in sports for persons with disabilities.

Common Goals of Sports Participation

As noted by Paciorek and Jones (1994), many sports opportunities throughout the United States and Canada are available to people with disabilities. Football, racquetball, softball, track and field, basketball, rugby, and tennis are just a few of the many wheelchair sports providing outlets for athletes with mobility limitations. People with visual impairments, sometimes using sighted guides, can participate in such sports as beep baseball, golf, archery, bowling, and many winter sports (Montelione & Mastro, 1985; Rarick, 1984; Spraggs, 1984). The Special Olympics offers opportunities for winter and summer competition among people with mental retardation. In addition, senior citizens with and without disabilities compete in the Senior Olympics. Each of these programs, as well as others providing sports competition for people with specific needs, makes unique contributions to participants. Each differs from the others in many ways, including administrative procedures, type of athletic contests offered, basic rules of competition, fund-raising techniques, and so on. Yet, there are a number of things that competitive programs for people with disabilities have in common. Most, if not all, of these programs, do the following:

- Provide a method of informing the public about the unique *abilities* that participants possess.
- Promote independence, sports skill development, and increased physical fitness among their participants.
- Promote maximum participation by offering local or regional events but also provide for recognition of outstanding performances through national and international competition.
- Have some system of classification, such as degree of disability, to make the competition in events as fair as possible.
- Use the classification system as a method of increasing participation opportunities among individuals with severe disabilities.

Criticism of Segregated Programs

In addition to sharing some common goals and procedures, sports programs for athletes who are disabled also receive similar criticism. One of the most frequent complaints about these programs is that they "segregate" participants who have disabilities from nondisabled athletes. Most of the programs mentioned previously have regulations that prohibit nondisabled participants from competing against athletes who have disabilities. Some authorities feel that the participants are denied significant social and psychological benefits that result from meeting, sharing, and becoming friends with nondisabled individuals who share similar interests in sport (Brasile, 1990; DePaepe & Bange, 1986). Although many segregated programs do include volunteers who socially interact with competitors who have disabilities, the role of a volunteer often places the person without a disability "above" the competitor. To be effective, social interaction between peers with and without disabilities should be on an equal level.

Advocates of programs for athletes with disabilities, however, counter the above criticism with several logical points. First, they note that sports programs are but one aspect of a person's life. Fundamental changes are needed in other societal institutions, such as education, and transportation, to promote integration of individuals with disabilities into society. In effect, sports programs for individuals with disabilities are a reaction to a segregated society, not a cause of it. Second, supporters of these programs contend that providing the athlete who has a disability with a fair chance for success in sporting events may require excluding individuals without disabilities from competition. Having peers who do not have disabilities serve as volunteers may also offer the chance for social interaction in a cooperative, rather than a competitive, situation. Third, advocates maintain segregated sports participation enhances the development of social and physical skills in an environment of acceptance and understanding. This social and physical development, which is enhanced by successful competitive experiences, promotes confidence and self-esteem among participants (Nettleton, 1974).

Brasile (1990), who is opposed to segregated sports competition among athletes with disabilities, has suggested that sports for persons with disabilities adopt a "reverse integration" approach whereby people without disabilities are integrated into sports activities that have traditionally been restricted to athletes with disabilities. Using wheelchair sports as an example, Brasile urged adding persons without disabilities to wheelchair basketball teams, thus fostering "an atmosphere for social integration in which all participants will be competing on an equal basis" (p. 4). Thibutot, Smith, and Labanowich (1992) agreed that for recreational sports activities, Brasile's ideas are logical and might facilitate inclusion of persons with disabilities into society. They disagreed strongly with Brasile, however, about using reverse integration in organized competitive sports for persons with disabilities. Thiboutot et al., noted that the primary emphasis of Brasile's reverse integration concept "appears to be rehabilitation, rather than competitive sports. As such, it represents a step backward for the wheelchair sports movement in the U.S." (p. 291). Lindstrom (1992) also took issue with inclusion of athletes without disabilities into competitive sports for athletes with disabilities. He stated, "If the meaning of integration is to equalize conditions of a minority group to those of a majority, then participation of able-bodied athletes in elite sports adapted for the disabled is an anomaly . . . participation of the able-bodied in elite sports in wheelchairs, with blindfolds, or with hands tied in the back is out of the question" (p. 58).

Rather than promoting reverse integration in competitive sports, many authorities advocate the use of "parallel" competition in which athletes with disabilities routinely compete against each other at the same time and in the same physical location as athletes without disabilities. This concept enables mutual sharing of the competitive spirit among *all* athletes but avoids the inequities that might result from direct competition between athletes with and without disabilities. McClements (1984) described Saskatchewan's effort to offer parallel competition among athletes with mental retardation and their nondisabled peers. He stated that parallel competition allows athletes with disabilities "a greater choice in athletic activities and programs and the opportunity to meet, interact with and most importantly, participate with their [nondisabled] fellow athletes" (p. 23).

Stan Labanowich, past Commissioner of the National Wheelchair Basketball Association, is a strong advocate for parallel competition in sporting events. He has observed (Labanowich, 1988) that one possible way to include athletes with disabilities in the Olympic games would be to provide for parallel participation. Such a scenario would include "modification of the rules to create a version of the sport to enable [athletes with disabilities] to participate separately" (p. 271). Parallel competition, unlike the "exhibitions" included in recent Olympiads (Crase, 1988) would be "accorded the same integrity and value as the nonmodified version of the sport" and represent "a highly acceptable form of integration of athletes with disabilities who are otherwise ruled physically ineligible to compete in the nonmodified version of a sport" (p. 271).

Fortunately, some progress appears to have been made toward parallel competition at the Olympic games. Lindstrom (1992) expressed hope that the work by the International Committee on Integration of Athletes with a Disability (ICI) "will speed up the process of including full medal events for athletes with disabilities in world competitions thus far reserved exclusively for able-bodied athletes" (p. 29). Lindstrom, himself an athlete with a disability, emphasized his support for parallel competition and stated that he "wants to see other athletes with disabilities in competitions for gold medals at the Olympic Games on their own conditions and with their own identities" (p. 58).

Competitive Programs

There are many sports programs offering a variety of competitive opportunities to people with disabilities. For example, the Committee on Sports for the Disabled, within the U.S. Olympic Committee, is composed of organizations that govern competitive sports for various disabling conditions. These organizations include the American Athletic Association for the Deaf, Dwarf Athletic Association of America, National Handicapped Sports, Wheelchair Sports, USA, Special Olympics International, Inc., United States Association for Blind Athletes, and United States Cerebral Palsy Athletic Association.

Obviously, it would be impossible to describe in this chapter all of the sports programs for athletes with disabilities throughout the United States and Canada; however, two widely known segregated programs have been selected to serve as examples: (1) wheelchair sports for people with mobility limitations; and (2) the Special Olympics for children and adults with mental retardation. In addition, the Barrie Integrated Baseball Association has been included to illustrate inclusion of athletes with disabilities into community sports programs. It is important for the reader to keep in mind that these programs are merely examples; therefore, each of these sports organizations has a unique history and organizational structure. Readers interested in further information on other sports organizations and programs should consult Paciorek and Jones (1994) and Kelly and Frieden (1989), listed in the references at the end of this chapter. In addition, selected sports organizations for persons with disabilities are included in Appendix B.

WHEELCHAIR SPORTS

Historical Development

The wheelchair sports movement in the United States owes its beginning and continued growth to three primary factors: (1) advances in medical technology, which have resulted in an increasing life expectancy for individuals with physical disabilities; (2) the competitive spirit and determination of athletes with disabilities who always manage to find ways to overcome personal and organizational difficulties to be able to participate in competitive sports; and (3) foresight among several determined professionals who have provided the leadership "spark" needed for establishment and continued expansion of wheelchair athletics.

Prior to World War II, wheelchair sports were virtually nonexistent. Although the needs of people with physical disabilities were becoming increasingly recognized by concerned United States citizens and organizations, few people thought that athletic competition was appropriate for so-called "cripples." By World War II, however, medical technology and battlefield evacuation methods had improved to the point where severely wounded soldiers were kept alive in increasing numbers. These soldiers, including young men with spinal cord injuries and amputations, would have died in prior wars, but now they returned home to veterans' hospitals throughout the United States. Despite their injuries, these men desired the same competitive sports opportunities that they enjoyed prior to going overseas.

The desire for competition in organized sports grew as these veterans, many of them athletes prior to injury, progressed from playing catch, table tennis, and bowling to the more active physical demands of water polo, softball, and touch football. But it was basketball that really caught the imagination and competitive spirit of these veterans. It was rough, strenuous, and highly competitive. Don Swift, one of the early wheelchair basketball players, described the game as "a combination of football and basketball in that there was considerably more contact than exists now . . . a much rougher game" (Labanowich, 1975, p. 34).

Soon just playing basketball against other patients within the hospital was not satisfying enough. By 1948, there were at least six organized veterans' teams in the United

States and the famous "Flying Wheels" from California began their cross-country tour playing wheelchair basketball against other teams. The wheelchair sports movement in North America was underway.

Formation of Associations

Among the many people who were aware of wheelchair basketball's start, as well as of the potential for other wheelchair sports, were Timothy Nugent and Ben Lipton. These two men, along with Sir Ludwig Guttmann in England, were to become the driving force for wheelchair sports as we know it today. Tim Nugent, from the University of Illinois, not only formed the first collegiate wheelchair basketball team in 1948, but he organized the first National Wheelchair Basketball Tournament in April 1949. This tournament provided the basis for development of the National Wheelchair Basketball Association (NWBA), which Nugent headed as commissioner for 25 years. When he retired as NWBA Commissioner in 1973, Tim Nugent could proudly boast that the modest beginning of six NWBA teams had grown to almost 100 teams throughout the United States.

While wheelchair basketball was blossoming in the 1950s, Ben Lipton, from Bulova School of Watchmaking, recognized the need for other types of competitive opportunities for individuals with disabilities. At the time, basketball was dominated by men, and ball-handling skills required fairly good use of most upper body muscles. Track and field events, table tennis, swimming, and other competitive activities, however, offered new avenues for women and individuals with high spinal cord injuries. In 1957, Lipton initiated the first U.S. Wheelchair Games. These games, which included many of the forenamed events, were a resounding success and Lipton became the chairman of the newly formed National Wheelchair Athletic Association (NWAA) in 1958. Like Nugent, Ben Lipton presided over the growth of the NWAA (now Wheelchair Sports, USA) for more than 20 years.

Thus, the development of organized wheelchair sports in the United States has been stimulated by two simultaneous but separate organizational movements: The National Wheelchair Basketball Association and Wheelchair Sports, USA. A brief examination of each organization's sports program will help explain the state of wheelchair sports in the United States today.

National Wheelchair Basketball Association

A complete picture of wheelchair basketball can only come from watching one of the fast and exciting games played between two highly skilled teams. Wheelchair basketball is played according to National Collegiate Athletic Association rules, although a few modifications to these rules are made to accommodate the use of wheelchairs. Each game is played on a full-sized high school or college court, and the baskets remain at the 10-foot level. The degree of strength and skill required by wheelchair basketball players can be easily demonstrated by trying to shoot accurately at a 10-foot basket from 15 feet away *while sitting on a chair!* But being able to shoot means very little if you cannot move the

In the 1950s, wheelchair sports events like track and field, table tennis, and swimming offered competitive opportunities for women with spinal cord injuries. Today, women with disabilities compete at a high level in all aspects of wheelchair sports programs. (Copyright Sports 'n Spokes/Paralyzed Veterans of America, 1993)

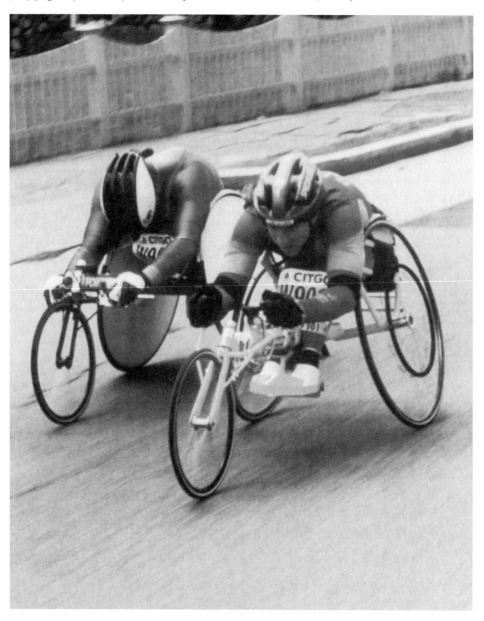

wheelchair with speed and agility. As one TV sports commentator noted, "I thought I was a pretty good basketball player but those guys (wheelchair team members) put me to shame. I was zero for twelve from the foul line, and they ran, er, wheeled circles around me on the floor."

Following are some important aspects of wheelchair basketball and the National Wheelchair Basketball Association.

Rules. As noted earlier, NCAA rules serve as the standard for wheelchair basketball, but modifications are made when special situations dictate. For example, contact between chairs was not originally considered to be a personal foul. Bob Miller, the first president of the NWBA, described the result:

> Wheelchair Bulldozers we called ourselves, the reason being that in those days before the rules were refined, you could ram a guy all you wanted—when you caught him sitting dead with the ball. You could ram into him and take the ball away from him. And so we picked the name Bulldozers—Wheelchair Bulldozers. (Labanowich, 1975, p. 34)

As a result of such tactics, the wheelchair is now considered to be a part of the player. Throughout the years, the sophistication of wheelchair basketball rules has increased to the point that today's *Official NWBA Rules and Case Book* is more than 30 pages long. The case book portion of this document gives rule interpretations for more than 50 actual game situations. See Figure 11.1 for a humorous look at wheelchair basketball rules.

Classification System and Team Balance. Wheelchair basketball requires a great deal of balance, upper body strength, and overall coordination. Players with lower spinal cord injuries (in general, the lower the injury, the more muscle function a player has) or disabilities only affecting the lower extremities (legs) usually have a competitive advantage over players with more severe disabilities. Despite prohibitions against minimal disabilities, including *temporary* disorders caused by injury, some wheelchair basketball players are able to walk unaided; however, on their feet they could not keep pace with players without disabilities.

To provide opportunities for individuals with severe disabilities to compete in basketball, a classification system was devised based on the athlete's level of spinal cord (or comparable) injury (see Fig. 11.2). Wheelchair basketball players are currently placed into one of three classes according to the following system:

> *Class I.* Complete motor loss at T-7 or above or comparable disability where there is total loss of muscle function originating at or above T-7.
>
> *Class II.* Complete motor loss originating at T-8 and descending through and including L-2 where there may be motor power of hips and thighs. Also included in this class are amputees with bilateral hip disarticulation.
>
> *Class III.* All other physical disabilities as related to lower extremity paralysis or paresis originating at or below L-3. All lower extremity amputees are included in this class, except those with bilateral hip disarticulation (see Class II).

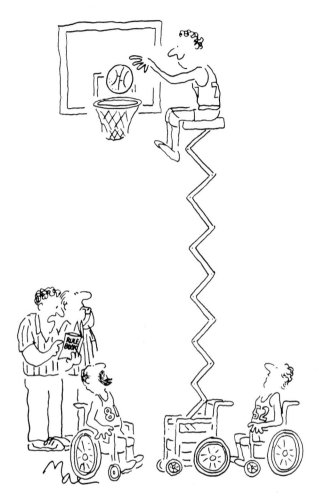

"Here it is, Nugent . . . rule 27, section 7: No player shall . . ."

Figure 11.2. Player classifications in the National Wheelchair Basketball Association are based upon each athlete's level of spinal cord injury or comparable level of disability. This diagram illustrates the three-level classification system used by the NWBA. (Originally appeared in *Palaestra,* Vol. 1, No. 2, 1985. Modified and reproduced with permission of Challenge Publications, Inc.)

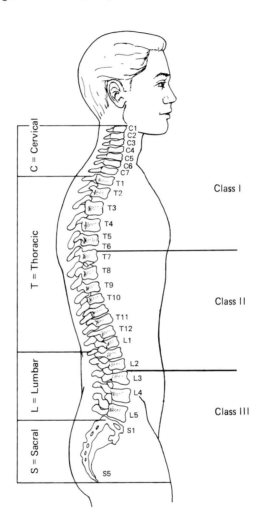

Basketball is a team sport, so merely classifying individuals according to the system on page 255 is not enough. Each classification (I, II, and III) is given a numerical or point value as follows:

Class I. 1 point
Class II. 2 points
Class III. 3 points

Current NWBA rules prevent a team from placing five players on the floor at the same time whose point totals exceed 12 points. Since no more than three Class IIIs are allowed at one time, many NWBA teams use three Class IIIs, one Class II, and one Class I. Thus, the more severely disabled Class I player is provided an opportunity to play because of the NWBA's team balance concept.

Scope. Although originally limited exclusively to males, NWBA teams have been open to participation by both sexes since 1974. Women may join any one of the teams in the association, which includes a number of all-women teams. In addition to the annual National Wheelchair Basketball Tournament for the final four top teams, the Association also helps to support the National Women's Wheelchair Basketball Tournament and the Intercollegiate Wheelchair Basketball Tournament. A youth division, chaired by Dr. Bob Szyman, St. Louis, Missouri, also provides support for youngsters who are learning the sport. Although most of the teams in the NWBA are located in the continental United States, there are also several Canadian teams that have chosen to affiliate with the association.

Democratic Representation. One of the more favorable aspects of the NWBA is its policy that the players establish all rules, including rules of play and the association's constitution and bylaws. This is accomplished at an annual meeting of team delegates at which all of the association's business is conducted. The idea of recreation consumer input from persons with disabilities is relatively new in the United States, but the NWBA has been practicing this policy since its formation in 1949.

Wheelchair Sports, USA (Formerly National Wheelchair Athletic Association)

The National Wheelchair Athletic Association (NWAA), now Wheelchair Sports, USA (WSUSA), was formed almost 10 years after the NWBA, but it quickly took on a very important role in wheelchair sports development. Because it was not limited to a single sport, the NWAA became the representative body for a varied group of competitors with disabilities. The following list of sporting events, currently governed by WSUSA, gives some idea of this variety: track events (100-yard dash to distance events), field events (shot put, javelin, discus), swimming, weight lifting, archery, and slalom (an obstacle course event in which competitors compete for the best time).

Under the leadership of Ben Lipton, the NWAA became the wheelchair sports organization that organized and supervised U.S. participation in most major international competitions. These international events, including the well-known "Paralympics," became a prized goal for every NWAA competitor. Jon Brown, holder of the world heavyweight weight-lifting record, underscored the personal importance of international competition by stating, "I don't remember walking. I've never climbed a stair. I've never run. So for me these games are a dream come true" (Weisman & Godfrey, 1976, p 121).

As with wheelchair basketball, Wheelchair Sports, USA and the events it governs have several aspects that should be highlighted.

Classification System. Since WSUSA events generally feature individual, rather than team, competition, some form of classifying the severity of a person's disability is essential. As noted previously, individuals with lower extremity injuries may have a competitive edge over those with injuries that also affect stomach, chest, back, or arm muscles. Currently, WSUSA uses a functional classification system modeled after the one used for international competition. This means that the athlete's "observed movement-patterns during sport performance (throwing a discus, racing in a wheelchair, or swimming in the pool), rather than neurological status, have become the major factors [in determining classification]" (Curtis, 1991, p. 45). This system overcomes some of the shortcomings of the previous, medically based system. As noted by Curtis, there are three distinct advantages of the current system. First, the functional system allows for sport-specific classification. Thus, the interaction between the requirements of a particular sport and the functional ability of the athlete is taken into consideration during classification. Second, the functional system makes it easier to classify persons with various disabilities. The previous system was based on complete spinal cord injury and required comparing the athlete's physical limitations with spinal levels of muscle innervation. Third, the functional system facilitates efficient organization of events by reducing the number of competitive categories, thus reducing the number of heats, trials, etc. The functional system, in various forms, has been used successfully in international competition for more than ten years. Still, as Lindstrom (1985) noted, "No classification system in competitive sports, for able-bodied or for disabled, will ever be totally fair to each individual: those being near the upper limit of the class definition will have an advantage over those being near the lower limits" (p. 48).

Scope. WSUSA's regional, national, and international competitive activities provide a wide range of events for many males and females with mobility limitations. Youth competitions, including the Junior National Wheelchair Games, have been part of the WSUSA since the mid-1980s. In the late eighties, WSUSA's sports competitions were "decentralized"; that is, the major U.S. championships in each sport (e.g., track and field, weight lifting) were held at separate dates and locations. Previously, most WSUSA sports held their championships at the National Wheelchair Games, located at a single site or area. It is unfortunate that decentralization of competitions has reduced some of WSUSA's camaraderie, but it was an inevitable outcome of the association's continued growth.

Unlike wheelchair basketball, WSUSA's format of individual competition offers almost unlimited competitive opportunities for persons with very high spinal cord injuries (quadriplegics). Individual competition also provides athletes with disabilities who live in rural areas an opportunity to compete, because team membership is not necessary.

Slalom Event. All of the events governed by WSUSA closely parallel the rules and format of sports for participants without disabilities, except for the slalom event. The slalom course requires a competitor to demonstrate exceptional wheelchair-handling skill by going over, under, and around numerous obstacles. Speed and wheelchair agility are the qualities needed to excel in this event, and the finalist in each class with the best time is declared the winner. Since this event is unique to wheelchair sports, it generates a great deal of spectator interest. It also provides many wheelchair athletes with the motivation to master difficult, but important, wheelchair-handling skills, for example, "wheelies" and curb jumping. The uniqueness of the slalom event has also resulted in criticism from some authorities because it is believed to violate the concept of normalization. Efforts to eliminate this event from wheelchair sports competition have not been successful, however, and the slalom continues to be a popular addition to most wheelchair games.

Benefits of Wheelchair Sports

There is no doubt that participation in organized wheelchair sports, whether through the NWBA or WSUSA, requires a large personal commitment—one involving time, effort, and *money*. The present cost of most sports-adaptable wheelchairs, which are lighter and more durable than conventional chairs, is more than $1,000.

The investment needed to establish a wheelchair basketball team may exceed $30,000, including wheelchairs, uniforms, equipment, and one season's travel and game expenses. Why, since it is so expensive, do individuals and some organizations provide their financial support to wheelchair sports? The answer to that question can be found in an explanation of three of the benefits that wheelchair sports offer. They are as follows:

1. *Participant Growth and Development.* Sports for individuals without disabilities are claimed to offer great physical and mental benefits. This claim is also made about wheelchair sports because athletes with and without disabilities share similar goals, objectives, motivations, and personal characteristics (Brasile & Hedrick, 1991; Coutts, 1986; Henschen, Horvat, & French, 1984; Ogilvie, 1990; Roeder & Aufsesser, 1986). Many studies and journal articles have stressed the importance of wheelchair sports for individuals with physical disabilities. Jochheim and Strohkendl (1973), for example, noted the physical problems caused by poor conditioning in paraplegia, and urged participation in several wheelchair sports events to overcome these problems. Stotts (1986) provided support for their contention. Comparing athletes and nonathletes with spinal cord injuries, she found that athletes had significantly less hospitalizations than nonathletes. Moreover, the illnesses reported by athletes were generally less serious than those reported by nonathletes. Loiselle (1979) also stressed the benefits of wheelchair

sports participation, with particular emphasis on the psychosocial effects. Research studies by Coutts (1986, 1988), Guttmann and Mehra (1973), Patrick (1986), Steadward and Walsh (1986), Zwiren and Bar-or (1975), and many others have provided evidence in support of participant benefits. Increased physical fitness and strength, a better self-concept and social adjustment, and greater awareness of the world through travel are all positive aspects of wheelchair sports participation.

2. *Public Awareness.* Wheelchair athletes often quote the expression, "It's ability, not disability, that counts," and wheelchair sports offer the individual who has a disability an excellent chance to display great skill and physical ability to the nondisabled public. Watching the exciting action of a wheelchair basketball game, or observing an athlete with a disability wheel more than 26 miles in a marathon event, cannot help but increase a nondisabled person's appreciation of people with disabilities. As found by Asken and Goodlin (1987), public attitudes toward sports for people with disabilities tend to be positive and supportive. The myth of "dependency" is quickly dispelled by watching displays of athletic skill, and the wheelchair sports spectator may walk away with a newly formed attitude of appreciation and respect toward people with disabilities. Hedrick's (1986) investigation of the effects of participation in an integrated tennis class provided support for this notion. He found that an improvement in perceptions among nondisabled subjects regarding sport-specific efficacy of peers with disabilities may generalize to improved perceptions of *general* physical competence among people who have disabilities. As Treischmann (1988) observed, wheelchair sports participants "have demonstrated to society that a full and rich life is available to all if one is willing to work for it" (p. 217).

3. *Motivation for Others.* The skill displayed by wheelchair athletes often provides much needed motivation for youth or individuals with recent disabilities. During the 28th National Wheelchair Basketball Tournament (NWBT) in Baltimore, for example, a large number of young people with physical disabilities attended the games. Later, the director of the tournament was informed by local school personnel that the 28th NWBT resulted in renewed enthusiasm for physical activity and adapted physical education programs. The publicity and excitement of the tournament was "just what the doctor ordered" for the youth of Baltimore. Today, several of the young spectators at the 28th NWBT are regulars on Baltimore's wheelchair basketball team.

Expanding Opportunities

The wheelchair sports movement has not only experienced phenomenal growth; it has provided the model for others to promote sports for individuals with disabilities who are ineligible for competition against, or not on a competitive level with, the "traditional" wheelchair athlete. Multiple disabilities or those affecting the upper extremities often limit or prevent participation in NWBA or WSUSA events. The National Cerebral Palsy Games, and their preliminary competition on local, state, and regional levels, have helped to fill the void in competitive sports opportunities for people with such disabilities. These games, held by the U.S. Cerebral Palsy Athletic Association, have classification categories for competitors who use wheelchairs, but also have classes for ambulatory and

"It's ability, not disability, that counts." Wheelchair basketball offers an athlete with a lower extremity disability the chance to demonstrate great skill and physical ability to the nondisabled public. (Courtesy of *PVA Sports 'n Spokes* Magazine)

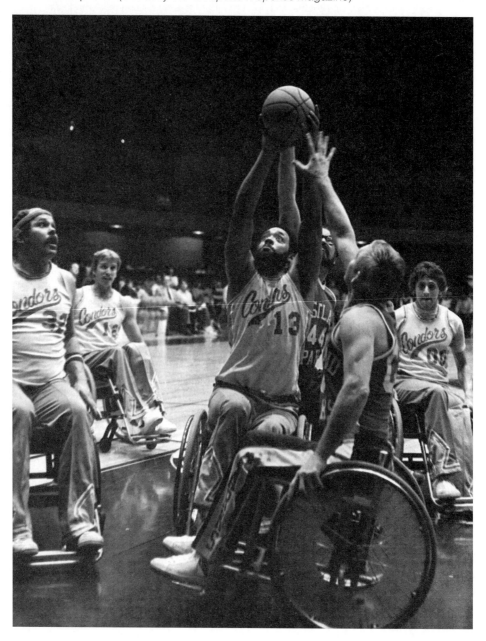

semiambulatory (users of crutches and other walking aids) competitors. Events held at these games include but are not limited to archery, horseback riding, weight lifting, table tennis, soccer, bowling, rifle shooting, and track and field.

The acceptance of competitive sports for all athletes, including those with severe and/or multiple disabilities, was evidenced by the success of the 9th Paralympic Games in Barcelona, Spain, in 1992. Approximately 3,000 athletes from 94 countries competed in these games, which encompassed 12 days of competition. As noted by Alger (1992), " 'Awesome' is the best word to describe the 1992 Paralympics" (p. 15)—more than 1.3 *million* spectators attended various Paralympic events and more than 35 TV and radio stations covered the events. "It was not unusual to see hundreds of spectators lined up outside the venues and down the street, hoping to get into one of the venues" (Alger, 1992). The United States team captured the most gold medals (75) and edged Germany for the largest total medal count (175 to 171). Canada's 143-athlete contingent set 14 world records, collected 28 gold, 21 silver, and 26 bronze medals, and finished a very respectable sixth place overall (Johnson, 1992).

Although spectacular in every respect, the 9th Paralympics, like most Olympic Games, were not without controversy. A cross-disability classification system was used for the first time, allowing athletes with different disabilities to compete in the same event. "Swimming was the main sport affected by the inclusion of all disabilities, and many gold-medal swimmers from years past returned home empty-handed, finding themselves victims of the new process" (Alger, 1992). In another controversy, the gold-medal-winning U.S. wheelchair basketball team was disqualified following the championship game when one of its athletes tested positive for a banned substance (dextropropoxyphene—a mild narcotic analgesic found in Darvon™). The drug is not considered to be performance enhancing and is commonly used by persons with incomplete spinal cord injuries to control pain; however, the U.S. team's appeal was denied and the entire team was disqualified. Despite these controversies, Juan Antonio Samaranch, president of the International Olympic Committee, observed, "The Paralympic Games have been as successful as the Olympic Games" (Johnson, 1992, p. 10).

An Era of Change

Sports 'n Spokes magazine is a bimonthly publication dedicated to wheelchair sports and recreation. The following chronology is modified and expanded from the 10th anniversary issue of *Sports 'n Spokes*. It illustrates some of the many dramatic events that occurred in wheelchair sports from 1975 to 1994.

1975   *Sports 'n Spokes* publishes its first issue.
       Bob Hall becomes the first wheelchair competitor in the Boston Marathon.
       First Women's National Wheelchair Basketball Tournament is held.

1976   Six countries decline to participate in the Toronto Olympiad because of South Africa's inclusion in the Games.

1977 First National Wheelchair Marathon is held in conjunction with the 81st Boston Marathon.
The Cerebral Palsy sports movement emerges and develops its own classification system.
First National Wheelchair Softball Tournament is held.

1978 First U.S. National Cerebral Palsy Games are held.
Canada's University of Alberta in Edmonton establishes a research and training center for athletes with physical disabilities.

1979 U.S. Olympic Committee forms Committee on Sports for the Disabled.
Peter Axelson develops first controllable sled for snow skiers with spinal cord injuries.

1980 First National Wheelchair Tennis Championships are held.

1981 First National Amputee Games are held.

1982 Amateur Racquetball Association's National Championships feature exhibition wheelchair racquetball division.

1983 U.S. Handicapped Ski Team is formed.
National Wheelchair Racquetball Association is founded.

1984 International Games for the Disabled are held in New York.
Wheelchair track exhibition events are held as part of the Olympic Games.
First National Junior Wheelchair Games are attended by youngsters from the United States and Canada.

1985 Mono-ski competition is included in the 14th National Handicapped Ski Championships.
First issue of *Palaestra: The Forum of Sport and Physical Education for the Disabled* is published.

1986 First National Triathlon for the Physically Challenged is held.

1987 Rick Hansen completes 29,901-mile "Man in Motion" tour around the world in a wheelchair. He is welcomed home to Vancouver, B.C., by 50,000 people.

1988 U.S. team nets most gold medals at Paralympics in Seoul, Korea.
First Quad Rugby Championships are held.

1989 National Wheelchair Games decentralize because of growth in competitors and spectators.

1990 U.S. wheelchair basketball team wins Gold Cup in Brugge, Belgium.
Wheelchair racquetball added to two major multiple-sports events.

1991 Ben Lipton, founder of the NWAA (now WSUSA), dies.

1992 U.S. team captures most medals in 9th Paralympic Games in Barcelona, Spain, despite disqualification of U.S. men's wheelchair basketball team.
Cross-disability classification system instituted for first time in Paralympics.

1993 NWAA changes its name to Wheelchair Sports, USA (WSUSA).
NWBA joins WSUSA as a member of the national governing body.

1994 Sharon Rahn Hedrick becomes first woman inducted in NWBA Hall of Fame.

The preceding chronology shows the diversity of wheelchair sports, as well as many of the changes that have occurred in recent years. One dramatic change not included in the list, however, is the evolution of the sports-model wheelchair. Prior to 1978, wheelchair athletes competed in "standard" wheelchairs with, at most, minor modifications such as smaller handrims and lowered seats. At the 22nd National Wheelchair Games in 1978, however, George Murray introduced two innovations that would forever alter the design and use of sports-model wheelchairs. LaMere and Labanowich (1984) noted that Murray modified the wheelchair to elevate "his knees excessively high to compensate for his lack of sitting balance owing to the [high] level of his [spinal cord] lesion. . . . Through compensating for his lack of sitting balance, Murray was able to generate a complete stroke and follow through" (p. 12). This alteration, plus Murray's use of steering handles on the front casters of his wheelchair, directly resulted in a liberalization of rules regulating competitive wheelchairs.

Today, there are about 25 manufacturers who produce quality sports wheelchairs that incorporate Murray's modifications, plus many additional innovative features. One of the most striking differences between present wheelchairs and those of the late '70s, however, is their weight. The wheelchair George Murray used in 1978 weighed about 50 lbs; today, his sports wheelchair probably weighs less than 11 lbs! Besides being lighter, modern sports wheelchairs incorporate a number of design features that increase their efficiency, including a three-wheel design. Even when differences in weight are taken into account, today's sports wheelchairs require close to 20 percent *less* energy to push than conventional wheelchairs (Hilbers & White, 1987).

Technological advances in the sports-model wheelchair, both in weight and design, have also helped to make life easier for nonathletes who use wheelchairs. Today's lighter and more maneuverable "standard" wheelchairs were made possible by advancements in wheelchair sports technology.

SPECIAL OLYMPICS

Historical Development

Unlike wheelchair sports, the Special Olympics was not formed because the participants themselves created a demand for the programs. The characteristics of mental retardation often prevent effective consumerism without the aid and assistance of "advocates" who do not have disabilities. These advocates work to ensure that the needs, desires, and rights of people with mental retardation are met within society. The formation of the Special Olympics is an example of such advocacy.

Early in the 1960s, President John F. Kennedy's administration stressed the importance of physical fitness activities for all U.S. citizens, and many studies were conducted that clearly established the need for such activities. By 1967, research on physical fitness revealed a lack of physical proficiency among people with mental retardation. The primary cause of this shortcoming was felt to be a lack of programs that stressed physical activities. Haskins (1976) noted that these studies revealed that 45 percent of schoolchildren in the United States who had mental retardation received *no* physical education instruction, and only 25 percent received as much as one hour per week. The Chicago Park District, responding to the obvious need for athletic programs for youth with mental retardation, developed the idea of a nationwide competition stressing track and field events.

In 1967, the Chicago Park District sought the assistance of the Joseph P. Kennedy, Jr. Foundation to finance their idea for a national track meet for youngsters who were mentally retarded. The idea was well received, no doubt in part because the Kennedy family had personal experience with metal retardation: A daughter of Joseph and Rose Kennedy has mental retardation. Rather than expending a lot of money and effort on a program that might not succeed, the Kennedy Foundation and the Chicago Park District agreed to test their new idea by holding and then evaluating the success of a single national meet. That meet, held in 1968, included participants from only 24 states, but the enthusiasm and enjoyment displayed by the 1,000 competitors overshadowed the failure of many states to organize teams. Mrs. Eunice Kennedy Shriver represented the Kennedy Foundation at that premier meet, and the joy she saw among competitors convinced her that the concept of a national sports program for people with mental retardation was a solid one. Following that first event, Special Olympics, Inc., was formed, with Mrs. Shriver serving as president. During the years that followed, the Special Olympics grew in participation, competitive events, and public recognition. Today, it is estimated that more than 1 million children and adults with mental retardation participate in Special Olympics programs throughout the world, and the number of local, chapter, regional, national, and international events exceeds 10,000 each year.

Organization and Events

Special Olympics competition is organized to ensure that as many people with mental retardation as possible get an opportunity to participate. Spring track and field competition, for example, is offered in a large number of "local" meets that do not require a lot of travel by participants. Holding local events close to the communities where the participants live means that event organizers are usually familiar with local agency or school personnel. Such agency or school professionals can be very helpful in recruiting and training Special Olympics competitors. For example, Special Olympics is recruiting local recreation professionals, through a formal partnership with the National Recreation and Park Association, to reach more eligible individuals within communities (Natalini, 1988). Thus, local rivalries may be promoted, local customs observed, and local resources used at this initial level of track and field competition. All of this helps to produce maximum participation among eligible citizens within the community.

Special Olympics has traditionally featured track and field competition, but the number of official Special Olympics sports and events continues to grow. (Photo by Greg Fredericks)

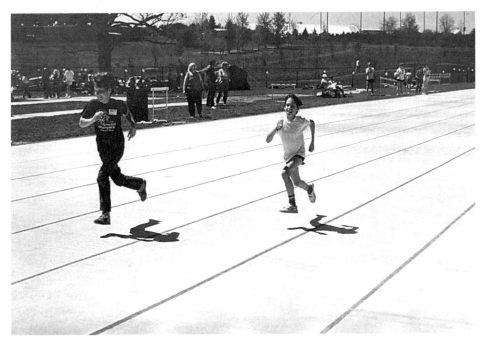

At the beginning of the 1990s, the number of competitive events in the Special Olympics grew dramatically. The traditional events are track and field activities, but Special Olympics now offers much more to athletes. Fall events and winter sports are becoming commonplace in many states, and the number of official Special Olympics sports and events continues to grow. Currently, official sports include aquatics (swimming and diving), athletics (track and field), basketball, bowling, cycling, equestrian sports, gymnastics, roller skating, football (soccer), softball, tennis, and volleyball. Demonstration sports feature badminton, golf, power lifting, table tennis, and team handball.

In addition to local events, Special Olympics offers a chance to participate in games that draw competitors from larger areas. These may lead to international competition, which is held every four years. The 1995 International Special Olympics Summer Games, for example, drew more than 7,000 competitors from 141 countries. Also in attendance were 2,000 coaches, 150,000 family members and friends of competitors, 116,000 volunteers, and more than 500,000 spectators. International Special Olympics competition is also offered in winter sports, and the 1993 Winter Games drew a record number of competitors from around the world.

Classification and Eligibility

Most sports programs for individuals with disabilities develop a competitive classification system that requires that participants compete in categories based on the degree of their disability (e.g., wheelchair sports programs). Although the Special Olympics does use the I.Q. score of an individual to establish eligibility for participation, no attempt is made to classify competitors according to their level of mental functioning. Instead, events are structured so that participants generally compete against others who are (1) the same sex, (2) similar in chronological age, and (3) at approximately the same level of performance. The last classification category is determined by examining actual scores, times, or distances recorded during prior meets or practice sessions. Thus, a 12-year-old girl with an I.Q. of 40 might compete in the same 50-meter dash as another girl of similar age but with an I.Q. that is 25 points higher. Despite this rather large gap in I.Q. level, the race should still be a close one because previous 50-meter dash times, not I.Q. test scores, were used to place these girls in the same race. Exceptions to the above three categories for equalizing competition may be made occasionally, but only to ensure that there are enough athletes to enable a sport or event to be held.

Special Olympics originally offered athletic opportunities exclusively for children with mental retardation, but today there is no upper age limit for participation. Competitive events are open to any individual with mental retardation who is 8 years of age or older. Eligibility for participation in Special Olympics is restricted to (1) persons identified by an agency or professional as having mental retardation, or (2) those found to have cognitive delays as determined by standardized measure or that require specialized instruction. Generally, Special Olympics competitors have I.Q. scores of 75 or less; however, some flexibility is given to local, area, and national organizations to determine eligibility for a given individual. Interestingly, athletes who are members of established interscholastic or intramural teams are not eligible for Special Olympics events. This policy does limit some youth with mental retardation who wish to take part in as many athletic opportunities as possible, but it is consistent with the concept of inclusion in "regular" programs and activities for those who do not require segregated experiences such as Special Olympics events.

Important Aspects

There are many aspects of Special Olympics that deserve special recognition. A few of these are as follows.

The 10 Percent Rule. Equality of competition is a very important part of Special Olympics sports and events. A closely matched contest provides a more exciting and enjoyable time for both spectators and athletes. But the reason for ensuring basic competitive equality goes much further than just enjoyment: The self-esteem of a participant may be harmed if he or she is entered against athletes at vastly greater skill levels. Even physical injury could result from such situations, particularly if the less skilled competitor tries to duplicate a difficult maneuver without prior experience and training. To avoid physically and psychologically harmful situations caused by competitive imbalance, Special Olympics has the 10 percent rule. Basically, this rule requires that participants should be matched for competition with other athletes who perform within approximately 10 percent of each other. A 15-year-old boy who usually throws the softball about 30 meters should be grouped for competition with boys of similar ability who generally throw approximately 27 to 33 meters. Although this rule is obviously a flexible guideline and cannot always be enforced, it serves as an excellent standard to alert event organizers to the importance of equality of competition.

Wheelchair Competition. Special Olympics does offer a chance for individuals with multiple disabilities to experience sports competition, and many of these individuals use wheelchairs for mobility. The wheelchair competition within Special Olympics should not be confused with wheelchair sports, however. The athletes participating in Special Olympics must conform to appropriate eligibility rules. Since the only restriction for participation in wheelchair sports is a lower extremity disability, Special Olympics wheelchair events offer a chance for *equal* competition for wheelchair users who have mental retardation that might not be available in conventional wheelchair sports programs.

Normalization Principles. One of the controversial aspects of Special Olympics is its traditional lack of conformity to the principles of mainstreaming and normalization (Hourcade, 1989; Wehman & Moon, 1985). The program emphasizes segregated competition by restricting participation to persons with mental retardation or cognitive delays. In addition, some professionals maintain that Special Olympics "does not develop life-long leisure skills or encourage athletes to participate in outside activities" (Klein, Gilman, & Zigler, 1993, p. 21). Although most agree that "Special Olympics is a normalized activity because it provides athletes with the opportunity to train and compete in athletic events," there is significant question about whether these services are provided in a normalized manner (Klein et al., p. 21). Face painters, clowns, and other well-meaning volunteers may also provide an atmosphere not normally associated with athletic competition, particularly adult competition. With the increasing professionalism of Special Olympics employees and volunteers, however, these situations appear to be changing. Dr. Tom Songster (1986), director of Sports and Recreation for Special Olympics, Inc., wrote that "the greatest challenge of all is to make Special Olympics a clear and open channel to the mainstream of society and not leave it as an end in itself. The athletes who participate in Special Olympics must be encouraged to enter regular school and community sports programs and to live as independently as possible" (p. 79). A 1993 study by Klein et al. indicates that Dr. Songster's words have been put into action. The study found that only 22 percent of experts surveyed felt that Special Olympics participation detracted from the goals of mainstreaming. In addition, it was reported that 95 percent of parents of Special Olympians indicated their child was actively involved in athletic activity beyond Special Olympics events. Thus, it appears that the concerns of some professionals that Special Olympics competition isolates participants from their communities are unfounded.

Unified Sports. The Unified Sports program of Special Olympics is intended to promote both competition and social integration by offering team-oriented sports for persons with and without mental retardation. As noted by Shriver (1990), Unified Sports "is designed to provide a new alternative for athletes with mental retardation, promote equality and teamwork, and certainly serve as a transition to community sports programs" (p. 10). Breaking from Special Olympics's tradition of offering only segregated competition, Unified Sports teams are comprised of approximately equal numbers of persons with and without disabilities. Participant selection is based on skill level and ability to contribute to the team's success, and teammates are grouped according to both age and performance (i.e., skill). Moreover, Unified Sports teammates are *required* to practice together on a regular basis. Unified Sports is established in five sports (basketball, bowling, soccer, softball, and volleyball), and pilot programs in several other sports are currently underway. Because the Unified Sports program is implemented in cooperation with existing community programs such as recreation departments and school districts, it responds to criticism that Special Olympics does not conform to normalization principles (see previous section). In addition, Unified Sports's community orientation helps to foster friendships between community residents with disabilities and those without disabilities. Competition, rather than community integration, is the primary focus of Unified Sports; however, inclusion is a "welcome by-product" of the program (Krebs & Cloutier, 1992). As noted by Krebs and Cloutier, "it is inevitable that increased understanding among individuals with and without mental retardation brought about through successful team sports reaches beyond the playing field" (p. 44).

Outcomes of Special Olympics

Special Olympics provides a unique training ground for children and adults with mental retardation. Through physical training and competition, particularly if these are conducted according to normalization principles, the participant learns behaviors that aid his or her adjustment in society.

Special Olympics has great potential for increasing physical fitness levels among participants. Although Pitetti, Jackson, Stebbs, Campbell, and Battar (1989) found no gains in fitness levels among their adult subjects as a result of Special Olympics participation, researchers at Texas Tech University (Bell, Kozar, & Martin, 1977) did note improvements among participants, particularly when year-round opportunities were available. The increasing number of physical education programs inspired by Special Olympics should result in future gains in this important area. But Special Olympics offers more than physical fitness. The chance to experience success is essential to everyone, and

Special Olympics offers successful experiences to many athletes with mental retardation, particularly those who work hard to get the most from their efforts. The following observation of one volunteer stresses the importance of effort and success:

> I remember one Special Olympian in particular. Her name was Christian. For an hour, from the time the games had begun at 9:15 A.M., she had been trying to complete a single [high] jump. After beginning her approach, she would stop two feet in front of the bar. There she stood, tense and rigid, either frightened or unsure, but always backing away, not attempting the jump. Other participants continued to take their turns. Some were successful, some weren't. And all the while Christian studied her jump. After an hour, she ran once more toward the bar with strong, even strides. She didn't balk this time. She jumped and cleared the bar, and the crowd roared its praise. Christian had cleared the high jump, a mere 1.1 meters (3' 7"), but the blue ribbon I pinned on her made her feel at least 1.9 meters (6') tall. (Cassell, 1981, p. 519)

Increased levels of fitness, plus recognition that effort and self-discipline lead to success, are valuable outcomes of Special Olympics participation. In addition, research has demonstrated that many Special Olympics participants show (1) more recreation participation after involvement in the Special Olympics (Rarick, 1978), (2) improvement in a variety of recreational skills, including throwing, running, and jumping (Bell, Kozar, & Martin, 1977), (3) a more favorable attitude toward school and physical education, (4) enhanced physical and social self-esteem (Gibbons & Bushakra, 1989), and (5) greater involvement with family members (Klein et al., 1993). Professionals and parents alike view Special Olympics as beneficial, particularly in terms of social adjustment and quality of life. It also has been identified as important for promoting public understanding and acceptance of individuals with mental retardation (Klein et al.).

Of course, not all aspects of Special Olympics are viewed as yielding positive outcomes for participants. Unless properly conducted, such programs may be more harmful than beneficial. Rarick (1978), for example, lists several undesirable features of Special Olympics, including: "(a) overemphasis by some on winning, with traumatic effects on the loser, (b) inappropriate grouping for competition, (c) program and meets being too long (inefficient administration), (d) inadequate safety precautions, and (e) parental apathy" (p. 245). Hourcade (1989) also criticized the traditional approach of Special Olympics, citing such problems as nonfunctional skill development, inefficient instruction, and patronization of participants. Miller (1987) found that almost one third of Special Olympics coaches did not consider themselves qualified to coach. As previously noted, however, Special Olympics leaders, under the direction of Mrs. Eunice Kennedy Shriver and Dr. Thomas Songster, have made much progress toward overcoming prior weaknesses in programs throughout the nation. The key to overcoming the problems noted here is effective volunteer training, and this is the thrust of current Special Olympics efforts. As Jim Schmutz, director of Sports and Coaches Education for the District of Columbia Special Olympics, noted, "Training volunteers is a critical element in creating a legitimate sports atmosphere for our athletes" (personal communication, November 22, 1989). Commenting

Skill development, under the guidance of qualified volunteers, is an important aspect of Special Olympics programs. Ice skating, for example, can be enjoyed after the competitive events are over. (Courtesy of Maryland National Capitol Park and Planning Commission, Special Populations Division; Photo by Steve Abramowitz)

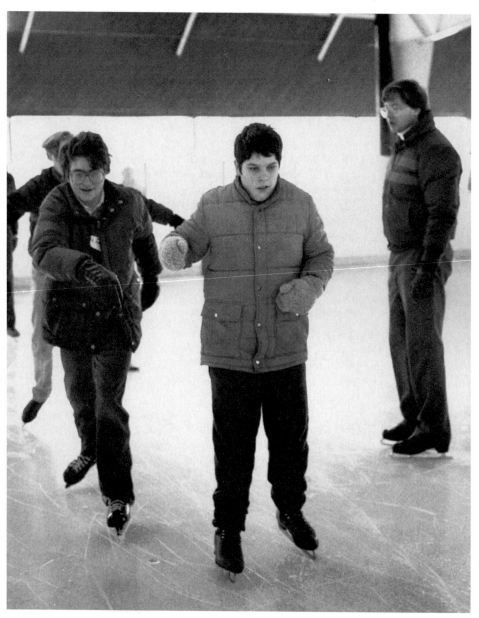

on efforts by Special Olympics International to upgrade volunteer coaches' training, Roswal (1988) observed that Special Olympics "has continually refined and upgraded training programs, resulting in a dramatic increase in the quality and number of training schools available" (p. 36). Such training schools for coaches, along with the training materials they use, should dramatically improve the quality of Special Olympics programs throughout the world. Despite some shortcomings, Special Olympics, Inc., is a rapidly growing organization that offers many valuable experiences to more than one million people with mental retardation.

BARRIE INTEGRATED BASEBALL ASSOCIATION (BARRIE, ONTARIO, CANADA)

It is unusual to find a community-based program that offers *both* social integration and genuine sports competition. The Barrie Integrated Baseball Association, however, is just such a program. Originally developed by the staff of Barrie and District Association for People with Special Needs, the Barrie Integrated Baseball Association is now an independent voluntary association that provides baseball competition to adults with and without disabilities in the Barrie area.

Historical Development

Started in 1988, the Association has grown from its original four teams to the present format that includes more than 10 integrated teams sponsored by local businesses and organizations. The growth in teams has been paralleled by an increase in the percentage of players without disabilities who compete in the league. Originally, 70% of the players had developmental disabilities (i.e., persons with mental retardation), and most of the players without disabilities were staff members of the Barrie and District Association for People with Special Needs. Now, however, more than 55% of players do not have disabilities, and the number of players from the community continues to grow. Of the 120 players without disabilities who participated in the 1993 season, only 20 were staff members of the Barrie and District Association for People with Special Needs.

Competitive Structure

The Association's competitive season runs from mid-May through mid-September, including play-offs, and each team plays approximately 15 games. The season also includes an All-Star game, and concludes with an awards banquet attended by more than 275 people. Players must be at least 16 years of age to be eligible for participation. Presently, more than 220 players, evenly divided between men and women, participate in the Association's competitive schedule.

Organizing and implementing an integrated sports activity that emphasizes competition is not an easy task. The Barrie Integrated Baseball Association's leadership is provided by four volunteer directors, plus a board of directors comprised of community members, players with disabilities, and professional staff from the Barrie and District Association for People with Special Needs. Primary concerns include financial support for the Association and public relations to ensure public acceptance of the Association's activities. In addition, the Association's leadership strives to ensure that competition takes place in an atmosphere of acceptance and respect for all players. Too much emphasis on winning can interfere with social integration (see Chapter 7). Not enough emphasis on winning, however, undermines the intent of competition and can lead to patronizing behaviors and attitudes among players without disabilities. "It is a hard balance to reach," stated Brett Millar, one of the founders of the Barrie Integrated Baseball Association. According to Millar, two factors are important in maintaining this balanced perspective on competition. These factors are: (1) strictly adhering to the Association's rules of play (see next section), and (2) maintaining a professional image. To ensure that a professional image is projected during games, all players wear complete baseball uniforms, umpires wear appropriate attire and are paid for their services, and public-address systems are used at each game to introduce players and make announcements.

Selected Rules and Regulations

The rules and regulations of the Barrie Integrated Baseball Association were developed to facilitate competition and ensure that all players participate to their maximum capabilities. More than 40 written rules govern play in the Association. The following are some examples of rules developed to facilitate integration:

Rule 1. Team ratio will be 50% special needs players[1] and 50% non-special needs players.

Rule 2. The *rover* is the 4th outfielder and can roam the entire outfield at will. All outfield players must remain on the grassy surface and cannot enter the infield to make a play.

Rule 3. A *buddy* may be added to the outfield only if the special needs player in that position is at risk under the following conditions:
   a) has very little or no knowledge of the game
   b) is physically unable to play the position alone
   c) is in danger of injury if left alone in the field
   d) would act out (become very upset) if left alone in the field
The relationship of the buddy and the special needs player is that of a *partnership*. . . . The buddy must ensure that the partner is involved in any play that he or she makes. Any play made by the buddy that does not involve the partner will be cancelled.

Rule 14. There must be a minimum of 3 special needs players on the field each inning (2 infield; 1 outfield).

---

1. The term *special needs player* is used by the Association to refer to players with disabilities.

The Barrie Integrated Baseball Association offers opportunities for persons with disabilities to compete on an equal level with persons who do not have disabilities. (Courtesy of Barrie Integrated Baseball Association)

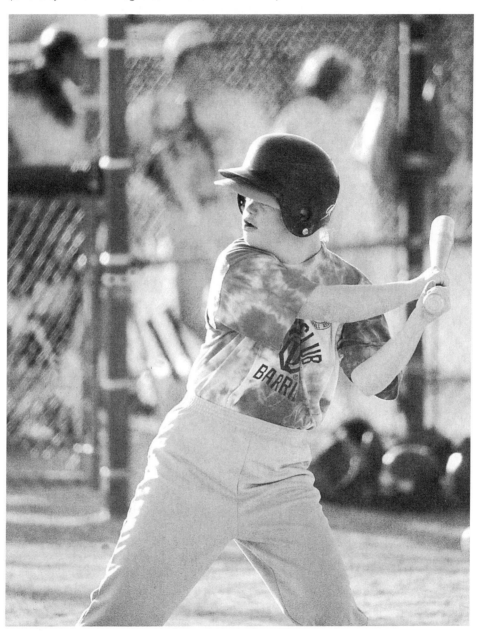

Rule 15. If a team cannot field 3 special needs players, then that team will forfeit the rover position until enough special needs players arrive.

Rule 25. Batting assistance at the plate will be permitted for those players who require it. The player *must* be given the choice of batting for him- or herself or having assistance.

Rule 32. All infield players must stay behind the baseline until the ball is hit by the bat. If an infielder is encroaching on the batter when the ball is hit into play, the batter will be awarded first base and all other runners will be awarded a free base.

Final Comment

The Americans with Disabilities Act is now a reality in the United States; therefore, communities must respond to the need for competitive sports programs that *include* persons with disabilities. The Barrie Integrated Baseball Association provides a model for communities to emulate. Its program, which maintains a balance in leadership between professional staff and community members (including persons with disabilities), demonstrates that social integration can take place within the context of competitive sports.

SUMMARY

Despite widespread emphasis on sports in North America, relatively little attention has been given to sports for people who have disabilities. One reason for this may be overemphasis on the rehabilitative benefits of sports participation, rather than recognition that the needs and motivations of *all* athletes are basically the same. Providing opportunities for parallel competition is one way to emphasize these similarities without creating inequities that might result from direct competition between athletes with and without disabilities. The phenomenal growth of programs such as wheelchair sports and the Special Olympics emphasizes the need for and benefits of sports competition among people who have disabilities. Opportunities for inclusion of persons with disabilities into a community's sports program, such as the Barrie Integrated Baseball Association, should also be provided.

SUGGESTED LEARNING ACTIVITIES

1. Observe (or participate in) a competitive wheelchair sports event, and write a two-page report on the experience. Try to include both positive and negative reactions.
2. Interview an athlete who has a disability and determine what personal benefits he or she attributes to sports participation.
3. Make a list of 10 topics that you would consider when preparing and training volunteers for a Special Olympics event.

4. Discuss the benefits of participation in competitive sports for individuals with disabilities.

5. Choose one undesirable feature of Special Olympics cited in the chapter, and determine at least three ways the problem could be resolved.

6. Using the cartoon pictured in Figure 11.1 as an example, create a cartoon illustrating sports for people with disabilities.

REFERENCES

Alger, S. L. Sports without limits: Barcelona '92. *Sports'n Spokes, 18*(4), 12–33, 1992.

Asken, M. J., & M. D. Goodlin. Attitudes toward disabled athletic competition: A preliminary inquiry. *Sports'n Spokes, 12*(5), 41–44, 1987.

Bell, N. J., W. Kozar, & A. W. Martin. *The Impact of Special Olympics on Participants, Parents, and Community.* (Research study funded by Special Olympics, Inc.) Lubbock, TX: Texas Tech University, 1977.

Brasile, F. M. Wheelchair sports: A new perspective on integration. *Adapted Physical Activity Quarterly, 7*(1), 3–11, 1990.

Brasile, F. M., & B. N. Hedrick. A comparison of participation incentives between adult and youth wheelchair basketball players. *Palaestra, 7*(4), 40–46, 1991.

Cassell, K. D. A special time for special children. *Phi Delta Kappan, 62*(7), 519, 1981.

Coutts, K. D. Physical and physiological characteristics of elite wheelchair marathoners. In C. Sherrill, Ed. *Sport and Disabled Athletes.* Champaign, IL: Human Kinetics, 1986, pp. 157–161.

Coutts, K. D. Heart rates of participants in wheelchair sports. *Paraplegia, 26,* 43–49, 1988.

Crase, N. Exhibitions at the Olympics. *Sports'n Spokes, 14*(4), 13–65, 1988.

Curtis, K. A. Sport-specific functional classification for wheelchair athletes. *Sports'n Spokes, 17*(2), 45–48, 1991.

DePaepe, J. L., & S. Bange. Mainstreaming disabled athletes. *Palaestra, 2*(4), 13–16, 51, 1986.

Gibbons, S. L., & F. B. Bushakra. Effects of Special Olympics participation on the perceived competence and social acceptance of mentally retarded children. *Adapted Physical Activity Quarterly, 6,* 40–51, 1989.

Guttmann, L., & N. C. Mehra. Experimental studies on the value of archery in paraplegia. *Paraplegia, 11,* 159–165, 1973.

Haskins, J. A. *A New Kind of Joy.* Washington, DC: Joseph P. Kennedy Jr. Foundation, 1976.

Hedrick, B. N. Wheelchair sport as a mechanism for altering the perceptions of the nondisabled regarding their disabled peers' competence. *Therapeutic Recreation Journal, 20*(4), 72–84, 1986.

Henschen, K., M. Horvat, & R. French. A visual comparison of psychological profiles between able-bodied and wheelchair athletes. *Adapted Physical Activity Quarterly, 1,* 118–124, 1984.

Hilbers, P. A., & T. P. White. Effects of wheelchair design on metabolic and heart rate responses during propulsion by persons with paraplegia. *Physical Therapy, 67,* 1355–1358, 1987.

Hourcade, J. J. Special Olympics: A review and critical analysis. *Therapeutic Recreation Journal, 23*(1), 58–65, 1989.

Jochheim, K., & H. Strohkendl. The value of particular sports of the wheelchair-disabled in maintaining health of the paraplegic. *Paraplegia, 11,* 173–178, 1973.

Johnson, S. Canada wins big at Paralympic Games. *Abilities,* 10–12, Fall/Winter, 1992.

Kelly, J. D., & L. Freiden, Eds. *Go for It.* Orlando, FL: Harcourt Brace Jovanovich, 1989.

Klein, T., E. Gilman, & E. Zigler. Special Olympics: An evaluation by professionals and parents. *Mental Retardation, 51*(1), 15–23, 1993.

Krebs, P., & G. Cloutier. Unified sports: I've seen the future. *Palaestra, 8*(3), 42–44, 1992.

Labanowich, S. *Wheelchair Basketball: A History of the National Association and an Analysis of the Structure and Organization of Teams.* Unpublished doctoral dissertation, University of Illinois, 1975.

Labanowich, S. A case for the integration of the disabled into the Olympic Games. *Adapted Physical Activity Quarterly, 5,* 264–272, 1988.

LaMere, T., & S. Labanowich. The history of sport wheelchairs: Part III. In *Sports 'n Spokes, 10*(2), 12–16, 1984.

Lindstrom, H. An integrated classification system. *Palaestra, 1*(2), 47–49, 1985.

Lindstrom, H. Integration of sports for athletes with disabilities into sport programmes for able-bodied athletes. *Palaestra, 8*(6), 28–32, 58–59, 1992.

Loiselle, D. Sport and the physically disabled. *Journal of Leisurability, 6*(1), 3–6, 1979.

McClements, J. Integration '84: Access to generic sports competition. *Journal of Leisurability, 11*(2), 20–23, 1984.

Michener, J. A. *Sports in America.* Greenwich, CT: Random House, 1976.

Miller, S. E. Training personnel and procedures for Special Olympics athletes. *Education and Training in Mental Retardation, 22,* 244–249, 1987.

Montelione, T., & J. V. Mastro. Beep baseball. *Journal of Physical Education, Recreation and Dance, 56*(6), 60–61, 1985.

Natalini, K. Going swifter, higher, and stronger with NRPA and Special Olympics. *Parks and Recreation, 22*(2), 24–27, 1988.

Nettleton, B. Self confidence and sport for the handicapped. *Rehabilitation in Australia, 11*(4), 7–11, October 1974.

Nugent, T. J. Precepts and concepts on research and demonstration needs in physical education and recreation for the physically handicapped. In *Study Conference on Research and Recreation for Handicapped Children* (proceedings), University of Maryland, 1969, pp. 20–23.

Ogilvie, B. C. Applications of sport psychology for the athlete with cerebral palsy. *Palaestra, 6*(5), 42–48, 1990.

Paciorek, M. J., & J. A. Jones. *Sports and Recreation for the Disabled: A Resource Handbook* (2nd ed.). Carmel, IN: Cooper Publishing Group, 1994.

Patrick, G. D. The effects of wheelchair competition on self-concept and acceptance of disability in novice athletes. *Therapeutic Recreation Journal, 20*(4), 61–71, 1986.

Pitetti, K. H., J. A. Jackson, N. B. Stebbs, K. D. Campbell, & S. S. Battar. Fitness levels of adult Special Olympics participants. *Adapted Physical Activity Quarterly, 6,* 354–370, 1989.

Rarick, G. L. Adult reactions to the Special Olympics. In F. L. Smoll & R. E. Smith, Eds. *Psychological Perspectives in Youth Sports.* New York: John Wiley & Sons, 1978, pp. 229–247.

Rarick, G. L. Recent advances related to special physical education and sport. *Adapted Physical Activity Quarterly, 1*(3), 197–206, 1984.

Roeder, L. M., & P. M. Aufsesser. Selected attentional and interpersonal characteristics of wheelchair athletes. *Palaestra, 2*(2), 28–32, 43–44, 1986.

Roswal, G. M. Coaches' training the Special Olympics way. *Palaestra,* ISSOG (Special Issue), 36–37, 41, 1988.

Shriver, E. K. Special Olympics . . . the Unified Sports program. *OSERS News in Print, 3*(1), 10–11, 1990.

Songster, T. B. The Special Olympics sports program: An international sports program for mentally retarded athletes. In C. Sherrill, Ed. *Sport and Disabled Athletes.* Champaign, IL: Human Kinetics, 1986, pp. 73–79.

Special Olympics. *Official Special Olympics General Rules.* Washington: Special Olympics, Inc., 1980.

Spraggs, S. Archery with the sightless sight system. *Palaestra, 1*(1), 38–39, 1984.

Steadward, R., & C. Walsh. Training and fitness programs for disabled athletes: Past, present, and future. In C. Sherrill, Ed. *Sport and Disabled Athletes.* Champaign, IL: Human Kinetics, 1986, pp. 3–19.

Stotts, K. M. Health maintenance: Paraplegic athletes and nonathletes. *Archives of Physical Medicine and Rehabilitation, 67,* 109–114, 1986.

Thiboutot, A., R. W. Smith, & S. Labanowich. Examining the concept of reverse integration: A response to Brasile's "new perspective" on integration. *Adapted Physical Activity Quarterly, 9,* 183–292, 1992.

Treischmann, R. B. *Spinal Cord Injuries: Psychological, Social, and Vocational Rehabilitation.* New York: Demos, 1988.

Wehman, P., & M. S. Moon. Designing and implementing leisure programs for individuals with severe handicaps. In M. P. Brady & P. L. Gunter, Eds. *Integrating Moderately and Severely Handicapped Learners.* Springfield, IL: Charles C Thomas, 1985, pp. 214–237.

Weisman, M., & J. Godfrey. *So Get On With It.* Garden City, NY: Doubleday, 1976.

Zeigler, E. F. *History of Physical Education and Sport.* Englewood Cliffs, NJ: Prentice-Hall, 1979.

Zwiren, L. D., & O. Bar-or. Responses to exercise of paraplegics who differ in conditioning level. *Medicine and Science in Sport, 7*(2), 94–98, 1975.

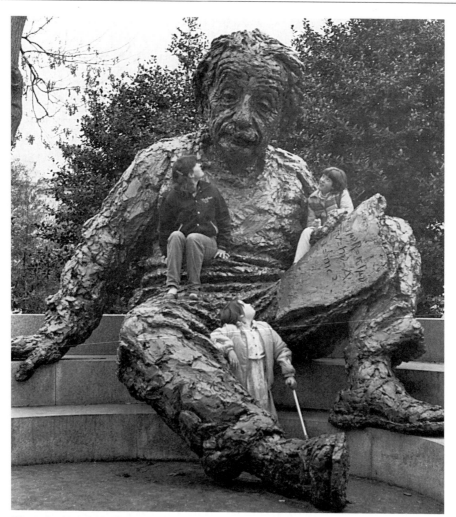

(Photo by Ralph W. Smith)

PART FOUR

RESOURCES AND TRENDS

The thought that communities are made up of individuals who function together in applying their resources toward the common good is basic to Chapter 12, Community Resources. A process by which citizens collaborate to bring about change in the well-being of the community, referred to as community development, is discussed in the chapter. Particular emphasis is placed on (1) community resources as they relate to recreation for persons with disabilities and (2) understanding the community from a sociocultural perspective.

In Chapter 13, Trends in Inclusive Recreation, an attempt is made to look into the future to understand how the area of leisure services for persons with disabilities will evolve. Drawing on the views of experts, the literature of the field, and personal intuition, trends for the future are discussed in terms of programming, new approaches, community relations, financial matters, and professional concerns. The chapter concludes on a positive note about increased acceptance of inclusive recreation services by those directing leisure service delivery systems.

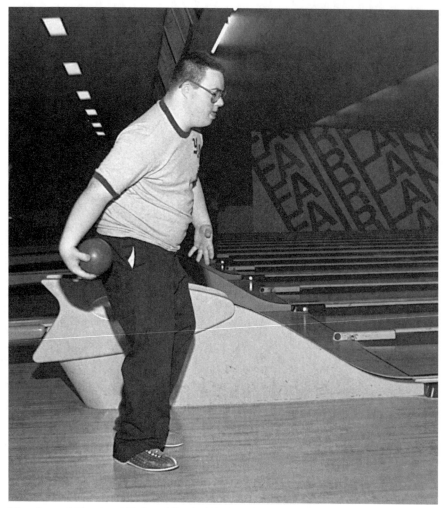

(Courtesy of Maryland-National Capital Park and Planning Commission, Special Populations Division; Photo by Steve Abramowitz)

12

Community Resources

. . .

What are community resources? How do community resources help provide for inclusive and special recreation services? What basic knowledge of and skills in community development are helpful in establishing community services for persons with disabilities? This chapter addresses these questions. Perhaps the best way to begin is by defining the term *community resources.*

The dictionary defines community as "a unified body of individuals." It goes on to clarify by stating that people in a community may have common interests, interact with one another, and live in a particular geographic area. Although the dictionary stipulates that the term may also be used to describe persons linked by a common interest (e.g., academic community, religious community), the term is not used in that sense in this chapter. Sessoms' (1980) sociologically based definition provides the most complete definition of community found in the recreation literature. He has written,

> Sociologists define a community as a collection of individuals who live within a specific geographical area, share a common bond of interdependency and commitment, and function as a group in achieving and fulfilling human needs and wishes. More simply stated, a community is people, geographically living and working together, sharing the benefits of their labor and other endeavors. (pp. 120, 121)

Resources, according to the dictionary, are "a source of supply or support: an available means." Resources are persons or things that can be drawn upon as they are needed in order to meet an end. They may include:

- human resources
- informational resources
- financial resources
- facility and equipment resources
- transportation resources

All these types of resources will be discussed in this chapter as they relate to a community providing special recreation services. Community resources, as used here, are those available means by which communities meet the recreational needs of persons with disabilities.

THE IMPORTANCE OF COMMUNITY RESOURCES

Why is an understanding of the community resources necessary for leisure service professionals? The answer to this question is simple. Resources are required to accomplish any goal the leisure service professional may have. Without a knowledge of potential resources and how to use them, it is unlikely that goals will be realized. Recreation and parks professionals need to develop a working knowledge of existing resources and to know how to draw upon these to achieve goals. The goal of fulfilling the recreational needs of *all* community members requires developing particular types of community resources.

HUMAN RESOURCES

Human resources that may be employed in conducting programs for persons with special needs include volunteers, existing agency staff, students completing professional field experiences, personnel from related agencies, and consultants who have skills that may add to the program. Some may assist with the special recreation program on a sustained basis; others may become involved only as they are needed. For example, some individuals may volunteer regularly to work with a particular activity or participate as a member of an advisory council. Others may become involved only with special events or those events that call for their particular skills.

Developing and cultivating human resources is a primary task of the professional coordinating community special recreation services. There are, of course, many ways to go about locating people who may serve as resources. Once an advisory council is formed, its members can be a ready source of information in identifying individuals to fulfill needed roles. Similarly, members of interagency councils can supply names of individuals who may be resources. In some communities, directories of social services are available. Contacts at colleges and universities are another source of human resources. Many colleges and universities have student volunteer bureaus. Faculty members may have students wishing to complete field experiences and may also serve as consultants, identifying human service personnel in the community. Labor unions and civic clubs offer additional sources of human resources.

No matter what approaches are used to identify human resources, the information collected should be organized in a way that is systematic and easily retrievable. Each time a person is identified, the individual's name, address, telephone number, and how he or she could be a potential resource should be recorded on a card or placed in a computer system for future reference.

Volunteers

Budget-conscious administrators may use volunteers to meet the needs of persons with disabilities while providing services under limited budgets. Volunteers offer a way to stretch an agency's resources. But volunteers supply far more than inexpensive labor in the absence of paid staff. They offer a wealth of diversity in backgrounds and skills that would rarely be available within a regular staff. Volunteers also share a dedication to service. Because of their diversity and dedication, they can accomplish tasks that would be difficult or impossible without their efforts.

Janet Pomeroy, founder and director of RCH, Inc. (formerly the Recreation Center for the Handicapped) in San Francisco, has spoken of the wide base of community support found on the original center's board of directors (Pomeroy, 1974). Among those on the board were

- several medical doctors
- a social worker
- several attorneys
- a real estate and insurance broker
- a superior court justice
- a recreation educator
- a physical educator
- a member of the Social Services Commission
- a food broker
- a product executive
- an architect
- other businessmen and businesswomen
- parents representing the center's auxiliary

Because of their diverse talents, the center's board members were able to take on a number of assignments including fund-raising, transportation, insurance, recruitment of staff and volunteers, reviewing legislation for funding sources, obtaining supplies and equipment, assisting with preparation of grant applications, and contacting city officials regarding contractual services for the center.

Every community has a number of persons who desire to volunteer their services to meaningful projects. These persons may wish to serve on a board or advisory council for the special recreation program, to do face-to-face leadership, or to work in a supportive capacity in administration, promotion, transportation, or some other aspect of the program.

Recruiting Volunteers. Pomeroy (1974) has employed a number of means to recruit volunteers at RCH, Inc. She feels that a primary means is to get potential volunteers to visit the center. Pomeroy states, "We can show the need for the program; we can demonstrate the benefits of recreation; and we can stimulate interest—all of which makes them want to help" (p. 11). Promotion is a second means Pomeroy uses to secure volunteers. The center provides presentations to service clubs, fraternal organizations, and other groups, and conducts planned campaigns in newspapers and on radio and television. Finally, program volunteers are recruited through contacts with junior high schools, hospitals, youth service agencies, volunteer bureaus, and participants in the center's program.

The concept of using volunteers from among the center's participants merits further discussion. Volunteer service can be an especially meaningful leisure pursuit for persons with disabilities, enabling them to give rather than receive. In addition to persons with disabilities, Tedrick (1990) has suggested other groups as sources of volunteers. These include preteens, older adults, and individuals who have been court-assigned to complete community service. Another source for volunteers is through corporate volunteer programs (Stensrud, 1993).

Keys to Successful Volunteer Programs.   Three key elements must exist in any successful volunteer program. These are (1) involving volunteers in the program; (2) recognizing the volunteers' contributions; and (3) providing proper training for volunteers. Volunteers must be made to feel a part of the program by being included in decisions. Volunteers, who give freely of themselves, do not wish to be "told what to do." They want to have a voice in the program. Volunteers also need to receive positive feedback when it is deserved. This praise should be given on a daily basis, with special recognition shown through an established awards program. Finally, volunteers must be provided with orientation and training to enable them to succeed.

An outline for the in-service training of volunteers is contained in the Project LIFE (Life Is for Everyone) resource and training manual produced at the University of North Carolina at Chapel Hill (Bullock, Wohl, Webreck, & Crawford, 1982, pp. 106, 107). Topics include

1. characteristics of various disabilities, noting possible limitations and special considerations (emergency and health care procedures should be outlined here also)
2. general activity and equipment modification techniques
3. overview of the least restrictive environment concept and how it is being implemented in the department
4. assessing existing attitudes of recreation professionals (and volunteers) toward individuals with handicapping conditions
5. creating peer acceptance
6. using instructional aides and volunteers
7. finding additional resource information for a specific disability

Henderson and Bedini (1991) have suggested 10 strategies for conducting successful volunteer programs.

1. *Carefully consider the tasks* to be completed by volunteers to ensure that each task is appropriate for a volunteer and that a good match is made between the individual and the assignment.

2. *Keep all staff informed* of how volunteers are to be used with the agency so that staff do not feel their jobs are threatened and understand the importance of volunteers.

3. *Match tasks with qualifications and interests of volunteers* by assessing skills and interests of volunteers and then placing each volunteer in a position whereby he or she may use existing skills or develop new ones.

4. *Acknowledge that everyone is a potential volunteer* in order to seek out not only individuals but civic groups who may volunteer as units for particular events.

5. *Give volunteers verbal feedback* on a regular basis to praise them for positive performances and to offer constructive criticism.

6. *Evaluate periodically* both individual volunteers and the overall volunteer program.

7. *Provide recognition in many ways* including daily social reinforcements (e.g., thank-yous, pats on the back) as well as formal recognition (e.g., awards, recognition nights).

8. *Stay up-to-date* on issues surrounding volunteering, such as liability insurance, tax deductions, and legislation.

9. *Recognize the connection between volunteering and leisure activity* because volunteering can be a positive leisure experience and an atmosphere provided by staff to foster leisure can enhance volunteer experiences.

10. *Provide appropriate training* so volunteers may feel comfortable in their roles and clients may enjoy maximum profit from the volunteers.

Existing Agency Staff

Existing agency staff can add greatly to programming for people with special needs. Of course, these staff members need to have an in-service training program similar to that outlined for volunteers in the preceding section. Schleien and Ray (1988) have written about the importance of providing regular recreation and park department personnel with such in-service training. They have stated, "An important element that should be present in any comprehensive inservice training plan is a segment devoted to delivery of leisure services to members of special populations" (p. 48). Schleien and Ray emphasized that such training should include exposure to the "experiences of others who have either had contact with potential consumers of community leisure services or who are themselves disabled" (p. 49).

Students Completing Professional Field Experiences

University departments providing professional preparation for recreation and parks services have students who are required to complete professional field experiences. These experiential learning opportunities may be part-time, usually accomplished during a few hours each week, or they may take the form of full-time internships. Such internships or field work experiences are often done over a quarter (10 weeks) or semester (15 weeks). University students can make valuable contributions, provided the agency is willing to offer professional supervision for them. While most students should have some educational preparation in special recreation, it is important that agencies complete an early assessment of each student's competencies so that appropriate responsibilities may be assigned, and gaps in knowledge or skills may be filled through additional training.

A student intern can be a valuable resource in any special recreation program. (Courtesy of Courage Center, Golden Valley, MN)

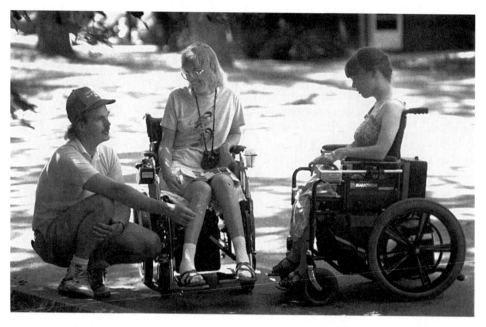

Contracting for Services

Another means of obtaining necessary human resources is to contract for the services of individuals who perform specific tasks. During the initial stage of program development, the most feasible approach may be contractual arrangements that include consulting with regular staff and actually conducting programs for people with special needs.

Consultation services can be arranged with administrators of existing recreation programs for persons with disabilities, with university faculty who have experience in working with special recreation programs, or with private consultants with expertise in community special recreation programs. Personnel from other community agencies often have the competencies necessary to provide direct service functions. These persons may be employed on a part-time basis to lead special recreation programs. For example, therapeutic recreation specialists for local hospitals or rehabilitation centers may be contracted to offer programs within community recreation and parks facilities.

Studies (Austin, Peterson, & Peccarelli, 1978; Edginton, Compton, Ritchie, & Vederman, 1975; Vaughan & Winslow, 1979) have identified the lack of trained program personnel as a major hurdle to clear in order to establish community special recreation services. The creative use of human resources may offer a vehicle by which to launch needed community recreation programs for people who have disabilities.

INFORMATIONAL RESOURCES

Many resources exist that can offer information valuable to establishing and developing community recreation services for people with special needs. These range from local resource persons to national computer retrieval systems.

Local Resources

In many communities, or in close proximity, will be colleges and universities that have faculty members with backgrounds in recreation for persons with disabilities. Second, therapeutic recreation specialists in local hospitals, rehabilitation centers, associations for retarded citizens, mental health centers, and other facilities are often anxious to assist in the development of special recreation programs. Finally, recreation and parks staff in neighboring communities or park districts may be able to share information concerning leisure services for persons with disabilities.

Literature

Only a few books have been published related to recreation for persons with disabilities, but several journal articles have appeared on the subject. Two journals—*Journal of Leisurability* and *Therapeutic Recreation Journal*—have frequent articles on the topic, and some magazines (e.g., *Parks and Recreation*) occasionally publish articles related to special recreation services. For those interested in sports and other active recreation for persons with disabilities, *Sports 'n Spokes* and *Palaestra* provide current and comprehensive coverage. Computer information retrieval systems offer a means to identify a full spectrum of articles, books, and papers that apprise the reader of recent developments. Most major university libraries have access to computerized retrieval systems through which may be obtained an abstracted list of publications in any area of interest. The National Rehabilitation Information Center (NARIC) also provides this service on a wide range of disability-related topics (see resources at end of Chapter 4).

Organizations

Another source of information on special recreation services is through various organizations. State and local professional recreation and parks societies often have committees or individuals who may provide information to practitioners. National professional organizations may also offer assistance. Two of the major organizations in the United States are the American Alliance for Health, Physical Education, Recreation and Dance (AAHPERD) and the National Recreation and Park Association (NRPA). AAHPERD has offered consultation and literature on programs for persons with disabilities. NRPA offers useful publications such as *Guidelines for Community Based Recreation Programs for Special Populations* (Vaughan & Winslow, 1979).

Athletic and recreational organizations for persons with disabilities, such as the National Wheelchair Basketball Association, National Wheelchair Athletic Association, Special Olympics, American Blind Bowling Association, and other similar organizations, offer information regarding their particular area of recreational interest. These organizations are listed in Appendix B. Appendix A lists selected organizations concerned with specific disabilities. Among these, several have been particularly active in promoting special recreation programs, including the American Foundation for the Blind, the Epilepsy Foundation of America, and the National Easter Seal Society. An example of the efforts of such groups has been the publication of *Recreation Programming for Visually Impaired Children and Youth* (Kelley, 1981), an extensive book produced by the American Foundation for the Blind. Finally, youth-serving agencies have attempted to serve the needs of special populations. Two examples are the Girl Scouts of the USA and the YMCA of the USA. Of particular note has been the Mainstreaming Activities for Youth (MAY) project, conducted by the YMCA Office of Special Populations, which brought together 10 youth-serving agencies in a collaborative effort to enhance their mainstreaming activities.

Conferences, Institutes, and Workshops

Continuing education opportunities abound today. The largest providers of conferences, institutes, and workshops are professional societies and universities. Both the AAHPERD and the NRPA annual conferences regularly offer educational programs on recreation for persons with disabilities. Universities also provide workshops and institutes for the development of community-based services for people with special needs. Recreation and leisure studies curricula are the usual sponsors of these programs.

While information on special recreation services has been relatively limited in the past, its growth has been inspired by the desire of many professionals and citizens to establish community-based programs. It is likely that the amount of information available will grow as interest in the area builds.

FINANCIAL RESOURCES

Perhaps no single resource area attracts as much attention as that of financial resources. Without adequate financial support, no program can continue to exist. Those concerned with developing programs for persons with disabilities must be knowledgeable about financial resources.

Vaughan and Winslow (1979) found that the major funding source for special recreation programs is the general tax fund. Slightly more than 87% of all recreation and parks agencies surveyed used the general tax as a source of funding. Fees and charges were the second greatest source, used by 44.2% of the agencies. Sources beyond these depended largely on the size of the community. Communities of less than 100,000 tended to fund 30% to 40% of their program from donations. Government grants were a major source of funding for those cities with more than 250,000 people. Other sources of funds were special taxes, private grants, and contractual agreements.

Vaughan and Winslow state that the major funding source for special recreation programs should be the general tax fund. We concur that special recreation programs should be supported to the largest degree possible through existing tax structures. However, in a time of budget limitations, professionals must be aware of alternative sources as well. This is particularly true when beginning new programs. Once established, special recreation programs usually are supported by the citizenry. Special appropriations may be needed, however, to initiate services.

Special Taxes. Park districts and municipalities in the state of Illinois have been highly successful in establishing special population programs. One reason for the success in Illinois has been legislation that allows park districts and other governmental bodies to cooperate by forming special recreation associations and to levy a special tax up to $.04 for $100 of assessed valuation for special recreation programs. Thus, at least one state has used legislation to establish financial means to support special recreation programs. Refer to Chapter 3 for more detailed information.

Fees and Charges. Fees and charges can provide another financial resource for special recreation programming. Just as other public recreation and parks programs are supported by fees and charges, programs for people with special needs can likewise receive support. Fees should, of course, be in line with other fees charged by the agency.

Contractual Agreements. Recreation and parks agencies can enter into contractual agreements with schools, nursing homes, and other agencies to provide recreation services for people with disabilities. Although contractual agreements are likely to be a minor financial resource, they do offer additional means of support.

Fund-Raising. Fund-raising projects are another means to obtaining revenue for special recreation programs. Many techniques may be used in fund-raising. These include governmental and foundation grants, memorial giving, house-to-house and direct mail solicitations, capital fund campaigns, and special events (Mirkin, 1972). Information on governmental and foundation grants is covered in the section that follows.

Grants. Grants may be made by a governmental agency or through a private foundation. In the past, federal grant monies have been available through a number of sources including Title IV of the Social Security Act for Aid to Families with Dependent Children, Title XIV of the Social Rehabilitation Act, the Developmental Disabilities Services and Facilities Construction Act (PL 88-164) and Amending Law (PL 91-517), the Architectural Barriers Act of 1968 (PL 90-480), and the Rehabilitation Act of 1973 (PL 93-112). Since the governmental grant picture is constantly changing, it is wise to refer to recent information sources when seeking grant funding. Community and university libraries (reference sections) can provide assistance with locating current resources on grants as well as guides or books to assist with proposal writing.

As we have seen, there are many different potential financial resources available for special recreation programs. Funding can come from general taxes, special taxes, fees and charges, contractual agreements, fund-raising projects, governmental grants, or foundation grants. The point should be reiterated, however, that the primary funding for special recreation programs should come from the normal funding source of recreation and parks, and not from grants or other special sources.

FACILITY AND EQUIPMENT RESOURCES

Potential facilities for special recreation programs include parks, forests, pools, community centers, gymnasiums, bowling lanes, athletic fields, and other places where organized recreation commonly takes place. Equipment includes lasting articles or apparatus needed to conduct programs. While adapted equipment is necessary for a few activities, standard recreational equipment is frequently employed in programs for people with special needs.

Facilities

The major facilities for inclusive and special recreation programs should be those controlled and programmed by the agency. Of course, existing facilities have to be evaluated to make certain they are accessible and usable by persons with disabilities before they are scheduled for programs.

Most communities have a wide array of potential facilities that may be used for inclusive and special recreation programs. In addition to those of the recreation and parks department, facilities may be made available through schools, voluntary and youth-serving agencies (e.g., YMCA, YWCA), bowling lanes, churches, hospitals, rehabilitation centers, and other public and private organizations. As a general rule, programs should be conducted in facilities normally used for programming by the recreation and parks department or park district.

A facility resource file should be maintained so that a current list of facilities is available. Included should be the name and address of the facility, the agency controlling it, accessibility information, special equipment available at the facility, any cost for use, the contact person, and a phone number. Many communities have published accessibility guides that would be useful in establishing such a resource file. Advisory councils and interagency councils are also potentially rich sources of information in identifying suitable facilities for special recreation programming.

Equipment

It may be necessary to purchase or construct adaptive devices or equipment for some recreation activities to be used by persons with disabilities. Adapted equipment, however, can take on a gimmicky quality if it is not well conceived. It is usually best to consult with an expert before purchasing or building equipment when unsure about the type of equipment or the necessity to have it. Therapeutic recreation specialists often can provide expert advice regarding adaptive equipment. Program participants may also have expertise regarding adaptive equipment.

Examples of adaptive equipment include handle-grip bowling balls (handles automatically retract to be flush into the ball when released), bowling rails to guide visually impaired bowlers, bicycle buddy bars (permit two regular bicycles to ride side-by-side), tricycle body supports (enable children with poor balance to use tricycles), and floor sitters (resemble chairs without legs that allow children to sit up during floor play) (Austin & Powell, 1980). There are, of course, scores of pieces of adapted equipment that may be purchased or constructed. A number of commercial suppliers list adaptive equipment in their catalogues (see Appendix C for a list of potential suppliers). In addition, ABLEDATA (contact the Adaptive Equipment Center, Newington Children's Hospital, 181 East Cedar Street, Newington, CT 06111) provides a computerized database of assistive devices, including many related to recreation participation.

TRANSPORTATION RESOURCES

Transportation of participants is viewed by many recreation and parks departments to be the greatest problem in providing special recreation programs (Vaughan & Winslow, 1979). Major resources suggested by Vaughan and Winslow to solve transportation problems include the following:

- *Car Pooling.* Participants, families, and friends may serve as resources for developing car pools organized by the recreation and parks system.
- *Service Clubs and Social Service Agencies.* Groups such as the Red Cross, Kiwanis, and Lions Clubs may provide transportation for participants. Service clubs may also possibly purchase vans for the recreation and parks department.
- *Federal Funding to Purchase Vans.* In the past, federal legislation has provided funding sources for transportation. The Federal-Aid Highway Act of 1973 (PL 93-87) and the Developmental Disabilities Services and Facilities Construction Act of 1971 (PL 91-517) are examples of federal laws for the allocation of funds for transportation.
- *Contractual Agreements.* Contractual agreements may be drawn with schools, health agencies, or other organizations. Such agreements have the added advantage of possibly bringing more participants into the special recreation programs from the contracting agency.
- *Public Transportation.* Current federal legislation calls for public transit systems to obtain accessible vehicles: therefore, mass transit offers a viable resource to assist in solving transportation problems for special recreation programs.

The effective use of existing community resources can enable the leisure service professional to meet the recreational needs of persons with disabilities. Creative use of community resources, of course, presumes a knowledge of available resources. The first, and largest, segment of this chapter has provided information for locating potential resources. The final portion of the chapter deals with the basic skills in and understanding of community development[1] that is needed to establish services for persons with disabilities.

---

1. The term *community development,* as used in this chapter, refers to the process by which citizens collaborate to take action to improve the well-being of the community.

Constructing adaptive equipment may enable persons with physical impairments to participate in some types of leisure activities. (Photo courtesy of Bradford Woods, Indiana University)

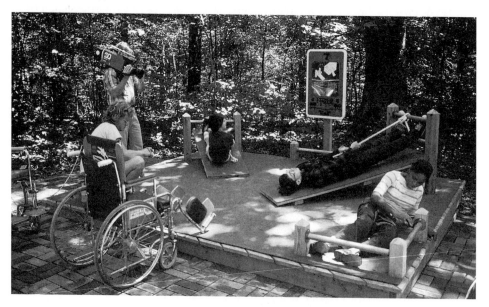

KNOWING THE COMMUNITY

Communities are diverse, each being unique from the next. The terms *sociocultural, demographic,* and *ecological* have been employed to categorize the essential features that make communities distinctive. Primary sociocultural variables are social organization and culture. Demographic variables include population size; age, sex, and race composition; birth and death rates; and migration to and from the community and within its boundaries. The ecological perspective is concerned with the interrelationship between the citizens of the community and the geographic setting (Edwards & Jones, 1976).

Sociocultural Variables

The material that follows deals with the sociocultural variables of concern to the leisure service professional wishing to initiate special recreation services. Analysis of the social organization and culture of the community is critical to success in working with structures that bring individuals, agencies, and organizations together to achieve common goals cooperatively.

Features of the social structure in the sociocultural facet of community life are social groups; social stratification; community subsystems such as the family, the economy, education, religion, government, and social welfare; and normative structures dealing with social norms and values (Edwards & Jones, 1976).

294

Social Groups. Groups can be formal or informal. Formal groups are those that have structural rules and regulations to govern relationships. Because of their structure, they can utilize formal communications systems that reach relatively large numbers. Examples of formal groups are labor unions, service organizations, and golf and tennis clubs.

Informal groups revolve around interpersonal relationships between group members. Informal groups are relatively small and allow members to meet emotional needs through intimate interactions. Examples are family groups and peer groups (Edwards & Jones, 1976).

Social Stratification. Social stratification deals with social prestige and power. Social prestige is concerned with social class structure. Power deals with the ability to control others and to effect change. Often those in the higher social classes have the most power, although there is not always a direct correspondence, since some of the "better" families (high social class) may not hold power because of diminished wealth and political influence. In most communities, however, those with the most influence are those in the upper social classes or those who hold high status in one of the subsystems such as government or religion (Edwards & Jones, 1976).

Three approaches may be applied to determine power holders in the community. These are the reputational, positional, and decisional approaches. To determine power by the reputational approach, one must ask the questions, With whom do you check before acting? What individual(s), formal groups, or informal groups do you consult on communitywide decisions? The positional approach assumes that those in positions of authority hold the power. Examples are the mayor and the superintendent of recreation and parks. The final approach, the decisional approach, takes for granted that those involved in making decisions for the community hold the power (Sessoms, 1980).

Sessoms has discussed two situations of power in the community. The first is the *power elite*. The power elite exists in communities where the power is in the hands of a few individuals. In contrast to this monolithic approach is the *multiple pyramid system* in which no single group holds power. Instead it is a pluralistic system in which the power is held by many.

Jewell (1983), in an article on power structures as they relate to the recreation integration of persons with disabilities, has discussed four types of communities originally proposed by McCarty and Ramsey (1971). These have been termed the (1) dominated or restricted power community, (2) factional or conflict-dissipated power community, (3) pluralistic or accordant power community, and (4) inert or power-avoidance community. Jewell has stated that the ability to analyze the community for these power structures is more important than any other aspect of community analysis.

The first of the community power structures presented by Jewell is similar to the power elite community discussed by Sessoms (1980). In the *dominated or restricted power community*, power is maintained by a single individual or a small group of people. Many times, the person or persons who are in control run an industry that dominates the community. Citizen boards simply "rubber stamp" the decisions made by the power elite, so the recreation and parks department is likewise apt to be under their control. In the case of the community with dominated or restricted power structure, it is necessary to gain the support of the power elite in a way that they will not perceive as threatening.

The second of the community power structures is the *factional or conflict-dissipated power community*. Under this structure, longstanding factions of the community constantly fight for power. Governing boards are split by factionalism and therefore have great difficulty agreeing on issues. This is a difficult power structure with which to work. The professional must attempt to make progress with both factions yet must not appear to be siding with one group. The creative professional can enable both groups to see how they would benefit from the new program so their support is guaranteed.

The *pluralistic or accordant power community* is similar to Sessoms' (1980) multiple pyramid system. Here Jewell (1983) states, "sanity and reason do reign and . . . issues and community welfare are important" (p. 27). Petty thinking does not override the decision-making process. Groups debate in a democratic manner to arrive at a consensus on what is best for the community. The leisure service administrator is likely to be viewed as a knowledgeable resource when making decisions. Therefore, the administrator should have thoroughly researched information on the establishment of community services for persons with disabilities so he or she can properly brief those in authority of the rationale and procedures for establishing the service.

The least common power structure is the *inert or power-avoidance community*. Both those in positions of authority and the citizenry are apathetic. Here the leisure service administrator ends up making decisions that are, in turn, "rubber stamped" by the board. The problem here is getting the community out of its dormant state and into something new. Even in the most inert of communities, there are a few individuals who are capable of responding, given the right motivation.

Knowing the likely community power structure allows the professional to choose the best strategy when approaching those who hold power. The professional who is not cognizant of the local power structure will likely have problems in establishing special recreation services, particularly when the integration of persons with disabilities into ongoing programs is a goal, since integration brings other participants into direct contact with individuals with disabilities.

Community Subsystems.   The third aspect of the sociocultural facet involves community subsystems such as the family, the economy, the government, religion, education, and social welfare. Those who hold high status in the various subsystems are likely to have influence within the community. Knowing these persons and their possible interest in community recreation for persons with disabilities can be very helpful in establishing new services. This is particularly true with the social welfare subsystem.

The social welfare subsystem, as defined by Edwards and Jones (1976), deals with three major types of community services. These are social work, health care, and recreation. Often social welfare agencies organize themselves for joint action. Community organization structures can take the form of wide-based cooperation such as a council of human service agencies. In other instances, agencies with particular thrusts may form councils. For example, a local recreation council may form. Recreation councils are usually made up of nongovernmental agencies such as Boy Scouts, Girl Scouts, YMCA, YWCA, Hebrew Association, and governmental agencies such as park districts, or city or county recreation and parks departments. In beginning special recreation services, it becomes necessary to know what councils exist in the community so that their support can be gained.

Smaller communities will be less likely to have coordinating councils. Nevertheless, individual social welfare agencies, churches, service clubs, educational systems, and advocacy groups (e.g., parents' groups) are potential allies to initiating special recreation programs. It is, therefore, just as important to understand these independent agencies as it is to be knowledgeable of coordinating councils in larger communities.

Normative Structures. The final aspect of the sociocultural facet is the normative structure of the community. Social norms are extremely important to the community, as Edwards and Jones (1976) state:

> The social structure of the community—as described above through social groups, social stratification patterns, and subsystems—gets its stability and order from the fact that it exists within a normative structure. The normative structure is made up of norms, i.e., rules and standards that define what people should and should not do in various facets of their community living; sanctions, in the form of penalties applied for violation of, and rewards offered for conformity to, the norms; and values that represent the priorities people attach to material and nonmaterial features of their culture. (p. 89)

Of particular importance to community development are the social norms and values of the community toward change. Some communities will be slower than others to accept any innovation. Resistance to innovation may be lessened if the change fits the existing community value system (Edwards & Jones, 1976). For example, a community that prizes athletic competition may be led to understand how persons with disabilities also need opportunities for sports participation and how the provision of such opportunities can strengthen the athletic image of the community.

Summary: Sociocultural Facet

The sociocultural facet of community life deals with informal and formal groups, social stratification and power, the varied community subsystems, and norms and values. The normative structure gives the community stability and order. It gives the community its "character." Actions leading to community development transpire through the social groups, social stratification patterns, and subsystems of the community. Familiarity with the sociocultural facet of the community can be of great assistance when initiating any new program, including special recreation services.

SUMMARY

This chapter has discussed community resources as they pertain to the provision of inclusive and special recreation services. Community resources, including human, informational, financial, and transportation, are necessary to accomplish any goal the leisure service provider may have. Thus, it is important that recreation and parks professionals be knowledgeable of such resources and know how to use them in achieving their goals. The use of volunteers and the seeking of additional funding are two aspects that are highlighted in this chapter. Also important to the establishment of special recreation services is understanding the community from a sociocultural perspective. Knowing the community power structures as they relate to the recreation integration of persons with disabilities enhances the capacity of the leisure service professional to provide services for all people, including those individuals who may have disabilities.

SUGGESTED LEARNING ACTIVITIES

1. Volunteer in a special recreation program. If this is for a single event (e.g., wheelchair basketball game), report your observations in class from your perspective as a volunteer. If you volunteer over a period of time, keep a log of your experiences and reactions. Prepare a brief report based on your log.
2. Interview a person with a disability who is volunteering. Ask how he or she became involved as a volunteer and the benefits derived. Bring your notes to class for discussion.
3. Invite several athletes who have disabilities to class to discuss sports organizations with which they are affiliated.
4. Compile a resource file on organizations in your home town that might have an interest in community recreation programs for persons with disabilities.
5. In a group, discuss why it is important for recreation professionals to be familiar with organizations related to people with special needs.
6. Interview a recreation administrator about funding for special recreation services. Take notes on your discussion and report to the class.
7. Work on the following problem in a small group. You are in charge of a camp that integrates campers with and without disabilities. What alternatives can you identify for funding your camp, in addition to having parents pay a fee for their child? Use library resources in preparing your response. Report your conclusions to the class.
8. Compile a resource file on national leisure organizations for persons with disabilities. To do this, divide the task among the class members. Organize the brochures and other items you collect so that they may be placed in the library for future reference by other students.
9. Working with a small group of students, analyze the community power structure in your home town, college community, or some other community chosen with your instructor. Write a report of no more than 10 pages on your findings. Then make a presentation in class to highlight your findings.

REFERENCES

Austin, D. R., J. A. Peterson, & L. M. Peccarelli. The status of services for special populations in the state of Indiana. *Therapeutic Recreation Journal, 12*(1), 50–56, 1978.

Austin, D. R., & L. G. Powell, Eds. *Resource Guide: College Instruction in Recreation for Individuals with Handicapping Conditions.* Bloomington: Indiana University, 1980.

Bullock, C. C., R. E. Wohl, T. E. Webreck, & A. M. Crawford. *Life Is for Everyone Resource and Training Manual.* Curriculum in Recreation Administration, University of North Carolina at Chapel Hill, 1982.

Edginton, C. R., D. M. Compton, A. J. Ritchie, & R. K. Vederman. The status of services for special populations in park and recreation in the state of Iowa. *Therapeutic Recreation Journal, 9,* 109–116, 1975.

Edwards, A. D., & D. G. Jones. *Community and Community Development.* The Hague, Netherlands: Mouton & Co., 1976.

Henderson, K. A., & L. A. Bedini. Using volunteers in therapeutic recreation. *Leisure Today: Therapeutic Recreation—Meeting the Challenges of New Demands.* In *Journal of Physical Education, Recreation & Dance, 62*(4), 49–51, 1991.

Jewell, D. L. Comprehending concepts of community power structure. Prerequisite for recreation integration. *Journal of Leisurability, 10*(1), 24–30, 1983.

Kelley, J. D., Ed. *Recreation Programming for Visually Impaired Children and Youth.* New York: American Foundation for the Blind, 1981.

McCarty, D. J., & C. E. Ramsey. *The School Managers.* Westport: Greenwood Publishing Corp., 1971.

Mirkin, H. R. *The Complete Fund Raising Guide.* New York: Public Services Materials Center, 1972.

Pomeroy, J. One community's effort. *Institute on Community Recreation for Special Populations.* North Texas State University and the Texas Recreation and Park Society, 1974.

Schleien, S. J., & M. T. Ray. *Community Recreation and Persons with Disabilities: Strategies for Integration.* Baltimore: Paul H. Brookes, 1988.

Sessoms, H. D. Community development and social planning. In S. G. Lutzin, Ed. *Managing Municipal Leisure Services.* Washington, DC: International City Management Association, 1980, pp. 120–139.

Stensrud, C. *A Training Manual for Americans with Disabilities Act Compliance in Parks and Recreation Settings.* State College, PA: Venture Publishing, 1993.

Tedrick, T. How to have the help you need. *Parks & Recreation, 25*(6), 64–68, 86, 1990.

Vaughan, J. L., & R. Winslow. *Guidelines for Community Based Recreation Programs for Special Populations.* National Therapeutic Recreation Society, a branch of the National Recreation and Park Association, 1979.

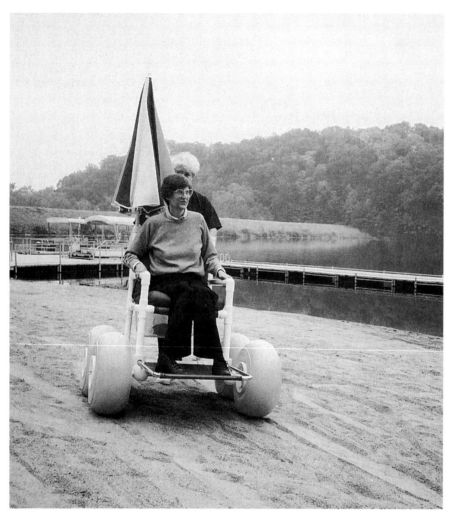

(Photo courtesy of Bradford Woods, Indiana University)

13

Trends in Inclusive Recreation

. . .

In this chapter, we attempt to peer into the future to catch a glimpse of what may unfold in inclusive and special recreation services. Knowing today's trends points the way to the world of tomorrow and provides us with visions of future realities.

We are living in a rapidly changing world. Computers, lasers, virtual reality, satellites, robots, space shuttles, rapid communication systems, and other signs of high technology are already a part of our culture. Naisbitt (1982) in his best-seller, *Megatrends,* reflects on the rapid changes in our society when he states: "Change is occurring so rapidly that there is no time to react; instead we must anticipate the future" (p. 18). In so doing, as Godbey (1989) has observed, "recreation, park, and leisure service professionals will be challenged, first and foremost, to be actors rather than reactors in the change process" (p. 57).

In the United States, one very real part of the future will be the Americans with Disabilities Act (ADA). This far-reaching law gives persons with disabilities the legal right to full inclusion into the mainstream of American society. This right extends to recreational and leisure opportunities for persons with disabilities. As Wehman (1993) has suggested, the wide scope of ADA extends far beyond architectural accessibility and will likely stimulate a great number of trends.

With this in mind, we reviewed the literature and questioned experts[1] for their thoughts regarding trends in inclusive recreation programs. The resulting compilation of trends is presented with the admission that, as a wag has said, those who live by the crystal ball must learn to eat ground glass. We shall probably digest our share.

---

1. Experts included Susan Drenkhahn, Carmel Community, Inc., Chandler, AZ; Jill Gravink, Northeast Passage, Durham, NH; Dr. Robin Kunstler, Lehman College, NY; Thomas McPike, Chicago Park District, IL; Dr. Lou Powell, University of New Hampshire; Don Rogers, Bradford Woods, IN; Lyn Rourke, Courage Center, Golden Valley, MN; Dr. Carla Tabourne, Dr. Stuart Schleien, Jonathan Balk, Ronald Jenkins, Jennifer Mactavish, and Kathy Strom, all of the University of Minnesota.

PROGRAM TRENDS

Outdoor Recreation Programs

Few activities cannot be entered into by persons with disabilities. Therefore, programs for people with disabilities are likely to follow societal trends. The rising interest in outdoor recreation pursuits among persons with disabilities reflects a societal trend. Perhaps amplifying this societal trend for persons with disabilities are recent improvements in outdoor recreation equipment and expansions in the accessibility of outdoor areas and programs.

Various terms such as *outdoor adventure, high risk,* and *stress challenge* are used to describe programs that offer participants new and challenging experiences in the outdoors. Caving, rappelling, traversing ropes courses, flying, parachuting, jet skiing, speed boating, scuba diving, and backpacking are examples of adventure activities enjoyed by many persons. Cold climate pursuits such as ice skating and winter camping are gaining popularity, as is snow skiing. In Canada and the United States, sledge hockey and ice picking, a form of speed skating, have developed. In Scotland, curling is a popular sport for persons with disabilities, including wheelchair users. Other outdoor recreation activities increasing in participation are sailing, fishing, gardening, archery, riding, road racing, biking, and nature study.

Indiana University's Bradford Woods outdoor education, recreation, and leadership-training center (5040 State Road 67 North, Martinsville, IN 46151) is a trendsetter in the provision of programming and training opportunities in outdoor recreation experiences for persons who have disabilities. Among its programs, Bradford Woods offers extensive camping and outdoor adventure activities for persons with disabilities. In addition, many training opportunities are provided through Bradford Woods. These include internships and an annual institute on innovations in outdoor recreation programming for persons with disabilities. Programs like Wilderness Inquiry, C. W. Hog, Northeast Passage, and POINT (see Chapter 9) continue to provide challenging outdoor experiences for persons who have disabilities.

Sports and Fitness

Competitive athletics continue to thrive under the auspices of traditional organizations such as the National Wheelchair Basketball Association, American Blind Bowlers Association, and Special Olympics.

Interest in such sports organizations has continued to expand. For example, the United States Cerebral Palsy Athletic Association was formed to fill the need for sports experiences for people with cerebral palsy who could not find equitable competition through other organizations. The NASCP now offers competition in a broad range of team and individual sports. Additional organizations have been formed for, among others, wheelchair road racers, wheelchair marathoners, wheelchair softball and tennis players, and skiers with disabilities.

Boat dock at Bradford Woods. (Photo courtesy of Bradford Woods, Indiana University)

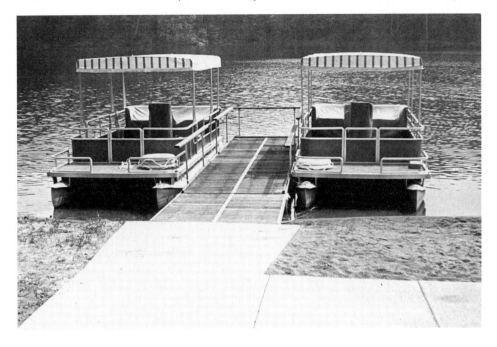

Although many of the athletic programs initially instituted were competitive sports for children and young adults, noncompetitive opportunities are beginning to develop for both children and adults. Many persons do not want competition but seek health and fitness through sports and exercise. One leader in this effort is National Handicapped Sports (NHS) (formerly the National Handicapped Sports and Recreation Association). Originally devoted exclusively to snow skiing, NHS has expanded to include other sports and a "Fitness Is for Everyone" program that promotes a total conditioning program for persons with disabilities. Working cooperatively with community recreation facilities, "Fitness Is for Everyone" uses videotapes, fitness-assessment procedures, and counseling techniques to encourage persons with disabilities to adopt healthier lifestyles. In 1989, clinics were offered in eight cities throughout the United States from Anchorage, Alaska, to Raleigh, North Carolina. These clinics have been cited as being successful catalysts for ongoing programs in cities where previous clinics were held ("Fitness Is for Everyone," 1988–89). "Fitness Is for Everyone" selects different training sites annually and offers its training videotapes for sale to interested individuals; thus, the program is accessible to anyone who has a disability.

Aerobic dance, karate, yoga, and weight lifting are also activities demanded by those in inclusive and special recreation programs. Still others desire to learn lifetime sports through adult leisure education classes. For example, in Indianapolis, bowling instruction is being provided to adults with disabilities under a program modeled after the President's Council on Physical Fitness and Sport.

Travel Programs

Travel programs that have a primary concern for persons with disabilities are growing in popularity. The publication *Directory of Travel Agencies for the Disabled* by Helen Hecker lists more than 350 agencies worldwide that specialize in travel arrangements for persons with disabilities. An example of expanding opportunities for travel is the success of Mobility International (MI). MI, which currently has offices in more than 25 countries throughout the world, was founded in London to integrate persons with disabilities into international educational exchange and travel programs. The United States Office (MIUSA, P.O. Box 10767, Eugene, OR 97440; (503) 343–1284) is directed by a person with a disability, Susan Sygall, and has organized successful exchanges to many countries, including China and Germany. Another successful agency has been The Guided Tour (555 Ashbourne Road, Elkins Park, PA 19117; (215) 782–1370) that was founded by a social worker, Irv Segal, in 1972. It specializes in providing travel experiences for individuals with developmental disabilities. It is obvious that there is a trend toward greater travel opportunities for persons with disabilities. It is likely that ADA requirements will even further enhance the popularity of travel by persons with disabilities.

Leisure Education in Schools

Children with disabilities too often do not have the same opportunities as other children to learn about leisure. A developing trend is toward using leisure education to help build leisure skills and attitudes. For example, the Northeast DuPage Special Recreation Association near Chicago has designed curricula to help teachers provide leisure education to children with disabilities. These curriculum materials have been eagerly accepted and widely used by teachers. Charles Bullock and his staff at the Center for Recreation and Disabilities Studies at the University of North Carolina at Chapel Hill have been national leaders in the development of leisure education curricula (*School-Community Leisure Link*, 1992).

With the implementation of the Individuals with Disabilities Education Act (PL 101-476), known as IDEA, recreation is not viewed by educators as simply a means to improve functional domains but as an important lifetime skill area in and of itself. This federal legislation recognizes that students with disabilities need therapeutic recreation services to develop leisure lifestyles for enhancing their quality of life. As a result of this legislation, it is anticipated that leisure education will continue to be an expanding area in the public schools.

Leisure Counseling

As inclusive and special recreation programs grow, greater numbers of individuals and families will require leisure counseling. Professionals competently prepared with counseling skills and a knowledge of leisure will advance the field of leisure counseling far beyond the relatively simple level of today's leisure counseling programs. Leisure services agencies offering leisure counseling services for people with special needs will be at the forefront of this effort. Advances will include higher levels of counseling skills and innovations in the use of computers in leisure counseling programs. A computerized resource center is currently being used by the Northeast DuPage Special Recreation Association to match client interests with available community leisure resources. The computer will play a larger and larger role in both leisure counseling and leisure education as computer programs are developed to teach people about leisure opportunities, to assess interests, and to catalog leisure resources.

Programs for Individuals in Group Homes

There is a continuing trend to provide community living situations for individuals who have been hospitalized or institutionalized, or who need an alternative to living at home. Group homes have been established by both private and public agencies for persons with disabilities who need living situations that approximate, as closely as possible, living experiences of other people. Group homes offer supervised community living in houses located in the residential neighborhoods of towns and cities.

Because of the advances of physical medicine, there is a growing population of persons with spinal cord injuries, head injuries, and developmental disabilities who require the community living opportunities offered by group homes. Some group homes are for individuals with disabilities who will reside in the homes on a temporary basis while building their independent living skills. An example of this type of service is ReMed Recovery Care Centers in Pennsylvania. These centers offer community-based services to individuals who have head (brain) injuries, and they focus on practical concerns of daily life. Individual recreation plans, designed by therapeutic recreation specialists, guide the person toward increased leisure independence within the community. As noted by David Strauss, ReMed's Clinical Director, "If an individual is learning to live in the community, then the community must be the classroom." Other homes provide more long-term living arrangements for adults who, while having mental retardation or another disabling condition, can function relatively independently but who may need some amount of assistance.

Some individuals residing in group homes need motor skill development. More common is the need to develop competencies related to social and leisure skills. Many special recreation programs have been created to help those living in group homes to develop motor skills and to have positive social and leisure experiences. Often these programs take place in the evening because participants normally are employed in the community, in a sheltered workshop, or in the group home. Some programs are conducted in the group homes, while others are offered in community recreation centers or human service agencies.

APPROACHES TO PROGRAMS AND SERVICES

Inclusion

Inclusion is the term adopted to describe the process by which persons both with and without disabilities are being served in one environment. Inclusive recreation reflects a program philosophy directed not just to the physical integration of groups of people but to embracing the needs of all within one environment. Inclusive recreation implies that persons with disabilities are actively involved with others and that there is an interaction pattern that leads people toward normative roles and relationships.

Programs designed to facilitate inclusive recreation, such as the Mainstreaming Initiative in Montgomery County, Maryland (see Chapter 8), are becoming integral parts of community recreation programs. Such opportunities have been shown to increase positive social interactions between participants with and without disabilities (Edwards & Smith, 1989). In addition, training programs and recreation-related literature are making recreation and parks professionals and students aware of their responsibility to provide inclusive recreation. Examples include the LIFE Project conducted by Dr. Charles Bullock and his colleagues at the Center for Recreation and Disabilities Studies at the University of North Carolina at Chapel Hill and *Community Recreation and Persons with Disabilities: Strategies for Integration* by Schleien and Ray (1988). Reynolds (1993) has suggested that attitudes toward persons with disabilities will become more positive as the general public has more opportunity to observe and interact with persons with disabilities in leisure activities.

The Americans with Disabilities Act (ADA) will likely play a large role in the development of inclusive recreation. Reynolds (1993) has stated that "the ADA may well result in a new era of leisure service provision, an era in which *all* Americans can work and *play* together" (pp. 231–232). First, more and more recreation facilities will become accessible to persons with disabilities. Not only public park and recreation areas but private sector theaters, museums, stadiums, hotels, and restaurants will become accessible to persons with disabilities. Private enterprise, including the travel and tourism industry, should be remarkably changed.

In addition to expansion in accessible recreation and leisure opportunities, the range of persons with disabilities served will greatly increase because ADA extends beyond individuals with visual or physical disabilities. Persons with mental impairments (e.g., individuals with mental retardation or chronic mental illness) are covered so that *programmatic accessibility* will have to be considered along with physical accessibility. It is also likely that greater programmatic and physical accessibility will encourage expanded family recreation. As more public and private facilities are made accessible, other family members will have increased opportunities to take part in recreation with family members with disabilities (Reynolds, 1993; Schleien, Rynders, Heyne, & Tabourne, 1995).

Levels of Programming

There exists a definite trend to establish several levels of programs within community services for persons with disabilities. For example, the Cincinnati Recreation Commission has a four-level system encompassing teaching sensory-motor and self-help skills (Level I), instructing basic activity and socialization skills (Level II), developing advanced recreation and socialization skills (Level III), and providing relatively independent participation where staff act as facilitators, trainers, consultants, liaison persons, and advocates (Level IV). Following these levels of programming, participants may become integrated into ongoing programs of the department (see Chapter 8). Another illustration is a model proposed by Hunter (1981). This model has five levels: (1) institutional and homebound one-to-one visitations, (2) developmental skill programming focusing on the acquisition of skills transferable to community recreation participation, (3) special interest groups where segregation is by choice for a particular activity such as wheelchair basketball, (4) integration with support (e.g., transportation, emotional support) to promote community involvement, and (5) direct independent participation in community leisure experiences. Throughout the five levels, leisure counseling and leisure education services may be provided to facilitate the participants' involvement. As programs grow in sophistication, more and more communities will adopt multiple levels of programming.

Therapeutic Programs

Closely related to the trend to offer various levels of programs is a trend toward the provision of therapeutically oriented programs. Community-based therapeutic recreation specialists are offering purposeful interventions for clients needing goal-directed programming. The therapeutic recreation process (assessment, planning, implementation, and evaluation) is being employed by skilled therapeutic recreation specialists to reach specified client outcomes. While the primary thrust of community-based special recreation programs will remain recreation participation, more therapeutically oriented programs will develop as therapeutic recreation specialists are employed by community leisure service agencies and public schools.

Campus Recreation Programs

A growing area of programming is found on college and university campuses throughout the United States and Canada. Students who have disabilities have made their needs for special recreation services known to campus administrators, who have begun to respond with a variety of leisure services. These services have included wheelchair user and non-wheelchair-user sports, outdoor recreation offerings, lectures, special events, and leisure counseling. Leisure services for students are sometimes administered by an office for disabled student services but are more often found in traditional campus recreational service systems, such as departments of recreational sports. We project that this trend will continue and that there will be increased cooperation between campus recreation providers and community recreation and parks departments as the recreational needs of young adults who have disabilities become more widely recognized.

High Technology

Today we may simulate real life through the technology of virtual reality (VR). VR uses a combination of visual, audio, and kinetic effects to create the virtual reality of going caving, hiking through the Grand Canyon, playing a round of golf at Pebble Beach, or any number of exciting recreational endeavors (Caneday, 1992). Caneday has suggested that persons with disabilities will be able to use VR "to enter an artificial universe and interact with other people, giving no hint as to their handicap" (p. 50).

As previously discussed, computers will be used extensively in leisure education and leisure counseling programs. Beyond this, however, computers offer many possibilities to enhance services for people with special needs. A software explosion is now upon us. Computer programs for scheduling, participant registration, and inventories are now available in recreation and parks. These will be applied to community recreation services. Computer games will also find their way into special recreation programming. These games are no longer just for children. Innovations provide interactive computer games that are stimulating for adults and may be played by almost anyone, including persons with severe physical disabilities. For example, flight simulator games allow players to land (or crash!) at dozens of airports across the United States. Games are not the only type of computer technology available to people with disabilities, however. Both software and hardware modifications have been made to enhance daily functioning (Burkhead, Sampson, & McMahon, 1986). Word processing, musical composition, and artistic endeavors are just a few examples of the software available to enhance leisure functioning of people with disabilities, including those with severe physical disabilities. An example of a hardware device is Head Master, which functions as a mouse emulator for IBM and Apple computers. Simply by turning their heads, users can position the cursor in the desired location on their computer screens. Then, through use of either an external switch or "puff" (mouth-activated) switch, a selection can be made. Another device, the FreeWheel, allows individuals who are paralyzed to wear a small passive reflector and use only slight head movements to operate a computer. The Aurora computer enhancement program allows an individual to produce typed words through a number of means, such as small head movements or the blink of an eye. AccessDOS permits persons who have difficulty pressing more than one key at a time to operate a

Computers are becoming widely used to enhance the leisure functioning of people with severe disabilities. (Courtesy of The League: Serving People with Physical Disabilities, Inc., Baltimore, MD)

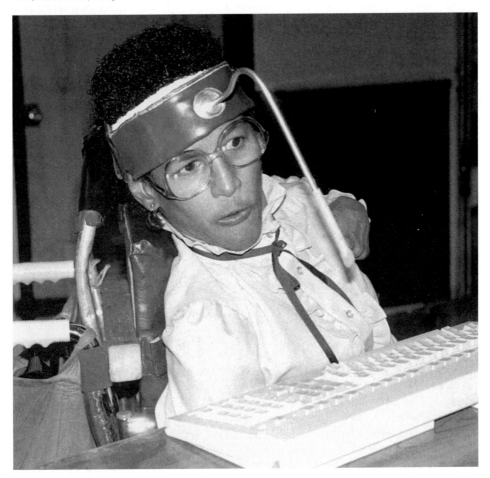

keyboard with only one finger. Screen Reader allows persons with visual impairments to use a computer as it "speaks" words that appear on the computer screen. Finally, Voice-Type is a 7,000-word speech recognition system for personal computers through which the user talks and the computer does the typing (Spede, 1993).

In the years ahead, technicians will also create new vistas for persons with disabilities through the production of innovative assistance devices, such as the computer hardware just described. For example, a great deal of progress has been made in developing communication aids for nonverbal individuals who have severe physical disabilities.

One device, the Autocom, has a portable board that is built into a wheelchair lap tray. A handpiece or headstick is used to point to vocabulary items on the board's surface, with a message appearing on an LED display or printed onto a paper roll. In England, Possum sells the Communicator, a device much the same as the Autocom. A father and mother whose 12-year-old son used a communication board reported to one of the authors that it had "opened new worlds" for the boy who, for the first time, was able to readily communicate with others. A similar device, the Touch Talker distributed by Prentke Romich Company, has received rave reviews from one mother. She wrote (March, 1989):

> Bryan desires to speak orally, but he is confronted with limitations in being understood hundreds of times a day. The Touch Talker provides a tool to break through the frustration created by these physical limitations. (p. 2)

Other examples of available technology include devices that send typed messages via telephone for people with profound deafness; computer terminals that print in Braille and speak in full-word synthetic speech; and portable, computer-based systems that read typeset or typewritten print and convert it into easily understandable synthetic speech for persons who are blind. In addition, the availability of computerized banking and shopping from the home in some areas of the country is expanding independent living opportunities to persons with severe mobility impairments. The number and variety of technological devices that are available for persons with disabilities is staggering. One computerized database (ABLEDATA) includes a list of 15,000 commercially available products useful to persons with disabilities. These products are categorized into 14 major categories, including recreation-related devices.

Today's assistive devices, and others in the planning stage, hold great potential to enhance the lives of persons with disabilities, particularly those with severe disabilities. We are a long way from many such aids being within the financial means of most persons, but there is some indication that improved manufacturing techniques and increased demand for these devices may make them more affordable (Allen, 1989). Recreation professionals, therefore, need to begin contemplating the possible effects of assistive devices, computers, and other types of new technology on programs and services. Readers interested in more information about technology and its impact on the recreational lives of persons with disabilities are directed to Dattilo (1994) and *Palaestra's* special issue on technology (published in summer, 1993). Technology is, unquestionably, a part of the future for *all* recreation professionals.

Changing Views Toward Sexuality

Traditionally, individuals with disabilities and older persons have not been perceived by many human service professionals to have sexual feelings or sexual activity. The traditional view has been that these individuals are asexual. In recent years, however, professionals have been undergoing substantial changes in their views toward the sexuality of both groups. Perhaps the "sexual revolution" has inspired a healthier view. Or it may be that society is finally beginning to perceive people with disabilities as persons with feelings and desires similar to those of others. Whatever the reason for the change, it seems there is a definite trend toward perceiving both persons with disabilities and individuals who are older as sexual beings who need to express their sexuality.

A handbook on sexuality and disabled persons (Cornelius, Chipouras, Makas, & Daniels, 1982) states that "sexuality can be defined as an integration of physical, emotional, intellectual, and social aspects of an individual's personality which expresses maleness or femaleness" (p. 1). Cornelius and colleagues later state:

> People do not express their maleness or femaleness only in the bedroom. Sexuality is a part of all the activities in which a person engages: work, socialization, decoration of one's home, telephone conversations, political discussions, expressions of affection, arguments, eating a meal, child rearing, walking down the street, watching a movie, etc. Sexuality, then, is an expression of one's personality and is evident in everyday interactions. (p. 1)

Recreation professionals are recognizing that persons with disabilities and individuals who are older should be free to express their sexuality just like anyone else. For example, progressive recreation professionals do not treat adults with mental retardation like children who are to be protected from sexuality. Instead, these adults are offered opportunities for learning and practicing social skills necessary to deal with their sexuality in appropriate ways. Such learning opportunities include education about the responsibilities that one accepts when he or she becomes sexually active. Responsible sexual behavior is especially important in an era overshadowed by the AIDS epidemic.

Progressive professionals offer opportunities for single adults and teenagers who have disabilities to mix with others in integrated recreation activities such as dances, parties, and corecreational sports. Through such healthy recreation, *all* participants can express their sexuality. Similarly, progressive professionals provide older persons recreational opportunities through which they may express their sexuality in social interactions with others with whom they share common interests.

In sum, there exists a trend for human service professionals, including recreation professionals, to accept the sexuality of persons who are older or have disabilities. These professionals provide opportunities within their programs for the normal expression of sexuality.

Outreach Workers

Outreach workers are being used by more than one agency to identify those who are homebound or for other reasons have not had the opportunity to become aware of programs and services for people with special needs. Outreach workers also develop referral systems with local hospitals and nursing homes that are returning clients to the community. Finally, these staff workers help refer those who contact the agency to appropriate programs and services. In short, it is the responsibility of the outreach worker

A preschool developmental play center in Tampa, Florida, designed to meet the needs of children with disabilities. (Design by Dr. Louis Bowers, University of South Florida; Photo by David R. Austin)

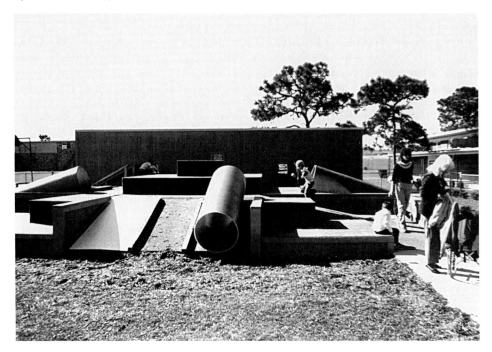

to contact persons who are newly disabled and those not traditionally served so that they may have the benefit of inclusive recreation programs and services. This may involve not only contacting and referring participants but also assisting clients to initially take part in existing programs. Outreach workers will become more widely utilized as agencies learn of their value.

Playgrounds

Traditional playgrounds have not been constructed to accommodate the needs of all children. Often barriers have excluded children with disabilities from playgrounds, creating feelings of social isolation. Today, however, there is a trend toward building and programming playgrounds to meet the needs of all children, including those with disabilities. Advancements in playground design are discussed in detail in Chapter 6. Far more will occur in playground design during the next decade as current knowledge becomes more widely disseminated and playground apparatus manufacturers include design features for children with disabilities.

TRENDS IN COMMUNITY RELATIONS

Community and Hospital Linkages

Community leisure service departments are building linkages between themselves and hospitals, institutions, and mental health centers. In doing so, networks are being developed to enhance the programs of all agencies involved. For example, the Cincinnati Recreation Commission has worked with state institutions to facilitate the transition of clients to the community. The arrangement allows Recreation Commission staff to meet individuals before they are released from the institution. The need for a close working relationship between institutions and community programs is likely to grow as institutions place more clients into alternative community living situations.

Volunteer Programs

Volunteers are extremely important to the success of special recreation programs. For this reason, the Cincinnati Recreation Commission has developed an awards program to formally recognize volunteers. Volunteers who give 50 hours of service are awarded an "I'm a TRiffic Volunteer" T-shirt. Other appropriate awards are given for all levels of service. Another trend is using special recreation programs participants as volunteers. In so doing, participants not only help the program but gain a sense of giving as well as receiving. RCH, Inc., in San Francisco has been a leader in this area. Finally, strong advisory councils and parents' groups have become essential to establishing and maintaining high-quality special recreation programs. The involvement of citizens is particularly necessary to securing appropriate community support and funding. It is likely that the trend toward expanded use of volunteers in many roles will continue and enlarge.

Cooperative Arrangements Among Leisure Service Agencies

The trend toward two or more leisure service agencies cooperating to meet the leisure needs of constituents with disabilities grew out of the frustrations of several progressive park districts and municipalities in Illinois during the late 1960s. Although efforts to serve persons with disabilities had been made in the form of summer camps and special events, the park districts and municipal recreation departments realized the limited nature of their programs and that they served only a small fraction of people with disabilities living in their geographic areas. Although recreation and parks personnel wanted to enlarge their services for persons with disabilities, their efforts were hampered by financial restrictions, low incidences of some disabilities in given districts, and a lack of trained professionals to design programs. Out of this situation arose the concept of pooling resources to establish special recreation cooperatives, each to be supported by several park districts and municipal recreation departments (Robb, 1976).

In 1970, the Northern Suburban Special Recreation Association (NSSRA) was formed by eight local park districts and community recreation departments in Cook and Lake counties. From the beginning, it was clear that the NSSRA was setting a trend for Illinois and the nation. The special recreation cooperatives in the Chicago area remain a vital part of each of their member districts and municipalities. This sentiment is expressed in the NSSRA *Policy Manual,* which states: "Rather than a separate program, the N.S.S.R.A. is an extension of its member agencies whose specific responsibility is to provide for the special population a program of recreation comparable to that which is offered the general public." Thus the cooperative associations are not "add-on" programs, but are a means for each park district and community to provide a comprehensive recreation program for its entire population.

The NSSRA began the trend toward cooperative ventures by park and recreation jurisdictions to establish special recreation services. From these pioneering efforts have come a concept and a model for cooperation that we hope will continue to grow throughout the nation.

FINANCIAL TRENDS

Fees and Charges

There exists a general trend within leisure service agencies to levy fees and charges for services. This trend is being followed within special recreation programs. Generally, fees charged for special recreation programs are comparable to those charged the general public. It is the feeling of administrators of special recreation programs that they should not place an unfair burden on their participants by charging them disproportionately higher fees than other citizens, even though special recreation programming is often more expensive to conduct. This trend is anticipated to persist as long as leisure service agencies continue to depend on the collection of fees and charges.

Fund-Raising

Fund-raising efforts have become widespread among special recreation programs. Approaches to fund-raising are varied. Illustrative of fund-raising projects are those of the Cincinnati Recreation Commission, which has developed a gift catalog, sponsored various 10K runs, and raffled tickets for a hot air balloon ride with a local celebrity. The Northeast DuPage Special Recreation Association has established the Cabin Foundation to help support the Cabin Nature Program Center, which offers integrated nature programs. Corporate sponsorship of major activities is also becoming a popular means of financing expensive events that include persons with disabilities.

These fund-raising projects are all positive efforts. Questionable fund-raising practices, such as promoting feelings of pity for children with disabilities, are on the decline. Positive, innovative means to fund-raising will be important for some time to come as a means to supplement tax funds.

PROFESSIONAL TRENDS

Continuing Education

Continuing education is an area that is growing today and will become larger in the future. General recreation staff will need to receive information on special recreation services. Among topics covered will be attitudes toward serving persons with disabilities and issues surrounding the integration of persons with disabilities into ongoing programs. Some staff will "retool" to facilitate mainstreaming. Programs on employee burnout will be provided for staff who need to develop new ways of coping with the demands of working intensively in special recreation programs.

Those concerned with continuing education will develop many alternatives to traditional staff workshops and state and national conferences. New types of training approaches, including computer programs, will replace conventional means to continuing education. Furthermore, universities and private consulting firms will make available an abundance of training packages on special recreation programming to local leisure service agencies.

Field-Based Research and Evaluation

Local leisure service agencies are beginning to enter into joint efforts with universities to answer applied research questions and to evaluate programs systematically. Both faculty and graduate students with research and evaluation skills are being called upon by agencies to conduct studies that are important to the agencies. For example, a graduate student in therapeutic recreation has conducted a study of a pilot program of the West Suburban Special Recreation Association near Chicago. Another therapeutic recreation graduate student investigated the efficacy of one of the Mainstreaming Initiative programs of Montgomery County, Maryland. As special recreation programs multiply and grow in sophistication, it will become established practice to conduct cooperative agency-university research and evaluation studies.

Further Definition of Inclusive and Special Recreators and Therapeutic Recreation Specialists

There is an emerging trend toward an identified area of specialization in inclusive and special recreation (Hamilton & Austin, 1992). Inclusive and special recreators will become recognized for their expertise in providing programs directed toward leisure experiences for persons with disabilities. Therapeutic recreation specialists will function in leisure service agencies only to conduct programs where clinical intervention is called for, and to assess participants referred to them. Inclusive and special recreators and therapeutic recreation specialists will continue to work with general recreators to include persons with disabilities in ongoing agency programs. Ramifications of this trend will be the establishment of at least one professional organization devoted to the concerns of inclusive recreation and to the development of university professional preparation opportunities specifically designed for students desiring careers in inclusive recreation. Hamilton and Austin have suggested that perhaps a branch of the National Recreation and Park Association, the National Therapeutic Recreation Society, will evolve as the professional organization that has as its primary mission championing the cause of inclusive recreation.

Methods and Materials to Interpret Programs to Community Officials

Means to interpret community recreation programs for persons with disabilities will be developed for use with elected and appointed officials and board members. Handouts, films, videotapes, and, perhaps, computer programs will become available to make officials sensitive to the leisure needs of persons with disabilities and knowledgeable about concerns in serving special populations. Since public officials continually change, and, because community special recreation services will remain a relatively novel concept, it will be necessary for agencies to have professionally prepared educational materials available for some time to come, interpreting inclusive recreation services to policymakers.

National Park Service

During the early 1980s, the National Park Service (NPS) initiated a concerted effort to improve accessibility to its facilities and programs for visitors with disabilities. A Special Programs and Populations Branch was established, under the direction of David Park, to facilitate NPS accessibility efforts. This division was given the responsibility of working closely with all units of the Park Service to identify and eliminate barriers to accessibility. In the late 1980s, with the cooperation of the NPS, Northern Cartographic completed a 464-page, large-format guidebook entitled *Access America: An Atlas and Guide to the National Parks for Visitors with Disabilities*. This useful book focuses exclusively on access in 37 of the United States' most prominent national parks. It constitutes a major step in helping visitors who have disabilities to take maximum advantage of national parks in the United States. Toward this end, the NPS has continued its efforts to correct accessibility problems, and many actions within the park system are clear signs of a trend toward making all of our national parks accessible to visitors who have disabilities. It is our opinion that the positive stance taken by the National Park Service will serve as a model to enhance accessibility efforts at state and local levels as well. NPS policies will positively affect accessibility in parks throughout America.

Greater Acceptance of Inclusive Recreation by Leisure Service Providers

People with disabilities have traditionally been underserved by leisure service providers. The Americans with Disabilities Act has forever changed the face of leisure services. As public and private leisure service organizations become more programmatically and physically accessible to persons with disabilities, leisure service providers realize the necessity of enlarging their roles to include the provision of services to persons with disabilities. They will have to modify facilities and equipment, ensure that facilities are accessible, and work with schools and human service agencies in order to meet the needs of people who are disabled (Reynolds, 1993). In short, leisure service providers in both the public and private sectors will take on the role of ensuring the rights of persons with disabilities to full inclusion into the mainstream of American leisure.

SUMMARY

It is evident that we strongly endorse the trend toward the provision of inclusive and special recreation services for those with disabilities. Persons with disabilities have the right to the same recreation and leisure activities that are available to the rest of the community.

The present period promises to be an exciting one in the history of community leisure service delivery systems in the United States and Canada. Progressive systems have already gone beyond the philosophical question of "Should we provide services for persons with disabilities?" to the question "How can we best serve the needs of persons who have disabilities?"

SUGGESTED LEARNING ACTIVITIES

1. In a small group, discuss the statement: "Few activities cannot be entered into by persons with disabilities. Therefore, programs for people with special needs are likely to follow societal trends." Agree or disagree with the statement. List reasons for your position. Then discuss these with the entire class.

2. Pick one type of activity listed in the chapter in which you have not previously taken part. Arrange to participate in this activity with persons who have disabilities. Write a one- to two-page paper on this experience, or give a report in class.

3. Survey several community parks and recreation departments or park districts to determine the type and extent of leisure education and leisure counseling programs serving persons with disabilities. These may be integrated or separate programs. Prepare a report on your findings.

4. Interview several persons with disabilities as to trends they see in programming. Then interview program directors or other recreation administrators from the same community. Compare the responses of the consumers and professionals. Report your findings in class.

5. Invite a therapeutic recreation specialist from a state institution into class to discuss the institution's community linkages. Question the specialist as to what would be ideal in terms of community linkages with leisure service delivery systems.

6. Debate the question in class as to whether participants in special recreation programs should pay fees equal to other citizens, even though special population programming is often more expensive to conduct.

7. Invite a therapeutic recreation specialist and a special recreator to class to discuss their roles and what they see as future directions for the therapeutic recreation profession.

REFERENCES

Allen, T. Technology and the marketplace. *AFB Newsletter, 24*(3), 11, 1989.

Burkhead, E. J., J. P. Sampson, & B. T. McMahon. The liberation of disabled persons in a technological society: Access to computer technology. *Rehabilitation Literature, 47,* 162–173, 1986.

Caneday, L. Outdoor recreation: A virtual reality. *Parks & Recreation, 27*(8), 48–51, 1992.

Cornelius, D. A., S. Chipouras, E. Makas, & S. Daniels. *Who Cares? A Handbook on Sex Education and Counseling Services for Disabled People* (2nd ed.). Baltimore: University Park Press, 1982.

Dattilo, J. *Inclusive Leisure Services.* State College, PA: Venture Publishing, 1994.

Edwards, D., & R. Smith. Social interaction in an integrated day camp setting. *Therapeutic Recreation Journal, 23*(3), 71–78, 1989.

"Fitness Is for Everyone" reaches 24 cities in three years. *Handicapped Sports Report, 8*(1), Winter, 1988–89.

Godbey, G. C. *The Future of Leisure Services: Thriving on Change.* State College, PA: Venture Publishing, 1989.

Hamilton, E. J., & D. R. Austin. Future perspectives of therapeutic recreation. *Annual in Therapeutic Recreation, 3,* 72–79, 1992.

Hunter, J. C. Leisure education: Its role in the recreation integration process. *Recreation Canada,* Special Issue, 76–81, 1981.

March, J. A parent's view. *PRC Current Expressions Newsletters,* 1–2, 6, Summer, 1989.

Naisbitt, J. *Megatrends: Ten New Directions Transforming Our Lives.* New York: Warner Books, 1982.

Reynolds, R. Recreation and leisure lifestyle changes. In P. Wehman, Ed. *The ADA Mandate for Social Change.* Baltimore: Paul H. Brookes, 1993.

Robb, G. M., Ed. *Guidelines for the Formation and Development of Special Recreation Cooperatives in the State of Illinois.* University of Illinois at Urbana-Champaign: Office of Recreation and Park Resources, Department of Leisure Studies and the Cooperative Extension Service, 1976.

Schleien, S., & M. T. Ray. *Community Recreation and Persons with Disabilities: Strategies for Integration.* Baltimore: Paul H. Brookes, 1988.

Schleien, S. J., J. E. Rynders, L. A. Heyne, & C. E. S. Tabourne. *Powerful Partnerships: Parents and Professionals Building Inclusive Recreation Programs Together.* Minneapolis: University of Minnesota, 1995.

School-Community Leisure Link. Chapel Hill, NC: Center for Recreation and Disability Studies, University of North Carolina, 1992.

Spede, J. F. Computers that make life possible. [Indiana] *University Computing Times,* 14,15, January–February 1993.

Wehman, P., Ed. *The ADA Mandate for Social Change.* Baltimore: Paul H. Brookes, 1993.

A

Selected Organizations Concerning Persons with Disabilities

For a listing of more than 550 disability-related organizations, consult the *Directory of National Information Sources on Disabilities* published by the National Institute on Disability and Rehabilitation Research (U.S. Department of Education, Office of Special Education and Rehabilitative Services). Information can also be obtained from the National Rehabilitation Information Center (NARIC), 8455 Colesville Road, Suite 935, Silver Spring, MD 20910–3310.

American Amputee Foundation
P.O. Box 250218
Little Rock, AR 72225

American Association on Mental Retardation
1719 Kalorama Road, N.W.
Washington, DC 20009

American Association of Retired Persons
1909 K Street, N.W.
Washington, DC 20049

American Diabetes Association
1660 Duke Street
Alexandria, VA 22313

American Foundation for the Blind, Inc.
15 W. 16th Street
New York, NY 10011

Arthritis Foundation
1314 Spring Street, N.W.
Atlanta, GA 30309

Association for Retarded Citizens of the United States
2501 Avenue J
Arlington, TX 76006

Autism Society of America
8601 Georgia Avenue
Suite 503
Silver Spring, MD 20910

Council for Exceptional Children
1920 Association Drive
Reston, VA 22091

Epilepsy Foundation of America
4351 Garden City Drive
Suite 406
Landover, MD 20785

Helen Keller National Center for Deaf/Blind Youths and Adults
111 Middle Neck Road
Sands Point, NY 11050

Learning Disabilities Association of America
4156 Library Road
Pittsburgh, PA 15234

Mainstream, Inc.
1030 15th Street, N.W.
Suite 1010
Washington, DC 20005

Muscular Dystrophy Association
3300 Sunrise Drive
Tucson, AZ 85718

National Association of the Deaf
814 Thayer Avenue
Silver Spring, MD 20910

National Easter Seal Society
70 East Lake Street
Chicago, IL 60601

National Head Injury Foundation, Inc.
1140 Connecticut Avenue, N.W.
Suite 812
Washington, DC 20036

National Multiple Sclerosis Society
205 E. 42nd Street
New York, NY 10017

National Organization on Disability
910 Sixteenth Street, N.W.
Suite 600
Washington, DC 20006

National Spinal Cord Injury Association
600 West Cummings Park
Suite 2000
Woburn, MA 01801

Research and Training Center on Community Integration
Center on Human Policy
Syracuse University
200 Huntington Hall, 2nd Floor
Syracuse, NY 13244–2340

Spina Bifida Association of America
1700 Rockville Pike
Suite 250
Rockville, MD 20852

United Cerebral Palsy Associations, Inc.
1522 K Street, N.W.
Suite 1112
Washington, DC 20005

U.S. Access Board
1111 18th Street, N.W.
Suite 501
Washington, DC 20036

B
Athletic and Recreational Organizations for Persons with Disabilities

American Athletic Association of the Deaf

1052 Darling Street
Ogden, UT 84403

American Blind Bowling Association, Inc.

411 Sherriff Street
Mercer, PA 16137

American Wheelchair Bowling Association

N54 W15858 Larkspur Lane
Menomonee Falls, WI 53051

Blind Outdoor Leisure Association

533 E. Main Street
Aspen, CO 81611

Canadian Association for Disabled Skiing

Box 307
Kimberly, British Columbia, Canada V1A 2Y9

Canadian Wheelchair Sports Association

1600 James Naismith Drive
Glooster, Ontario, Canada K1B 5N4

Cooperative Wilderness Handicapped Outdoor Group

Idaho State University
Box 8118, Pond Student Union
Pocatello, ID 83209

International Wheelchair Aviators

1117 Rising Hill Way
Escondido, CA 92025

Mobility International USA

P.O. Box 3551
Eugene, OR 97403

National Amputee Golf Association

11 Walnut Hill Road
P.O. Box 1228
Amherst, NH 03031

National Foundation for Wheelchair Tennis

940 Calle Amanecer
Suite B
San Clemente, CA 92672

National Handicapped Motorcyclist Association

35-34 84th Street #F8
Jackson Heights, NY 11372

National Handicapped Sports
4405 East-West Highway
Suite 603
Bethesda, MD 20814

National Ocean Access Project
410 Severn Ave.
Suite 107
Annapolis, MD 21403

National Wheelchair Basketball Association
2850 N. Garey Ave.
P.O. Box 6001
Pomona, CA 91769

National Wheelchair Softball Association
1616 Todd Court
Hastings, MN 55038

North American Riding for the Handicapped Association, Inc.
P.O. Box 33150
Denver, CO 80233

Ski for Light
1400 Carole Lane
Green Bay, WI 54313

Special Olympics, International
1350 New York Avenue, N.W.
Suite 500
Washington, DC 20005

U.S. Association of Blind Athletes
33 N. Institute, Brown Hall
Suite 015
Colorado Springs, CO 80903

United States Cerebral Palsy Athletic Association
34518 Warren Road
Suite 264
Westland, MI 48185

United States Deaf Skiers Association
56 West 84th Street
New York, NY 10024

U.S. Quad Rugby Association
2418 West Fallcreek Court
Grand Forks, ND 58201

Wheelchair Sports, USA
3595 E. Fountain Blvd.
Suite L-10
Colorado Springs, CO 80910

Wilderness Inquiry
1313 Fifth Street, S.E.
Suite 327A
Minneapolis, MN 55414

C

Assistive Sport Resources

Archery

Shooting Releases. Enables individuals with limited finger and hand function to draw bow string to anchor point. Tru-Fire Corporation, 7355 State Street, North Fond du Lac, WI 54935. (414) 923–6866.

Splints, Braces, Cuff. Enables quads (C-5 and up) with physical function to hold bow and draw bow to shoot. Fred Sammons, Inc., Box 32, Brookfield, IL 60513. (800) 323–5547. Or Access to Recreation, Inc., 2509 E. Thousand Oaks Blvd., Suite 430, Thousand Oaks, CA 91362. (800) 634–4351.

Bow Stand. Holds the bow. For individuals who have only limited function on one side. Excellent for individuals with severe C.P. Courage Center, REHAB Technology Dept., 3915 Golden Valley Rd., Golden Valley, MN 55422. (612) 520–0811.

Mouth Release. Enables individuals with use of one arm to shoot a bow, using the mouth to draw the bow string to anchor point. Courage Center, Sports, Physical Education and Recreation Department, 3915 Golden Valley Rd., Golden Valley, MN 55422. (612) 520–0476.

Billiards

Billiards Accessories. Flaghouse, Inc., 150 N. MacQuesten, Mount Vernon, NY 10550. (800) 221–5185.

Rollers/Cuffs. Access to Recreation, Inc., 2509 E. Thousand Oaks Blvd., Suite 430, Thousand Oaks, CA 91362. (800) 634–4351. Or Fred Sammons, Inc., Box 32, Brookfield, IL 60513. (800) 323–5547.

Note: This section was adapted from a handout prepared by Lyn Rourke, Sports Physical Education and Recreation Department, Courage Center, Golden Valley, MN.

Blow Darts

Blow Darts. Target shooting with a blowgun that does not require any hand function. BATAVIA, 700 Seventh Street, S.W. #813, Washington, DC 20024. (202) 863–2783.

Bowling

Bowling Ball Holder Ramp. For wheelchair bowlers. Safely holds ball while moving chair up to foul line. Access to Recreation, Inc., 2509 E. Thousand Oaks Blvd., Suite 430, Thousand Oaks, CA 91362. (800) 634–4351.

Bowling Ball Ramp. Ideal for persons with little or no use of their arms. The ramp is placed in front of the lane, and an assistant places the ball on the frame. Access to Recreation, Inc., 2509 E. Thousand Oaks Blvd., Suite 430, Thousand Oaks, CA 91362. (800) 634–4351.

Ball Pusher. A long-handled device for pushing and guiding bowling ball down alley. Use from wheelchair or standing position. Access to Recreation, Inc., 2509 E. Thousand Oaks Blvd., Suite 430, Thousand Oaks, CA 91362. (800) 634–4351.

Handle Grip Bowling Ball. Unique handle permits bowler to grasp ball without the usual fingerhold grip; simply grasp the handle, roll the ball, and the handle retracts when released. Access to Recreation, Inc., 2509 E. Thousand Oaks Blvd., Suite 430, Thousand Oaks, CA 91362. (800) 634–4351.

Bowling Ramp. BRIGGS, 7887 University, P.O. Box 1698, Des Moines, IA 50306. (800) 247–2343.

Bowling Ball Pusher. BRIGGS, 7887 University, P.O. Box 1698, Des Moines, IA 50306. (800) 247–2343.

Handle Grip Ball. SPORTIME, 2905 E. Amwiler Rd., Atlanta, GA 30360. (800) 444–5700.

Two-Piece Steel Bowling Ramp. SPORTIME, 2905 E. Amwiler Rd., Atlanta, GA 30360. (800) 444–5700.

Bowling Ball Holder Ring. A third hand for the wheelchair bowler. Safely holds the bowling ball while you push to the foul line to bowl. George Snyder, 5809 N.E. 21st Ave., Ft. Lauderdale, FL 33308.

Bowling Ball Pusher. A long-handled device for pushing and guiding bowling ball down alley. Use from wheelchair or standing position. Extension handle lengthens for use. Shortens for transportation. Maddak, Inc., Pequannock, NJ 07440. (800) 443–4926.

Bowling Ball Ramp. Allows disabled persons to participate in the regular game of bowling. The ramp guides the ball toward the pins with minimal skill and effort by the player. Easily stored and quickly set up. J. A. Preston Corp., 60 Page Rd., Clifton, NJ 07012. (800) 631–7277.

Bowling Ramp. Ideal for persons with little or no use of their arms. The ramp is placed in front of the lane, and an assistant places the ball on the frame. Maddak, Inc., Pequannock, NJ 07440. (800) 443–4926.

Third Hand. For wheelchair bowlers. Safely holds ball while moving chair up to foul line. Has steel ring and heavy-duty aluminum attachment. No nuts or bolts. Attaches to most chairs. Maddak, Inc., Pequannock, NJ 07440. (800) 443–4926.

Handle Grip Bowling Ball. Unique handle permits bowler to grasp ball without the usual fingerhold grip. Simply grasp the handle and roll the ball, and the handle retracts when released. Maddak, Inc., Pequannock, NJ 07440. (800) 443–4926.

Bowling Equipment. Recreation Unlimited, 830 Woodend Rd., Stratford, CT 06497. (203) 377–8976.

Mahler's Standard Bowling Rail. Serves as a bannister guide for blind bowlers. Type four balls fit in formed metal bars. Comes in two parts. No attachments to alleys for return racks are necessary. Replacement parts available. American Foundation for the Blind, Consumer Products, 15 West 16th Street, New York, NY 10011.

Bowling Sticks. Phillip Faas, 3226 Bayou Placido Blvd. N.E., St. Petersburg, FL 33703. (813) 526–6588.

Bowling Aids. FLAGHOUSE, Inc., 150 North MacQuesten Pky., Mount Vernon, NY, 10550. (800) 221–5185.

Craft Aids

Needle Threader. Useful for those lacking fine motor dexterity. Access to Recreation, Inc., 2509 E. Thousand Oaks Blvd., Suite 430, Thousand Oaks, CA 91362. (800) 634–4351.

Embroidery Hoop. Enables persons with use of only one hand to knit, crochet, embroider, and darn socks. Access to Recreation, Inc., 2509 E. Thousand Oaks Blvd., Suite 430, Thousand Oaks, CA 91362. (800) 634–4351.

Knitting Aid. This aid holds a knitting or crochet needle firmly, allowing those with only one hand to knit confidently. Access to Recreation, Inc., 2509 E. Thousand Oaks Blvd., Suite 430, Thousand Oaks, CA 91362. (800) 634–4351.

Knitting Needle Holder. Clamps with quick-release device to chair arm or table. Snail clamp holds needle firm for one-handed use. Fred Sammons, Inc., Box 32, Brookfield, IL 60513–0032. (800) 323–5547.

Needle Threader. Fred Sammons, Inc., Box 32, Brookfield, IL 60513–0032. (800) 323–5547.

Embroidery Hoop. Enables person with use of only one hand to knit, crochet, embroider, and darn socks. Fred Sammons, Inc., Box 32, Brookfield, IL 60513–0032. (800) 323–5547.

Exercise Equipment

Rickshaw Rehabilitation Exerciser. This lightweight, compact rickshaw is ideal for individuals in wheelchairs to develop strength. Access to Recreation, Inc., 2509 E. Thousand Oaks Blvd., Suite 430, Thousand Oaks, CA 91362. (800) 634–4351.

Therapeutic Weight Belts. Wrist and ankle weight belts that have been color-coded and marked in pounds. Access to Recreation, Inc., 2509 E. Thousand Oaks Blvd., Suite 430, Thousand Oaks, CA 91362. (800) 634–4351.

Beej Rollers. Double roller system to accommodate wheeling in place for road racing training and exercise programs. IDEA (Innovator of Disability Equipment and Adaptations, Inc.), 1393 Meadowcreek Drive, #2, Pewaukee, WI 53072. (414) 691–4248.

Fist Grip Cuff. This cuff with velcro closures is useful in any situation where a good fist grip is required. Cuff can be used for weightlifting, boat rowing, fishing, and racquetball. IDEA, 1393 Meadowcreek Drive, #2, Pewaukee, WI 53072. (414) 691–4248.

Rowcycle. This was designed after the number 1 chosen equipment by the Surgeon General, the rowing machine. This Rowcycle is excellent for cardiovascular, muscle tone, and calories burned. The results will be a lean, hard body. ROWCYCLE, 3188 North Marks, #120, Fresno, CA 93722. (209) 268–1946.

Saratoga Cycle. The first truly accessible fitness system allowing you to exercise arms or legs without body transfers or "set up help." Three handgrip options are available to accommodate full, limited, or even nonexistent hand grasp. Saratoga Access and Fitness, Inc., 6 Birch St.—P, Saratoga Springs, NY 12866. (518) 587–6974.

Upper-Max Exerciser. Designed by a quad for wheelchair users. Roll under and exercise arms, shoulders, etc., The Creative Shop, P.O. Box 7, Leoma, TN 38468.

UBE Ergometers. Upper body workout machine. CYBEX, Division of Lumex, Inc., 2100 Smithtown Avenue, P.O. Box 9003, Ronkonkoma, NY 11779. (800) 645–5392.

Uppercycle. High tech bike for your arms. Garvey Company, 816 Transfer Rd., P.O. Box 4306, St. Paul, MN 55114. (800) 832–6407.

Paragym 1000. Wheelchair persons can enjoy exercising in their home with more than 21 exercises, including special exercises for the lower back, abdomen, and neck. PARAMED, P.O. Box 48168, Jackson, MS 39204–8168. (800) 526–7272.

Pedal-in-Place Exerciser. Exercise your legs and strengthen your upper body and arms all at the same time. Thoele Manufacturing, Route 1, Box 116, Montrose, IL 62445. (217) 924–4553.

The Big Roller. Two drum sports model, Sportsmodel wheelchair roller for perfect workout weather anytime. Mclain Cycle Products, 1718 106th Avenue, Otsego, MI 49078. (616) 694–9704.

Flexiceser. High-quality electrical motor with a speed control. Can be used for passive or resistive workouts. Richer Life of Iowa, Box 12, Boyden, IA 51234. (712) 725–2334.

Multi-Exerciser. Exercise in your own home, independently, and at your desired level of intensity. It provides high-quality exercise with low-impact resistance. Strength and aerobic workouts are optimized, with less stress to ligaments and joints. Easy Access Corp., 912 Drew Street, Suite 103, Clearwater, FL 34615. (813) 441–EASY.

Hardbody Fitness Bar. The bar is constructed of lightweight, durable materials, assembles in seconds, and is ready for immediate use. The latex tubing provides adjustable resistance for all stages of body development, reportedly allowing the performance of more than 20 exercises that work all muscle groups. Hardbody Fitness Systems, Mfg., 22600 B Lambert Street, Suite 807, El Toro, CA 92630. (714) 768–8070.

Weight Training Equipment. Universal exercise machine that can be used from a wheelchair; manual dexterity not required. Helm Distributing, Box 878, Polson, MT 59860. (406) 883–6206.

Nautilus Independence Line. Nautilus Sports/Medical Industries Inc., announces the independence line of wheelchair-accessible exercise equipment. Nautilus Sports/Medical Industries, Inc., P.O. Box 809014, Dallas, TX 75380–9014. (800) 874–8941.

Workout Programs

Armchair Aerobics. "Armchair Aerobics" is an exercise program designed to increase fitness while sitting in a chair. Participants are guided through a 30-minute workout, but the developer of the video indicates that the exercises can be done for as long a time as levels of fitness permit. The Fitness Firm, Linda Chaloupka, P.O. Box 367, Port Washington, WI 53074. (800) 545–4141, Ext. 344. Or (414) 375–2502.

Armchair Fitness. "Armchair Fitness" is an aerobic workout in a chair for people who avoid vigorous activity because of preference, life-style, age, or disability. The workout includes three 20-minute stretching and strengthening routines, to the accompaniment of big band-style music. CC-M Productions, Inc., P.O. Box 15707, Chevy Chase, MD 20815. (202) 291–3884.

Exercise Video Series. The Amputee Sports Association has produced a new exercise video series that is available in VHS format. Included on the tapes, approximately 45 minutes in length, are aerobics (land and aquatic), flexibility and strength exercises (free weight and Nautilus), and suggestions about other sports that contribute to general fitness and health. There is no cost for rental of the videotapes; however, the cost of return shipping is the responsibility of the borrower. Distribution is made on the priority basis established by the Amputee Sports Association. Amputee Sports Association, George C. Beckmann Jr., P.O. Box 60412, Savannah, GA 31420–0412. (912) 927–5406.

"Fitness Is for Everyone!" This program featuring six 30-minute exercise tapes is sponsored by Invacare Corporation, Elyria, OH, and produced by National Handicapped Sports (NHS). The exercise tapes include four 30-minute aerobic dance routines (which may be purchased individually or as a set) and two routines for developing strength and flexibility (which are available only as a set). The routines are led by professional fitness instructors and demonstrated by disabled athletes: an amputee, a paraplegic, a quadriplegic, and a person who has cerebral palsy. NHS/IN-VACARE, c/o Wyse Public Relations, 24 Public Square, Cleveland, OH 44113. (800) 468–2227.

Keep Fit While You Sit. "Keep Fit While You Sit" features a professional aerobic instructor, a physically limited actress, and two disabled athletes. Designed by a licensed physical therapist, the video shows how to have a good workout in a sitting position. Slabo Productions, Alexander Slabo, 1057 South Crescent Heights Boulevard, Los Angeles, CA 90035. (213) 935–8624.

Nancy's Special Workout for the Physically Challenged. Created by a registered occupational therapist from Michigan, "Nancy's Special Workout for the Physically Challenged" starts with a warm-up, moves to a challenging aerobic segment, and ends with a cool-down period, all to original, upbeat music. The aerobic program is appropriate for those with multiple sclerosis, muscular dystrophy, cerebral palsy, spina bifida, amputations, blindness, mental retardation, spinal cord injuries, head injuries, and other physical disabilities. Nancy's Special Workout, Nancy J. Sebring, O.T.R., P.O. Box 2914, Southfield, MI 48037–2914. (313) 682–5511.

Reach for Fitness. This custom workout, created by media personality Richard Simmons, is designed to address the fitness needs of people with a wide range of physical disabilities. The workout was created with the assistance of specialists at Los Angeles Orthopedic Hospital as well as physical therapists throughout the country. Karl-Lotimst Home Video, Anna Snepp, 17942 Cowan, Irvine, CA 92714. (800) 624–2694. In California, (714) 474–0355. In Canada, (416) 842–6860.

Sit and Be Fit. Designed and instructed by kinesiologist Karen Wilson, "Sit and Be Fit" is a vigorous workout for sitting people of all ages. It provides a complete upper-body conditioning program, scientifically designed for safety and results. Sit and Be Fit, Karen Wilson, 7908b E. Chaparral, Suite 105, Scottsdale, AZ 85253. (602) 990–9005.

Wheelchair Workout with Janet Reed. This exercise program was developed by Janet Reed, who is a paraplegic, in consultation with a registered physical therapist and a clinical professor of neurosurgery. The 30-minute program can be done from a wheelchair or other sturdy chair. The audiocassette has exercises narrated to music on one side and music alone on the other side. The workout emphasizes upper-body movement and is designed for people of all ages. Sister Kenny Institute, Publications/Audiovisuals Office #1, 800 East 28th St., Minneapolis, MN 55407. (612) 863–4175.

Wheelercise. "Wheelercise" consists of a beginner (10 minutes) and advanced (20 minutes) workout for upper-body strengthening. Created by physical therapist Maura Casey, this video is designed for wheelchair users to increase cardiovascular fitness level and joint flexibility. Scott & K.C. Enterprises, Inc., P.O. Box 443, South Bound Brook, NJ 08880. (201) 725–5552.

Fishing

Royal Bee Electric Reels. A system of gears tie into the gears of the existing spool and a motor switch in the back drives the gears attached to the trigger system to reel in the line. Access to Recreation, 2509 E. Thousand Oaks Blvd., Suite 430, Thousand Oaks, CA 91362. (800) 634–4351.

Van's EZ Cast. Cast and reel independently even with no wrist or finger movement. Access to Recreation, 2509 E. Thousand Oaks Blvd., Suite 430, Thousand Oaks, CA 91362. (800) 634–4351.

One-Handed Fishing Vest. Lightweight vest and harness holds a fishing rod to allow the user to reel with one hand. Access to Recreation, 2509 E. Thousand Oaks Blvd., Suite 430, Thousand Oaks, CA 91362. (800) 634–4351.

Electronic Fishing Reels. Rods for trolling, jigging, and bottom fishing. Miya Epoch, 1635 Crenshaw Blvd., Torrance, CA 90501. (213) 320–1172.

Fishing Pole Holder. This metal hook is attached to any lightweight fishing pole having a cork or foam handle. IDEA, 1393 Meadowcreek Drive, #2, Pewaukee, WI 53072. (414) 691–4248.

Rods, Reels, Holders, Knives, etc. (All products to assist the disabled sports enthusiast.) Write to get this catalog from J. L. Pachner, Ltd., 33012 Lighthouse Court, San Juan Capistrano, CA 92675. (714) 661–2132.

Handi-Harness. A lightweight harness constructed to hold your rod. For more information, contact Mike Russell, 126 Chesterfield Dr., Amherstview, Ontario, K7N 1M2 CANADA.

Royal Bee Fishing Equipment. Royal Bee Corporation, P.O. Box 2000, Pawhuska, OK 74056. (800) 331–7629.

One-Hand Fishing. Lightweight harness acts as a second hand. Fashion Able, 5 Crescent Ave., Box 5, Rocky Hill, NJ 08553. (609) 921–2563.

The Free Handerson Recreation Belt. The harness and attached hardware allow the user to bait a hook, cast, troll, and reel entirely with one hand. The Free Handerson Co., P.O. Box 4543, Helena, MT 59604. (406) 449–2764.

Expandable Fishing Rod. A compact 15″ length for storage but springs into a 5′6″ rod when called into action. The Lankford Company, P.O. Box 2714, Abilene, TX 79604-2714. (915) 672–1046.

Frisbee

Flying Disc. Frisbee designed with hooks so quads can throw it. IDEA, 1393 Meadowcreek Drive, #2, Pewaukee, WI 53072. (414) 691–4248.

Quad Bee. Looks like any ordinary Frisbee but has two adaptive clips mounted where the thumb would naturally be placed. Access to Recreation, Inc., 2509 E. Thousand Oaks Blvd., Suite 430, Thousand Oaks, CA 91362. (800) 634–4351.

Hunting

Rifle Rest. The Free Handerson rifle rest allows one-armed operation of a rifle. Comfortable and stable, the rifle rest lets you shoot quickly and accurately. The Free Handerson Co., P.O. Box 4543, Helena, MT 59604. (406) 449–2764.

Trigger Finger Brace. A metal brace attached to index finger enables user to pull a gun trigger. IDEA, 1393 Meadowcreek Drive, #2, Pewaukee, WI 53072. (414) 691–4248.

Wooden Vehicle Window Gun Support. This device is intended only to support the end of a small-caliber rifle or pistol. IDEA, 1393 Meadowcreek Drive, #2, Pewaukee, WI 53072. (414) 691–4248.

Shoulder Harness with Butt Placement Sleeve. Ron Adams, Director of Therapeutic Recreation and Adapted Physical Education Services, Children's Rehabilitation Center, University of Virginia Medical Center, Charlottesville, VA 22901.

Shooting Rest. Mechanical rest for high-level quadriplegics. Bob Bowen, 363 Maple Street, Chadron, NE 69337.

Remote Electronic Trigger Mechanism. National Wheelchair Shooting Federation, 545 Ridge Rd., Wilbraham, MA 01095. (413) 596–4407.

P.V.A. Trap Aid. Therapeutic Recreation Systems, 1280 28th Street, Suite 3, Boulder, CO 80303. (303) 444–4720.

Kite Flying

Go Fly a Kite. By supporting the wheelchair frame so that one rear wheel can spin freely and attaching this spool to the spokes of the Freewheel, the relaxing enjoyment of flying a kite is possible. IDEA, 1393 Meadowcreek Drive, #2, Pewaukee, WI 53072. (414) 691–4248.

Photography

Camera Mount. Camera mount allows expert picture taking with increased stability and one-handed ease of operation. Ball-and-socket joint allows you to choose camera angle. The Free Handerson Co., P.O. Box 4543, Helena, MT 59604. (406) 449–2764.

Universal Support Arm. Camera mount is attached to the universal support arm with standard 1/4–20 that fits all 35mm camera thread wells. Access to Recreation, 2509 E. Thousand Oaks Blvd., Suite 430, Thousand Oaks, CA 91362. (800) 634–4351.

Camera Holder. Camera holder attaches to your wheelchair; fits any wheelchair. It attaches with Donaldson clamps. Access to Recreation, 2509 E. Thousand Oaks Blvd., Suite 430, Thousand Oaks, CA 91362. (800) 634–4351.

Bodypod. A lightweight, adjustable camera mount designed for people with limited mobility. Bodypod, Vic Crowley, 1431 Main Street, Gresham, OR 97030. (503) 665–4958.

Racquet Holder

Fist Grip Cuff. This cuff with Velcro closures is useful in any situation where a good fist grip is required. IDEA, 1393 Meadowcreek Drive, #2, Pewaukee, WI 53072. (414) 691–4248.

Grasping Cuff. Designed for those with good arm function and limited hand function. Fred Sammons, Inc., Box 32, Brookfield, IL 60513–0032. (800) 323–5547.

Sport Grip: Orthotic Racquet Holder. The sport grip will give you a firm grip on the racquet. They are currently being used in spinal injury tennis competition. Access to Recreation, 2509 E. Thousand Oaks Blvd., Suite 430, Thousand Oaks, CA 91362. (800) 634–4351.

Table Tennis

Table Tennis Cuffs. Enables those with little or no hand or wrist function to play table tennis. Paddle is held securely in palm. Fred Sammons, Inc., Box 32, Brookfield, IL 60513. (800) 323–5547.

Table Tennis Cuffs. Access to Recreation, Inc., 2509 E. Thousand Oaks Blvd., Suite 430, Thousand Oaks, CA 91362. (800) 634–4351.

Tables. Flaghouse, Inc., 150 North Macquesten Pkwy., Mount Vernon, NY 10550. (800) 221–5185.

Tricycles

Adult Tricycle. For handicapped adults and grown children. All standard full-sized bicycle components including ball-bearing wheels. Handlebar brakes and extra-large seat. Rear platform supports a large basket. J. A. Preston Corp., 60 Page Rd., Clifton, NJ 07012. (800) 631–7277.

Irish Mail. An appealing substitute for children who are unable to pedal a standard tricycle. The Irish Mail moves when the handle is pumped back and forth. Comfortable front bar for resting feet. Extra large vinyl seat with a body support to ensure correct posture. Available without body support. J. A. Preston Corp., 60 Page Rd., Clifton, NJ 07012. (800) 631–7277.

Irish Mail. In child and adult sizes. Rugged vehicle has padded, tractor-type seat. Offers development exercise involving arm, upper torso, and leg movements. Adjustable seat. Body torso support and special pedals available. Other models also. Beckley-Cardy, 114 Gaither Dr., Mt. Laurel, NJ 08054. (800) 227–1178.

Terrier Chain-Drive Tricyle. Similar to a regular tricycle with standard bicycle-type chain and chain guard. All wheels have safety rims. Handbrake mechanism on right handlebar. Available with or without body support and foot attachments. J. A. Preston Corp., 60 Page Road, Clifton, NJ 07012. (800) 631–7277.

Trainer Bicycle. Has adjustable wheels for various stages of balance ability. Equipped with adjustable spring saddleseat, handlebars, coaster brake, and puncture-proof tires. Available with or without body support and foot attachments. J. A. Preston Corp., 60 Page Rd., Clifton, NJ 07012. (800) 631–7277.

Maddacycle Hand-Propelled Tricycle for Handicapped Children. Seat tricycle with chair drive and steering mechanism. Rear wheel is an independent swivel wheel. Motive power is transmitted from the hand cranks to the front wheels. Suitable for indoor use for children from 2 to 7 years of age. Maddak, Inc., Pequannock, NJ 07440. (800) 443–4926.

Rifton Tricycle. Valuable aid to the mobility of the handicapped child. Includes adjustable handlebar, seat, and padded backrest with belt, a pair of upright handles, and a pair of sandals. Community Playthings, Rifton, NY 12471. (914) 658–3141.

Torso Support Tricycle. Has motorcycle-style back support made of steel tubing. A curved foam backrest with a broad nylon belt gives adjustable support. Available with standard or upright handlebars. For children who require such support. G. E. Miller, Inc., 484 South Broadway, Yonkers, NY 10705. (914) 969–4036.

Snow Skiing

Shadow Ski. Magic in Motion, 239 W. Stewart Ave., Puyallup, WA 98371. (206) 848–6845.

Ski Bras/Ski Handle. Ski Ease, 4401 Devonshire, Lansing, MI 48910. (517) 882–4608.

Out Riggers. LaCome, 3103 W. 48th Ave., Denver, CO 80221. (303) 480–5268.

Arroya Type Sit-Ski. Dallas Dietrich, 4533 S. Canyon Rd., Rapid City, SD 57709. (605) 394–4915.

GLF Mono-Ski-Bob. The mono-ski is a fiberglass sitting unit, or pod, on leaf spring suspension and single ski. Innovative Recreation, Inc., 623 Valley Oak, Newbury Park, CA 91320.

Mono-Ski by GFL. Mobility Systems, 861 Robinwood Court, Traverse City, MI 49684. (616) 941–4626.

Skiing on One Ski with One Up. J. M. Industries, Inc., P.O. Box 93, Newtown, PA 18940. (215) 860–1718.

Mountain Man. Sit-ski for mobility impaired. Mountain Man, 720 Front St., Bozeman, MT 59715. (406) 587–0310.

Unique. Sit-Ski. Enabling Technologies, 2411 N. Federal Blvd., Denver, CO 80211. (303) 455–3578.

Skiing. National Handicapped Sports of Northern California, 5946 Illinois Ave., Orangevale, CA 95662.

Swimming

Hoyer Swimming Pool Lifter. Ted Hoyer & Co., Inc., 2222 Minnesota Street, P.O. Box 2744, Oshkosh, WI 54901. (414) 231–7970.

Beachmaster Aquatic Wheelchair. Beach Wheels Inc., 1555 Shadowlawn, Naples, FL 33942. (813) 775–1078.

Waterproof Cushion. Access to Recreation, Inc., 2509 E. Thousand Oaks Blvd., Suite 430, Thousand Oaks, CA 91362. (800) 634–4351.

Noland Pool Lift. Access to Recreation, Inc., 2509 E. Thousand Oaks Blvd., Suite 430, Thousand Oaks, CA 91362. (800) 634–4351.

Hoyer Pool Lift. Access to Recreation, Inc., 2509 E. Thousand Oaks Blvd., Suite 430, Thousand Oaks, CA 91362. (800) 634–4351.

Danmar Swim Aids. (Delta Swim System, Pad Plus, Sectional Raft, Swim Rings, Head Float, Stabilizer Bar, Comfort Mat, Dolphin) Access to Recreation, Inc., 2509 E. Thousand Oaks Blvd., Suite 430, Thousand Oaks, CA 91362. (800) 634–4351.

The Sand-Rik. Enables elderly and disabled persons easy access to beaches and other rough terrain previously inaccessible to them. Access to Recreation, Inc., 2509 E. Thousand Oaks Blvd., Suite 430, Thousand Oaks, CA 91362. (800) 634–4351.

Flotation Devices. Danmar Products, Inc., 2390 Winewood Ave., Ann Arbor, MI 48103. (313) 761–1990.

Waterskiing

Kan Ski. Innovative Recreation, Inc., 623 Valley Oak, Newbury Park, CA 91320.

Manta-Ray-Water Skiing Alternative. A new recreation product that allows you to sit or lie down as you glide across the water. Access to Recreation, Inc., 2509 E. Thousand Oaks Blvd., Suite 430, Thousand Oaks, CA 91362. (800) 634–4351.

INDEX

. . .